W9-CJM-913

VALUES IN HEALTH CARE:
CHOICES AND CONFLICTS

VALUES IN HEALTH CARE:
Choices and Conflicts

By

JOHN G. BRUHN, PH.D.

The University of Texas Medical Branch at Galveston
Galveston, Texas

and

GEORGE HENDERSON, PH.D.

The University of Oklahoma
Norman, Oklahoma

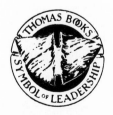

CHARLES C THOMAS • PUBLISHER
Springfield • Illinois • U.S.A.

Published and Distributed Throughout the World by

CHARLES C THOMAS • PUBLISHER
2600 South First Street
Springfield, Illinois 62794-9265

© *1991 by* CHARLES C THOMAS • PUBLISHER

ISBN 0-398-05741-9

Library of Congress Catalog Card Number: 91-586

With THOMAS BOOKS *careful attention is given to all details of manufacturing
and design. It is the Publisher's desire to present books that are satisfactory as to their
physical qualities and artistic possibilities and appropriate for their particular use.*
THOMAS BOOKS *will be true to those laws of quality that assure a good name
and good will.*

Printed in the United States of America
SC-R-3

Library of Congress Cataloging-in-Publication Data

Bruhn, John G., 1934–
    Values in health care : choices and conflicts / by John G. Bruhn
and George Henderson.
        p.   cm.
    Includes bibliographical references and index.
    ISBN 0-398-05741-9
    1. Allied health personnel and patient.   2. Values.   3. Medical
ethics.   I. Henderson, George, 1932–   .   II. Title.
[DNLM: 1. Attitude of Health Personnel.   2. Ethics, Medical.
3. Social Values.   W 50 B892v]
R727.3.B78   1991
174'.2—dc20
DNLM/DLC
for Library of Congress   91-586
                                                                        CIP

FOREWORD

E very one of us has moral convictions and commitments. Some of these are widely shared by others, some less so, and yet others are a source of contention. This holds true in virtually every sphere of social life—work, play, politics, religion. Health care is no exception. Here as elsewhere in our pluralistic society, moral consensus is hard to come by. We disagree, sometimes heartily, about what are acceptable risks to health, about where health belongs in the larger scheme of things that we value, and about what quality of life is worth living. Because professional health care practice is personal, it is value laden, and increasingly, prone to conflict. This being so, health care professionals are expected to be knowledgeable about the ethical dimensions of their practice. This book will increase their awareness of those dimensions.

To value something—in this case, health—is to prize it, to consider it worthwhile and worth preserving. Health care ethics is reflection upon and deliberation about the value of health and the sorting out of choices and conflicts in health care. The authors remind us that health is not of absolute value. There are other things in our lives that we may care about as much or even more. Health is, nonetheless, valuable. When it is severely compromised, so is our ability to do many other things that matter to us in life. This book contains useful advice about how health care professionals can help give substance to the otherwise abstract idea of health. By connecting the idea to day-to-day decisions made by individuals about such things as life style and work habits, each of us may be encouraged to assume responsibility for our health.

When individuals fall ill or suffer injury, the range of health care professionals' responsibility extends beyond prevention, cure and rehabilitation to the relief of distress and the provision of comfort and encouragement. Furthermore, these various responsibilities must be carried out by the professional with due respect for the patient's integrity. This means that if a sick person is to make wise choices under the usually stressful conditions of illness, he or she must be suitably informed of the risks and benefits of a proposed course of treatment and made aware of the advantages and liabilities of alternative courses of action. Appropriately informing patients of these options is, the authors contend, "one of the health care provider's major ethical responsibilities."

Members of the helping professions have always been expected to provide competent, humane care. To carry out that responsibility in our time requires special attentiveness to values in health care. This book will guide the reader in developing such attentiveness.

RONALD A. CARSON
Director
Institute for the
Medical Humanities
University of Texas
Medical Branch at Galveston

PREFACE

This book is concerned with values as they apply to health care. Health values influence human conduct in the context of health care practice, policy, and relationships. More specifically, values affect the behavior of health care professionals in health care situations, and the impact of their actions on other persons as individuals or as members of groups.

One reason for studying health values is that health care professionals increasingly find themselves in conflict, torn between the professional ideals and values that they have learned in training and the values that they are expected to pursue on the job. As a result, health professionals frequently find themselves in a double bind. For the individual who is ill equipped to handle it, this double bind can produce fear, anger, self-pity, and outrage. These reactions cannot help but influence how health professionals relate to their peers and to patients. A second reason to study health values is that advances in medical science and the emergence of the patient as a consumer have heightened the moral and ethical dimension of health care decisions. A third reason for the need to examine health values is health care's moral quandary. Often, there is the absence of a clear moral standard to guide health care decisions, an uncertainty in defining rights and responsibilities, and a poorly defined concept of moral accountability. Decisions that any health professional would make are largely determined by values. When we value something, we view it as having worth. Hospital rules constitute a value; so do compassion for the patient and patient autonomy.

In choosing personal and professional goals, in selecting the means to attain them, and in resolving conflicts, we are influenced by our conceptions of what is preferable and important. The quality of our relationships with others, the way in which we conduct ourselves professionally, the degree of respect we have for others and ourselves, and all of the aspects of our daily lives are influenced by our system of values. Each of us has a value system that differs somewhat from anyone else's. Nonetheless, our individual values arise from the core values of our culture. How health is viewed and valued in our culture and how each of us personally values health affect how we live, how we relate to others, and how we practice our professions. As health professionals, and as citizens, we need to develop an awareness and sensitivity to our own values, as well as the values of others. This book addresses some of the major values that come to play in the life and practice of health care professionals today.

Topics discussed briefly in the first few chapters are treated in greater detail in later chapters. This should not be thought of as needless repetition; rather it is a way of expanding on relevant issues. This approach is in harmony with the psychological principle that growth and learning are continuous.

We hope this book will be useful, especially for students in medicine, nursing, and allied health. The book may also be a resource for students in fields not directly associated with hands-on patient care, such as public health, health education, medical sociology, medical psychology, medical anthropology, and social work.

No single source can identify or deal with all of the social, moral, ethical, or legal aspects of health or health care. While the chapters in this volume obviously reflect the concerns and interests of the authors, the selection of the topics was influenced greatly by the frequency with which questions or problems have arisen in these areas as students go through the process of becoming a health professional. We hope this volume will stimulate both the curiosity and sensitivity of students to the human dimensions and changing complexities of being a health professional.

The motivations for choosing to become a health professional are not always fully known until the student graduates and begins to function as a professional. What keeps a health professional going, what gives a health professional personal satisfaction, and what does a health professional do to replenish his/her vessel when it has been drained by giving? The answers to these questions lie in the value system of each individual health professional. We hear of great scientists and teachers, but rarely do we hear of the on-line health practitioner who provides exemplary care on a daily basis extolled. Perhaps this reflects a deficit in our culture's value system. One is reminded of Will Rogers' quotation, "It's great to be great, but it's greater to be human."

JOHN G. BRUHN
Galveston, Texas

GEORGE HENDERSON
Norman, Oklahoma

ACKNOWLEDGMENTS

We are grateful to Paula Levine for her editorial assistance, constructive criticism, and for constructing the index. Also, we thank Lucretia Scoufos for her editorial assistance.

Prologue

I WONDER WHAT HE WAS LIKE?

ANDREW F. PAYER[1]

It was Monday morning, my weekend was a disaster, my secretary was late, my schedule was full for the day, and I was really feeling sorry for myself.

The door to my office swung open wide and a bright-eyed young man entered radiating with happiness and a lively step. He asked me if I was the doctor who ran the body donation program for the medical school. I acknowledged that I was in charge of such a program, but expressed that it might be a bit early for him to be thinking about donating his body for medical education and research. He smiled and said that he was only 28 years old, but that his time was very near.

I gave him the official form to complete for my records. As he was filling out the form, he proceeded to tell me that he had a terminal form of brain tumor. He was going in for surgery this coming Friday for the "last time" and was told he would not survive much longer. Suddenly, he switched the topic and began asking about me and how things were going at work and home. He was politely amused to find out that I raised tortoises. It was evident that he sensed my "sad" state of mind and tried to cheer me up.

He began to tell me more about himself. He was spending time visiting terminally ill patients at the hospital and trying to help them through their own ordeals. He was very worried about his mother, and wanted to ensure that all would be taken care of so she would not have to deal with the final details. He asked if he could use my phone to confirm his meeting with his lawyer. "You know how messy the legal details can get in settling the affairs of one's estate."

[1]Andrew F. Payer, Ph.D., is associate professor of anatomy and neurosciences at The University of Texas Medical Branch at Galveston, and director of UTMB's Willed-Body Program. Reprinted with permission of the author.

I told him that he was handling this situation much better than me. He smiled and said, "I have had my bad moments, but as I look back, I was very lucky to have had a life filled with the love of my family and friends. I have accepted my fate and am just luckier than most to know when the event will most likely happen."

We continued to talk. Emotions began to swell up inside me. My terrible day was not as bad as I originally thought. I caught myself feeling selfish because I wanted to go outside to feel the sea breeze, go home and kiss my wife, work out the problems I had with a faculty colleague, and tell my secretary to take the day off!

As he walked down the hall from my office, his step and movements were as lively and happy as when he entered. He turned with a smile and said: "I would like to ask one favor. When those medical students are looking down at my remains and getting the nerve up to make the first cut, tell them that I was a nice person who loved life and his fellow man. Tell them that they should not feel bad about what they are about to do. Finally, tell them that they got a damn good specimen and they should be able to learn a lot of anatomy from me!"

He died peacefully at home several weeks later.

That fall was the beginning of medical school for a new group of students. I was at the dissecting table that held his remains as the four medical students looked at their cadaver and pondered about what to do next. I heard one of them ask another: "I wonder what he was like?"

CONTENTS

VALUES IN HEALTH CARE:
CHOICES AND CONFLICTS

Chapter 1

VALUES FOR HEALTH PROFESSIONALS

Man's chief purpose ... is the creation and preservation of values: that is what gives meaning to our civilization, and the participation in this is what gives significance, ultimately, to the individual human life.

Lewis Mumford, *Faith in living,* 1940.

B ecause the values of health care professionals influence their medical decisions, biomedical ethics is "applied" ethics. It is a multifaceted discipline employed to examine medical decision making across the broad spectrum of health care, focusing on medical practice, health care delivery, research, and public policy. Contraception, consent to treatment, allocation of funds, genetic engineering of the germline, abortion, and euthanasia are some of the particular biomedical issues that affect almost every life and are often the occasion of bitter disputes (Beauchamp & Childress, 1979; Engelhardt, 1986). The problems associated with the biomedical sciences and health care have called philosophy, with its rigorous methodology, back into prominence. Historically, philosophers have studied three primary values: (1) the good, (2) the true, and (3) the beautiful—other values are subsumed under them. However, there is now, and probably will continue to be, disagreement about what people accept as legitimate moral dicta as they are derived from secular philosophy in contradistinction to religious beliefs.

Questions for Life

Living as we do in a world of secular societies, with a broad plurality of views, makes reaching a working consensus in matters of health care an almost insurmountable task. To succeed, we must consider the relevant values and reexamine their cultural foundations. This will require mutual respect and peaceable negotiations. Philosophical reflections have been directed to values and ethical decision making in health care because major and rapid changes in technology call into question under-

3

lying assumptions of established medical practices; rising health care costs place scrutiny on the allocation of available resources; pluralistic values of patients are often in conflict with their health care professionals; and legal decisions have expanded the publicly recognized right of self-determination in medical matters.

In Biblical times, a man's wealth was measured not only by his flocks and his herds, his ingots of gold, his menservants and maidservants, but also by his offspring—his sons and daughters and their sons and daughters. Today, in many places of the world, particularly in underdeveloped nations, the equation of wealth remains basically the same. Consequently, the ancient norm of having many children has turned into a contemporary nightmare: there are too many people in the world. Resources are not available for the treatment of all human beings. Therefore, we must decide on what principles should health care be allocated. Should it be on the basis of which patients have the best chance to survive or, instead, which patients' treatments will be shorter and cheaper? Or should we make our decision from a genetic perspective; that is, which patients will most likely make the greatest contribution to the general societal welfare? Boxill (1985) summarized the issues thusly: "Does the right to the highest possible quality of life outweigh the right to life itself?" (p. 97). Or stated another way, does mere biological life with the yet unrealized capability to share in truth, beauty, pleasure, achievement, and love have value? If it has value, is that life equal in value to that of a patient who has already contributed to the lives of others? Is the health care professional's duty to preserve the right of life equal to his or her duty to preserve the right to the highest quality of life?

Values that affect the answers to these questions must be examined and reexamined to determine the very best medical-ethical decisions possible, for these decisions will shape the direction of our individual destiny and our collective future. The objectives of this chapter will be to explore the meanings of value; to examine briefly the history of ethical systems that have influenced Western ethical systems; to make the application of those ethical systems to health care in general and, specifically, to medical practice; to examine health care as a right; and to explore medical decision making and motivations that prompt it.

Values

Each person is born into a community in which people share values that provide them with a sense of which behaviors will be tolerated. We acquire our sense of what is socially important in life from our community, with the family and church being the foremost arbiters of norms and values. Values should not be confused with facts. Facts tell us what *is* and values reflect what *ought to be*. Different community standards of accepted truth and moral principles make difficult the decision to carry out freedom of choice within health care settings.

To be free to choose among alternatives is both a blessing and a curse. The thought-feeling or valuing-analyzing process of selecting values from among alternatives is an on-going human activity (see Table 1-1). As an illustration, a doctor may tell a patient with a heart disease that he ought to have surgery, but the science of medicine says no more than that, in the case of this particular heart disease, a particular surgery might have effects A, B, C, and the decision not to undergo the surgery might have effects X, Y, Z. The patient cannot know whether he ought to consent to surgery without appealing to a general value, namely, that of health. Only if he wants to be healthy ought he make the appropriate decision. In an ideal situation, if we choose well we can take credit for our great insight, and if we choose poorly we have only ourselves to blame. Not all of our choices are clear-cut. In fact, most of our value decisions are intricate because we are responsible to other people. Without common values there can be no society, no world community, and conceivably no true individuality. It is unclear what form these common values will take as we move closer to the 21st century.

The study of values in the field of philosophy is called *axiology*. Two of the major concerns of axiology are: (1) what is the good life? and (2) what should we do to achieve it? Since the 19th century, philosophers have become increasingly fascinated with the questions that arise from examination of personal values derived from global human relationships. This growing interest has been brought about largely by television, which acquaints us instantaneously with the values accepted by people in other nations. Focus has been placed on values because of the wide disparity of attitudes within all societies concerning what the good life is and how we can achieve it. The dissemination of value information about other people, here and abroad, has multiplied and accelerated many times over. In addition to television, the radio, telephone, space satellites, and

Table 1-1. Subprocesses of valuing

Subprocess	Indicators
1. Choosing beliefs and behaviors	Choosing from alternatives Choosing after considering consequences Choosing freely
2. Prizing beliefs and behaviors	Cherishing Publicly affirming
3. Acting on beliefs and behaviors	Taking action Internalizing a consistent and repetitive pattern of action

advanced modes of transportation that speed the print media make action and response almost simultaneous. The values of the peoples of the world are inextricably interwoven in this modern age because we are interdependently related to each other not only in communication but also in commerce, transportation, economics, natural disasters, ecology, and research undertaken to advance health care. Edwards (1985) observed that value or ethical conflicts between individuals are more easily resolved if they are based on factual differences, but not if they are based on differences in moral principles after factual beliefs have been accounted for. Consider the following case cited by Myers (1969):

> The child's arm flailed, her head wobbled, and her eyes rolled. Before her, on the school recreation table, were the sickening shambles of a lunch. The table had been crowded around by many children. Now every one of them had beat a retreat and clustered again at a safer distance, to watch and even cruelly to mimic the helpless youngster routing so dreadfully in her food.... Bits of cookies, sandwich, fruit littered the table, and the little girl gagged like a little beast. (p. 59)

Would it have been best for all parties concerned to allow genetically defective Girl X to die during her mother's pregnancy? In this situation, the issue of abortion is further complicated by the issue of physical disability. And they are both complex value issues. Values concerning abortion and physical disability usually stem from a variety of sources, including religion, politics, science, philosophy, social structure, and medicine. Some values, particularly religious values, support the *sanctity* of life; other values favor *quality* of life, while yet other values advocate *respect* for all life. There is the need for medical science to find an acceptable value framework for the very difficult everyday decisions patients and caregivers must make (Almond, 1988). Most individuals who have addressed such problems have given considerable weight to the practical consideration that these arguments are not merely theoretical, but that they have serious consequences in the lives and happiness of ordinary people and can change the direction of such things as world demographics.

To arrive at a starting point, is it better to initiate a value system from the macroperspective of philosophers or from a microscale more in keeping with the medical perspective? If there must be a consideration of practical curative consequences, surely this consideration can incorporate concern for producing both the best and happiest outcome possible in a given circumstance. We need to remember that most of our value pronouncements concerning prolonging or taking life were formulated in religions long before the technological advances that have increased the choices and procedures now at our disposal. Along with technological advances in health care have come the ethical dilemmas we now face.

Those who defend freedom of choice in abortion, for example, often contend that this question was answered when the Creator gave humans free will, without which there can be no moral responsibility. This is a potent argument. Many people are not willing to jeopardize free will in other areas of their lives by agreeing to give it up to legislation in the matter of abortion. People who adopt this view argue that pro-choice leaves the sanctity of free will expression with the individual. Antiabortion advocates, they argue, not only signify their choice but they also impose it on the rest of the population. Further, pro-choice proponents argue that they do not try to legislate against the excesses of those who over-populate the world. As a matter of fact, their taxes are appropriated to feed and care for those excesses. Antiabortion devotees counter the pro-choice position by stating that they have a right to impose their interpretation of values on others because the Mosaic Decalogue decrees that the word of God demands, "Thou Shalt not Kill." Yet the act of killing during war is a moral imperative for many antiabortion advocates.

The highest values of most people are such that they seek both individual and community good. We never experience existence or essence in complete isolation. The values that we learn from our parents, our culture, and our unique circumstances within that culture combine with the values of other people within their cultures to form the warp and woof that pattern the tapestry of our society and the world. Edwards (1985) presents findings which suggest that people from different cultural traditions can understand and respect each other's ethical values because, while they rank them differently, their overall values are basically the same.

When we make value judgments, most often we prefer our own local standards or norms. As responsible people, we are forced by societal mores to consider whether our own standards are compatible not only with our personal goals but with the goals of others (Duff & Campbell, 1980). Fortunately, or unfortunately, values vary so vastly among cultures that we feel compelled to contemplate the notion that there may not be an absolute standard of value measurement, but customs that have been devised from many sources to fit the circumstances of the valuer. This is called *moral relativism.*

Values are derived not only from facts but from feelings. Therefore, we are moved to ask whether we are attracted to something because it is valuable, or whether it is valuable because we find it attractive? If the value of something does not depend on our subjective response to it, then the value is "objective." Objectionists believe that value is intrinsic—it resides in the objects of our experience. If, on the other hand, the value of a thing depends on our attitude toward it, then it is "subjective." Subjectivists believe that value resides in our responses rather than in objects. Most reasoning people would accept the view that all things have either an objective attraction or a subjective attraction that in turn affects their value.

Besides objectivism and subjectivism, there is a middle ground compromise, the *relationist theory,* which proposes that values are the result of a relationship between people and actions or objects. All three positions—objectivism, subjectivism, and relationism—agree with the notion that a value is inclined to reflect what "ought to be," while a fact reflects what "is." Some of the more modern philosophers take a linguistic approach and propose that it is foolish to discuss values until a semantic clarification has established the meaning of value and the significance of terms such as "good" and "evil" and "right" and "wrong."

Utilitarianism supports the thesis that something is right or good because it benefits the greatest number of people. For example, application of utilitarianism to the medical profession would make it imperative that pain relief be provided for hundreds of thousands of arthritic sufferers rather than performing heart transplants that would help considerably fewer patients (Eliopoulos, 1988). Under this system, a utilitarian society would be inclined to provide the highest economic rewards to caregivers who have the largest number of patients.

Egoism is a value position that considers doing what is best for oneself as the right action. An example of this might be private hospitals that, even though able to provide health care, would transfer indigent patients to public hospitals that are already overburdened. In this illustration, the fiscal well-being of the private hospital takes precedence over the well-being of indigent patients who are summarily turned away.

Naturalism is another value system that encompasses two sets of beliefs regarding ethical actions. On the one hand, advocates of this position hold that something is right if it has a positive outcome. For example, immunization is right because it diminishes the spread of disease. On the other hand, this value approach defends the position that something is right if an objective person assesses it to be so. An example would be the U.S. Supreme Court's decision that it is right and reasonable that there should be a job guarantee during maternity leave for female employees. All value systems have conflicts.

Value Conflicts

Conflicts concerning values have negative effects on medical personnel and patients alike. Unresolved value conflicts are likely to cause some health professionals to withdraw from stressful situations. However, this seldom completely insulates them from feeling stressed. Denial is another negative result of value conflicts. Sometimes patients and health care providers deny their own conflicts and focus on other people's problems. Contrary to popular opinion, simply to avoid distasteful personal choices is not healthy. People who avoid or deny their own conflicts are prone to deliberately withhold information from others if it is thought to be too upsetting or controversial.

Rigidity is another consequence that results from conflicts in values. Most of us at sometime in our life have attempted to impose our values on other persons with little regard for the autonomy of the persons being imposed upon. Rigidity also results in strict conformity to rules and guidelines. For example, in hospitals rigidity can take the form of discharging on the tenth day all patients who have had heart attacks, regardless of mitigating circumstances, because practitioners have been told this is the limit of the patients' insurance or Medicare reimbursement.

Clearly, values that are rigidly imposed can sometimes compromise the health care that is expected of medical institutions and professionals. Poorly timed termination of the caregiver-patient relationship can be devastating, particularly when value decisions are not negotiable or amenable to compromise. In these instances, health care professionals display attitudes and behaviors that cause patients to believe that they are not valued. Of course, there are times when patients may become so obnoxious the weary practitioner believes it is in the best interest of all parties to end the relationship. This can be another form of avoidance.

Reading about cultural philosophies, religions, and other values can assist both patients and caregivers in clarifying their own beliefs as well as gaining an insight into the beliefs of others. And multidisciplinary conferences to discuss ethical issues can also be of assistance. But there is no substitute for getting to know people on a one-to-one basis. Relatedly, decision making in health care tends to be best done by practitioners knowledgeable about values. Succinctly stated, to "value" something means *to prize, esteem, or appreciate it and to give it worth.* Therefore, values are uniquely human concepts that cause people to contemplate the wonders of the universe and their purpose, or lack of purpose, within it. From such a perspective has emerged health care ethics. Perhaps the issues we have been discussing can become more sharply focused by asking ourselves the following questions:

- Do I value all lives equally? If not, what causes the differences?
- How much responsibility should each of us assume for other people?
- If all patients in need cannot benefit from available medical resources, should any patient benefit? How should the decision be made to determine who does or does not receive treatment?
- Is it acceptable to commit a minor wrong to bring about a great benefit?
- Should I perform an act that is contrary to my value system if that act will benefit a patient?

Medical Ethics: From Greek to Christian

Ethics is one of the five divisions of classical philosophy, the other four being aesthetics, epistemology, logic, and metaphysics. We will focus on ethics: *the science of values of human life.* It concerns itself with conduct and character that is acceptable or unacceptable, that is approved or disapproved, that is esteemed or disesteemed. Ethicists depend for their judgment on all the biologic and social sciences for reliable input of facts concerning human nature and behavior. Their positions are based on the belief that humans are voluntary creatures constantly facing choices among alternative values. In ethics two questions consistently arise: (1) What is the highest good? (2) What is the supreme principle of valuation? Most Western ethics are derived from the ancient Greek philosophers and Christian theologians.

Medical ethics is not merely a list of physician-patient rights and duties; it is also the study of the reasons for those rights and duties (Veatch, 1989). Formal codes of medical conduct or ethics were recorded long before the so-called Hippocratic ethics and the Oath attributed to Hippocrates (see Appendix A). Historically, medical codes have incorporated ethics and etiquette. *Medical ethics* focus on moral principles that form the basic obligations of caregivers to patients and society. Medical etiquette delineates appropriate professional behavior between caregivers, and proper behavior when interacting with patients. The Egyptian papyri (16th century B.C.) were the first known documents to mention the moral aspects of priest-physician healing processes. The papyri outlined methods of (1) establishing diagnoses, (2) deciding whether to treat a patient, and (3) appropriate therapy. Physicians who followed the outlined methods were not held culpable when their patients died. But those who did not follow the rules were held culpable and, if the patient died, they could forfeit their own lives. Thus, from early times, physicians have been concerned with the moral aspects of healing.

It is generally accepted by medical historians that most of the works attributed to Hippocrates were written by scholars in the Alexandrian library around 430 B.C. (Heschel, 1975). It is of interest to note that Hindu physicians were taking an oath 1500 years before Christ. Relatedly, the Hammurabi Code (2000 B.C.) and Hindu or Susruta Code (5th century B.C.) focused on doctor-patient relationships. Hammurabi created an elaborate code of laws, which set surgical fees according to the social status of the patient and also prescribed punishment for poor technical performance. The Hindu oath of initiation into the medical profession required: "Day and night, thou shall endeavor for the relief of patients with all thy heart and soul. Thou shall not desert or injure the patient even for the sake of thy living." Chinese medicine has over a thousand years of precepts similar to the Hindus', Babylonians', and Greeks'. The medical profession's current concern with morality in preference to morbidity is, however, directly traced to the Judeo-Christian philosophy of life and its attitude about death. Even so, the Greek influence on ethics is undeniable.

Socrates, an early Greek philosopher who is considered to be the father of moral philosophy, moved Greek thought from the study of nature to self-evaluation. He proposed that self-understanding is our greatest need, and when people understand themselves, they may then be able to achieve their greatest good. He stressed the importance of universal principles and emphasized the value of rational judgment. Plato, who was Socrates' pupil, placed the idea of good or the principle of value as the highest of all cosmic principles. "Is it for the best?" was the crucible question Plato asked in order to examine the worth of any thing, any process, or any project. He believed the three cardinal virtues are temperance, courage, and wisdom.

Plato's most prominent student was Aristotle. The principles of Aristotelian ethics are derived from his biologic and psychologic studies. He proposed that we could call anything good that performs well in its characteristic function. Aristotle believed nature and humans are most apt to attain perfection and thus happiness by progressively converting their potentialities into actualities. But Aristotle admonished his followers to avoid extremes and maintain balance. He recognized the social aspect of ethics throughout his works. In the social application of ethics, Aristotle supported the close relationship of persons. Applying his principle to friendship, he described true friendship as a communion of persons moved by mutual respect and devotion, with each eliciting the best in the other. This could well be applied to the health care professional-patient relationship, where the mutual objective is healing.

The Christian foundation for ethics was laid by the pre-exilic prophets—especially Amos, Jeremiah, and Isaiah—who extolled the virtues of observing the law but also reaching, of our own volition, beyond it to serve humanity. Amos (5: 23–24) summarized this ethical position thusly:

> Yea though ye offer me burnt-offerings
>   and your meal-offerings
> I will not accept them . . .
> Take thou away from me the noise
>   of thy songs;
> And let me not hear the melody
>   of thy psalteries.
> But let justice well up as waters

And righteousness as a mighty
stream.

The Hebraic ethical tradition of *righteousness* and *justice*, which centered on religion and was begun by Amos in the 8th century B.C., has had a profound influence on modern concepts of *morality* and *ethicality* (Chapman, 1984). From this early beginning, rabbis were expected to go beyond their routine professional roles and render righteousness to those whom they served. The combined roles of rabbi and physician has been a Jewish tradition from the giving of the Torah. The Book of Leviticus describes the rabbi's early religious role in the temple, as well as his role in quarantine, diagnosis, and treatment of leprosy. And this tradition was carried on by Elijah, Jesus, Sforno, Nachmanides, Yehuda Halevi, and Maimonides (Braverman, 1987). Like the priest-doctor, the rabbi-doctor became a new profession.

Christian-medieval ethics moved from the rigidity of Jewish law observance to focus on an ensouled spirit of loving devotion. This conversion-of-life outlook proceeded from secular improvement through intellectual enlightenment, to spiritual redemption and, finally, regeneration. Trust, humility, meekness, mercy, forgiveness, purity of heart, peacemaking, devotion, faith, hope, and love became the new touchstones of healing. Supreme exaltation of love replaced the cardinal virtues of classical ethics. St. Thomas Aquinas put forth the most important medieval doctrine of ethics: a system of Christian-Aristotelian rationalism that moved the ultimate goal of humans beyond the reach of reason into the realm of *faith*. The ultimate ethic, Christian blessedness, is to be achieved by faith, hope, and love—the greatest of all human expressions. Exercise of these values is the precursor of ethics in health care.

Moral Reasoning

Medical morality and ethics have evolved slowly, following a long, circuitous pathway. Today, medical practitioners and the rest of society must solve an array of complex ethical problems—each precipitated by scientific advances, public literacy, and the spread of participatory democracy. Revisions in medical and allied health associations' codes of conduct reflect heightened sensitivity to the needs, wants, and legal rights of patients. Indeed, there is an almost frantic drive within some associations to preserve in the codes those guidelines that are helpful and to add new ones. But general guidelines do not resolve all of the specific health care problems characterizing modern medical practice. Beauchamp and Childress (1979) presented the following interesting hierarchical approach to moral reasoning in biomedical deliberation and justification:

4 Ethical Theories

3 Principles

2 Rules

1 Judgments and Actions.

Judgments about what ought to be done in a particular medical situation are based on moral rules, which in turn are supported by principles and ultimately lead to ethical theories. In this instance, we are concerned only with situations that clearly involve moral dilemmas that can be cast in the following forms: (1) There is some evidence that act X is morally right, and some evidence that it is morally wrong, but the evidence on both sides is inconclusive. (2) It is clear to health care professionals that on moral grounds they both ought and ought not to perform act X. Performing amniocentesis is such a dilemma for some physicians:

> A physician who refuses to perform amniocentesis (a process of withdrawing fluid from the amniotic sac of a pregnant woman in order to test for congenital disease) may hold that it is morally wrong intentionally to kill innocent human beings. When pressed, he may justify the proclaimed moral rule against killing innocent human beings by reference to a principle of the sanctity of human life. Finally, the particular judgment, the rule, and the principle may be grounded in an ethical theory (a theory that for many people may be only implicit and inchoate). (Beauchamp & Childress, 1979, p. 5)

Medical *judgments* are decisions or conclusions about a particular action. Although the distinction between rules and principles is imprecise, *moral rules* require that certain actions ought (or ought not) to be done because they are right (or wrong). In regard to truthtelling, the rule could be, "It is right to tell the truth to the patient." *Principles* are more fundamental than moral rules; they serve as the foundation for specific, concrete rules. Principles provide answers to the question of why we believe a particular decision is right, good, or appropriate. The principle of respect for each patient, for example, can be the foundation for truth-telling. Finally, *theories* are collective rules and principles that are systematically related. These include principles and rules about what to do when there are conflicts in medical situations. In most respects, biomedical ethics is similar to political ethics, business ethics, and jurisprudence. The same general moral principles apply.

The difficulty of making moral judgments can be seen in the following case: Baby Jane Doe was born with severe handicaps: spina bifida, or an open spinal column; hydrocephalus, excess fluid on the brain; microcephaly, an unusually small head and brain, and an improperly formed brain stem. Physicians conclude that with conservative treatment Baby Jane Doe could live up to 2 years. With surgery she might live up to 20 years but would be paralyzed from the waist down and would have no awareness of her environment. We can offer six different reasons to not allow Baby Jane Doe to die. Some of the reasons are moral; others are nonmoral but could be stated in a way that would make them moral. The major issue is not how much weight to give these reasons in our decision making, but whether they are moral reasons. We could postulate the following reasons:

1. We should not allow Baby Jane Doe to die because similar individuals have been treated in the past, and the decision to terminate her life would be arbitrary and capricious.

2. We should not allow Baby Jane Doe to die because imminent death is not certain. With proper care, she might live a reasonably good life.

3. We should not allow Baby Jane Doe to die because public knowledge of our action would negatively affect the hospital's effort to raise money for much needed equipment.

4. The hospital is bound by its own code of ethics to maximal treatment of all patients.

5. It is against the law to allow Baby Jane Doe to die.

6. The Bible says that we should value all human life; therefore Baby Jane Doe should not be allowed to die.

The first two reasons are moral. However, it is unclear without additional information whether they are compelling enough to justify not allowing Baby Jane Doe to die. The other reasons (3–6) are nonmoral. But as noted earlier, each of them could be stated in ways that would make them moral. For example, we could connect the reason which holds that it is against the law with the reason that we have a moral obligation to obey the law and the combined statements become a moral statement.

When considering actions that will affect the welfare of others, it is important to note that the welfare of all parties must receive the same weight. Which is the greater morality: to enhance significantly the lives of a few individuals or to improve slightly the living conditions of a whole society? In the case of health care, the question becomes: Is it moral to deny health care to people living in abject poverty if this would lead to a better standard of health care for the majority of nonpoverty-stricken people? With a growing concern about the future of humankind, traditional beliefs are being questioned, including the notions that (1) scientific progress is automatically good, (2) what is medically benefi-cial for one person is necessarily good for society, and (3) scientists know best how to improve humanity. The range of questions to be answered is broad: Does a dying person have the right to ask not to be treated? What are the rights of society when caregivers, funds, hospital beds, and technology needed for terminal patients are in short supply? Implicit in the questions is the assumption that we must find a way to enhance our empathy and kindness without destroying our evaluative and selective processes. Of course, there are moral instances when some individuals must be sacrificed for the sake of others. But who should decide?

Ethics in Health Care

Health care is concerned with life and death, the correlative extremes of values in human existence. Since health care professionals are the medical brokers of both the living and the dying, patients and their families accord them extravagant awe and esteem, but they also transfer with these attitudes the crushing weight of both adulation and culpability. When physicians and other health care personnel are successful, they are elevated to the status of saints; when death is the victor (and ultimately it will be), they languish in the monotone of excruciating defeat. Mendelsohn (1980) concluded that this result is deserved because of the arrogance, paternalism, authoritarianism, fear and guilt transmission, jargonism, and mercenary priorities that infect medical and allied health professions. His assessment has been challenged by those who believe health profes-sionals do remarkable things to heal people. In any case, health care jobs are among the most stressful, time-demanding, and self-abnegating professions.

While evaluators of ethical systems in health care take into account the moral character of practitioners, the nature of their motives, and the quality of their effort, they are most heavily persuaded by the results of the action taken. Most members of humankind shun death as the final abyss of evil. Those who stand in the presence of death are not completely consoled by the explanation that death is the liberator of humans who deserve to be released from suffering, and whom physicians cannot cure and loved ones cannot adequately comfort or console. Despite a pragmatic attitude of surrender, death to most human beings remains the attacking vanquisher, and health care is the last citadel to protect them from the impotence of extinction. Treating AIDS patients brings health care professionals face-to-face with their own mortality, and the experience can be the most traumatic of their careers.

Confronted with this disparity of attitudes regarding life and death, it is little wonder that health care is an area fraught with ethical dilemmas. Scott's review (1987) of the development of modern medicine shows that where once medical decisions concerning disease were made by rational inference, now this method has been supplanted by pathological anatomy, the dissecting of the body. This change of perspective from the rational to the empirical has brought about a change in language that has moved more closely to what "is" rather than to "what ought to be," and the shadow of this change has altered the subtleties of ethics.

Physicians and those who support them are daily faced with decisions concerning euthanasia, abortion, pharmaceutical affiliation, tissue transplants, gene splicing, organ donations, access to health care, fraud and abuse, and selection of procedures, to mention but a few. Developments in medical technology over the last two decades, as well as changes in laws, have placed within the province of health care professionals the ability to play God: "Life may be created in the laboratory test-tube. The nature of that life can be altered by gene-splicing. Those who reach a point of death through the deterioration of a vital organ may have their lives prolonged by organ transplantation; those unable to eat and unable to breathe may be intravenously fed and artificially respirated; and when death is inevitable, the process of dying may be indefinitely prolonged" (Almond, 1988, p. 173).

Now let us explore in greater detail what ethical dilemmas such technological developments may mean to the practice of medicine.

Ethics in Medical Practice

Individuals delegated to formulate ethics in medicine face the quandary of scientific minds attempting to accommodate spiritual needs both in themselves and in their patients. Indeed, there are many ethical questions begging to be addressed that are not amenable to scientific proof. So, in keeping with Pascal's wager of faith, what we cannot *prove* we must *decide*. Prudence in making these critical decisions can advance or retard a higher quality of ethics in patient-care responsibilities.

One of the major changes in medical ethics is an attitudinal one. In recent years there has been much criticism of the blatant paternalism of past times when physicians and other health care providers told patients very little concerning their conditions and made all the medical decisions themselves (Long, 1987). The new trend is for practitioners and patients to come together in a partnership of joint power and joint responsibility both before and during the regimen when medical options must be exercised. When pursuing this partnership, we must keep a proper focus. Caregivers and patients are fundamentally *unequal in the* relationship—the former are expected to be better trained in medical facts and procedures. Nor are caregivers required to accept medically inappropriate opinions and desires of patients. The salient question becomes not *who* should make health care choices but rather *what* will facilitate the new ethic of caregivers and patients deciding together.

Another ethical question that confronts those in medical and allied health fields is protection for human-research subjects. In the final analysis, new treatments for human beings must be tested on human subjects (Abram, 1983). Decisions in this area involve informed consent. There always exists the possibility that an unscrupulous health care professional eager to try a new procedure or intent upon realizing economic gain may present the situation to patients in such a way that they are not fully informed and, if they were, would deny their consent to participate in breaking the new medical ground. Also, there is the question of equity. When hundreds of thousands of government dollars will be spent for treatment of a single patient, who will be chosen for treatment and what criteria will determine that choice? It should be noted that there are exceptions like, for example, Barney Clark, the first recipient of an artificial heart, when informed consent was legitimately given and the patient gave his life knowingly to advance medical knowledge.

While it is deemed proper to transplant hearts, livers, and kidneys that have been reaped from the recently deceased, a question still unresolved rages concerning whether medical practitioners should use the tissue of the unborn. It is possible that Parkinson's disease, diabetes, sickle-cell anemia, strokes, and some forms of cancer could be dramatically reduced by implanting certain tissues from dead fetuses that have been removed from a patient during an abortion (*Newsweek*, 1987). Is this ethical? Further, if fetal brain cells can establish new connections in the optical system, is it unethical to use them if they could one day restore sight to the blind? Some alternative protocols are inferior, e.g., use of adult bone marrow. Fetal tissue is favored because it and the cells do not pose the problem of triggering an overreactive immune response.

Those who stand against abortion as an immoral act give forth a resounding "No" to the question of fetal tissue use. Others as devoutly dedicated to life-saving submit that a fetal cadaver should be treated the same as any other cadaver so long as society continues its approval of organ transplants. This thorny issue resides squarely within the purview of medical ethics. Some guidelines have been offered by medical researchers and ethicists alike. First, they propose a ban on the sale of fetal tissue and, second, they propose prohibiting women from having any role in the decision of choosing who will receive tissue from their aborted fetuses. Yet another proposal would confine the use of fetal tissue to medical centers of high integrity that have been recognized for their impeccable standards in both basic and clinical research. There seem to be more questions than answers.

Technological advances have increased the already burgeoning ethical questions that are now swamping the medical profession. Scientific breakthroughs that reveal the secrets of the genetic apparatus of the cell will soon place us in the position of designing the technology for the final cure of many diseases. Such a discovery could also lead to a molecular genetics that will enable us to do molecular surgery that will make physicians and biomedical scientists virtual masters of human existence. The power to design human combinations through gene splicing will be attended by enormous responsibility. Imagine being able to delete undesirable genes, insert others, and mechanically or chemically transform still others. Someday, we may be able to predetermine the physical, mental, and racial characteristics of fetuses. Or imagine what would happen if we were able to reproduce complete individuals identical to living ones. *Cloning,* as the process is called, has awesome implications. Fanatics and criminals, as well as humanitarians and saints, could be duplicated. Again we ask: "Who should make the decisions?"

In a preliminary request to a National Institutes of Health subcommittee in March, 1990, federal researchers were refused permission to perform the first U.S. gene therapy experiments on humans (Weiss, 1990). The proposal called for injecting therapeutic gene-altered cells into children with a life-threatening deficiency of the immune system. In this same meeting, some of the researchers who had proposed the gene therapy did receive permission to infuse cells bearing nontherapeutic genetic alterations into an expanded number of patients with malignant melanoma. Because momentous decision making will be required, some experts believe medical students very early in their training should be taught medical ethics as a basic part of their curriculum. Has any person the truth, the beauty, and the goodness to become the creator of both the form and content of a new human race? This is the question that only a noble ethic, equal to the profundity of the problem, will be able to resolve.

Mortality or Morbidity?

While medical practitioners would generally agree that healing, helping, comforting, and acting with compassion are the basic components that guide their practice, there still remain many unresolved ethical decisions. One such decision is whether the health care professional's primary focus should be on mortality or morbidity. If we elect to concern ourselves primarily with mortality, we would give priority to combating diseases with high mortality rates (Neki, 1979). But if the focus is to be on morbidity, emphasis would be on chronic conditions which cause more extended and intense distress to humankind. Obviously, if mortality is chosen, the fight cannot be won; it can merely be postponed—death is inevitable. If we opt for morbidity as a priority, chronic diseases such as mental illness and arthritis would have to be given more urgent attention.

Decision making becomes even more acute as our population increases. It is apparent that as this occurs there will be less money to address the needs of each individual. Is it ethical to allow health care to become contingent upon the ability to pay? That is, is it ethical to spend excessive amounts of public money on new technologies that only the rich can afford? The weight of this ethical responsibility cannot fall upon the medical community alone, especially not solely upon physicians. They, too, are human beings with ambitions, with appetites and vulnerabilities to the same infirmities that afflict the rest of the population. So large looms the crisis of ethics in medical practice that the patient population is going to have to accept a partnership role in decisions concerning their own physical and mental well-being, and they must seek legislation or new guidelines to establish and ensure their equitable rights.

Some of the decisions that patients can help make include abortion, living wills, differential access to health care, genetic screening and engineering, reviving the impaired and dying, initiating and withholding treatment, AIDS disclosure, exporting FDA rejected food and drug products to Third World countries, surrogate motherhood, animal organ research, and withholding food and fluids from the terminally ill. While these decisions need to be made from a personal perspective, one hopes from a humane perspective that they will be made with due consideration for the betterment of society as a whole. But therein lies the problem: "The concepts of value are profound and difficult exactly because they do two things at once: they join men into societies, and yet they preserve for them a freedom which makes them single men. A philosophy which does not acknowledge both needs cannot evolve values, and indeed cannot allow them" (Bronowski, 1965, p. 55).

Health Care as a Right

No matter which view one holds concerning the right of each individual to have adequate medical treatment and the means by which such treatment will be delivered, there can be very little doubt on one point: The world is facing a crisis in health care. On the one side, there are those who can afford the services of physicians and hospitals or clinics; on the other side, there are those who cannot afford such services and thus face a future made bleak by chronic illness. Currently, there are between 35 million and 40 million Americans who would be medically unprotected should they require extended nursing home and home care services (Ginzberg, 1988). It appears that our society places a higher priority on providing "the best that money can buy" for people who have access to health care than on expanding access to health care (Taylor, 1989).

Despite progress during the past 20 years, the United States still has a long way to go before all of its citizens achieve equitable access to health care. Although we spend more than other nations for health care (see Table 1-2), the services are unequally shared. Some of the best medical treatment in the world is available in the Mayo Clinic in Minnesota, Johns Hopkins Hospital in Maryland, Methodist Hospital in Texas, Stanford University Hospital in California, and Columbia-Presbyterian Medical Center in New York. Yet, only a few miles away from these fine facilities, thousands of low-income people receive almost no health care.

Table 1-2. Health care outlays as a percentage of gross domestic products, 1960–1986

Country	Year		
	1965	1980	1986
Australia	4.9	6.6	7.2
Canada	6.1	7.4	8.5
Denmark	4.8	6.8	6.1
France	5.2	7.4	8.5
Germany (West)	5.1	7.9	8.1
Italy	4.0	6.8	6.7
Japan	4.5	6.6	6.7
The Netherlands	4.4	8.2	8.3
New Zealand	4.3	7.2	6.9
Norway	3.9	6.6	6.8
Sweden	5.6	9.5	9.1
Switzerland	3.8	7.2	8.0
United Kingdom	4.1	5.8	6.2
United States	6.0	9.2	11.1

The advances in health care have not accrued to black Americans as a whole. On the contrary, their health conditions have declined. A good measure of overall health is "life expectancy." According to the National Center for Health Statistics, in 1984, the life expectancy was 75.3 years for white Americans and 69.7 years for black Americans. In 1988, the rates were 75.6 years for whites and 74.9 years for blacks. The life expectancy for blacks was 75 years in 1987. When we add to these statistics large annual increases among blacks in the number of deaths from infant mortality, motor vehicle accidents, homicides, and AIDS, we are confronted with a national crisis. But it is not only blacks who lack adequate health care. Nonwhites, in particular, are disadvantaged by poverty, racial discrimination, and other barriers to adequate health care. To most low-income nonwhite Americans, stories about cancer and drug research, and birth control clinics are akin to fairy tales. Low-income nonwhite babies die at a rate 90 percent higher than for white babies, and nonwhite mothers die during childbirth at a rate four times that of white mothers. In fact, the nonwhite American deaths at birth and during infancy are worse than the record of most of the world's urbanized nations. Clearly, the major issue for low-income nonwhite Americans is not tax reform or welfare checks—it is survival. Considerably fewer lives would be lost if nonwhite Americans had better access to health care (Blendon et al., 1989).

The burden of chronic illness is borne most heavily by low-income elderly (Jennings et al., 1988). After 1940, the United States, like an individual who had just taken a good look in the mirror, realized that it was no longer as young as it used to be. We are no longer primarily an under-thirty-years-of-age population. Indeed, a large number of Americans fit Shakespeare's description of an older person: "sans teeth, sans eyes, sans taste, sans everything." The result was a feeling of shock, followed by an earnest search for remedies to the problems of age. In 1985, only 45 percent of the health care costs of older Americans were paid by Medicare (Roemer, 1988). From 1975 to 1983, the proportion of low-income citizens covered by Medicaid dropped from 63 percent to 46 percent (Butler et al., 1987). What happened to the so-called "safety net" for the poor? The Medicaid program was established as a federal-state system of personal medical treatment for the poor under which the federal government would match from 50 percent to 78 percent of the total program cost, depending on the per capita income of each state.

Several states, particularly those in the South, have never contributed the necessary amount to receive the maximal federal contribution. In 1986, for example, the annual Medicaid expenditures amounted to $951 per recipient in West Virginia and $993 in Mississippi, while such expenditures amounted to $3,541 in New York and $3,675 in New Hampshire (Ginzberg, 1988, p. 3310). In 1990, a family of three living in Alabama earning more than $1,416 annually—about 13 percent of the federal poverty level—could not qualify for Medicaid. Especially in rural areas, low-income families who have no medical coverage experience even greater health care problems than families living in cities with more hospitals, physicians, and other professionals. This is akin to geographical death sentences. Medicaid data document the lack of access to top-quality health care. Most Medicaid recipients use hospital outpatient departments and emergency rooms as their regular source of care (Howell, 1988).

The health care difficulties of low-income adults in the United States are formidable, and they are overwhelming for our nation's children. Our inner cities are becoming populated with unemployed migrant people. They are people of many colors—white, brown, black, red, yellow, and combinations of them. More important than their diverse colors is their common condition of poverty. These people sleep in dilapidated structures that usually lack adequate heat, refrigeration, and sanitary facilities. Or they sleep in no structures at all. In addition, they walk and play on garbage-strewn grounds infested with internal parasites, and they drink polluted water. The children of the poor are infected with intestinal parasites, have chronic skin infections and dental and hearing problems. Malnutrition and diseases leave most of them unable physically or mentally to compete with their affluent peers. Only about one-third of poor children under eighteen years of age have any private insurance, despite the fact that two-thirds of them reside with families in which at least one member is employed during the year (Butler et al., 1987).

The United States is one of the last developed countries that does not guarantee access to basic medical care for its citizens. As Berenson (1989) put it, "We have simultaneously created a crazy-quilt, public-private bureaucratic maze that frustrates patients, doctors, and usually the bureaucrats themselves" (p. 14). The crucial question about health care was asked by Ruddick (1989): "Is there—for everyone—a general right to health care, prior contract or legislation? A right which derives from other rights and duties or general features of humanity or society?" (p. 161). Whether we answer this question affirmatively or negatively, we must deal with it, for it would seem that any plan for national health care will stand or fall on the answer.

According to several international declarations, health care *is* a social right. The Universal Declaration of Human Rights adopted by the United Nations General Assembly in 1948 states: "Everyone has the right to a standard of living adequate for the health and well-being of himself and of his family, including food, clothing, housing and medical care and necessary social services . . . " The International Covenant on Economic, Social, and Cultural Rights, drafted pursuant to the International Declaration of Human Rights, recognizes "the right of everyone to the enjoyment of the highest attainable standard of physical and mental health." And the World Health Organization declares that "the right to a long life, which might theoretically be averaged at 100 years, is a basic human right of every individual."

Along this line of reasoning, health care has been called an "instrumental right," for it is a means to other things a democratic society considers major values, including autonomous functioning. Freedom means very little if disease or disability prevents us from achieving our optimum potential. A liberty that does not include the material and health conditions necessary for being a productive citizen is as good as no liberty at all (Churchill, 1987). Given a right to health care based on need, then such a right means equitable access based on need alone to effective care that society can reasonably afford. Equity based on "need alone" means that no one has a prior entitlement based on status, ethnicity, income, or other social differences. A certain level of health is necessary if equity is to be granted by any society which claims to value human life. A similar philosophical argument has been constructed by writers who maintain that every human being has the right to "primary goods"—those things which are necessary for achieving other goals in life.

Democratic societies assume that each citizen has a right to earn a living. They also assume that each person has certain duties connected with citizenship, e.g., voting in public elections. However, these rights and duties are meaningless unless people are physically able to assume them. If we are without medical care when ill, we do not have an equal opportunity to exercise our citizenship (Moody, 1989). Conceivably, a right to health care is derived from the American Declaration of Independence, since it declares that "all people are endowed by their Creator with certain unalienable Rights, that among these . . . are Life, Liberty, and the Pursuit of Happiness." Nevertheless, in the early part of this century, it was generally held that the Constitution contained no provision, either in its main body or in the Bill of Rights, that supported a claim to the right of every citizen to health care.

Medical-Ethical Decision Making

In a consideration of medical-ethical decision making, there are many conflicting views. Some people believe guidelines should be developed by the medical community, other people are adamant that medical-ethical guidelines should be imposed from outside medical institutions, perhaps by behavioral scientists; still others contend they should be developed by medical educators as a part of medical and allied health curricula. Self (1979) suggested that the first step in solving a medical dilemma should be to identify a central issue. This is usually accomplished from the perspective of the physician, but such a frame of reference would tend to discourage the inclusion of nonphysicians', particularly patients', values.

A more proper identification of the relevancy of decisions might be to pose the question: Will the decision improve the quality of the patient's life? From this perspective, the choice of treatment, whatever the value stance of the physician, would be determined by considering diagnostic possibilities, as well as the therapeutic modalities, with the patient being the locus of concern (Pinkus, 1981). Once a decision has been reached, consideration must still be made as to the best person available to perform the chosen therapeutic intervention—whether another practitioner with more technical expertise or experience should be summoned. The quality of the remaining life of the patient should also be weighed, as well as whether the patient is capable of comprehending the implications of the procedure to be performed. Value judgments and ethics will enter into the questions asked and the answers given. And these should be given sensitive and careful attention to best help patients and members of their family cope with medical problems. Health care professionals must carefully weigh their own values, too (Duff & Campbell, 1980). In the not-too-distant past medical-ethical decisions relied too heavily on outdated medical standards.

The goals, temperament, and technological orientation of doctors make them the least likely to make patient-benefiting medical decisions. Mendelsohn (1980) stated if 90 percent of modern medicine disappeared— including doctors, hospitals, drugs, and equipment, the effect on our health would be beneficial. To support this argument, he cited the following statistics: In 1976 in Bogota, Colombia, during a 52-day period when only emergency treatment was given, the death rate went down 35 percent; when doctors went on a strike in Los Angeles County in 1976, there was an 18 percent drop in the death rate (during this same time, 60 percent fewer operations were performed); in 1973 during an Israeli doctor's strike for a month (which reduced patient load from 65,000 to 7,000), the death rate dropped 50 percent. These data notwithstanding, few people really want most of modern medicine to disappear.

Some credence can be given to the suggestion that we need to review medical-ethical decision making by doctors who, as a statistical group, have incidences of psychological maladjustment, chemical addiction, and burnout higher than most other professionals. The suicide rate of doctors is twice the average for all professionals. Also, because many doctors tend to limit their closest friendships to other doctors, this places them in a position of rarely having to defend their medical ethics among people who might hold a different view. Indeed, physician values and decision making are seldom challenged because they are formed almost exclusively within a myoptic medical circle of peers. We should not dismiss too lightly the suggestion that if medical-ethical decision making is to improve, pressure for change must come from outside: Medicine is not likely to cure itself because its prescriptions come from its own system of values (Mendelsohn, 1980).

The Challenge

Futurists, appealing to common sense logic, predict that substantial global changes in lifestyle will make drastic changes in moral values an absolute necessity. Many of the basic issues in ethics and morality we face today were recently outside the domain of science because many of the crises that we face are recent scientific phenomena. AIDS is such an example. Yet, we seem determined to kill ourselves in order to improve our sciences. Medical researchers and practitioners are debating the morality of placing costly machines, medications, and space-age technologies needed for optimum health care beyond the means of the great majority of the peoples of the world. This is a debate that must be concluded soon. Our future is being decided now, and medical-ethical decisions must be made about which values are best for the creation of a world community where all people can live in dignity and die a timely death.

Human values pertaining to survival can be viewed as universal determinants of moral decision making. Global health problems, for the most part, are human engendered and can be addressed in terms of human values. To effectively remedy global health problems, care providers must be proactive and prevent illness rather than waiting for it to occur. There is no reason to expect members of the scientific community to step aside and let other persons take the lead in delineating and prioritizing ethical issues focusing on medical problems. Besides, many medical ethicists assert that they have already made the changes necessary to mediate health problems. This is more than a struggle for pedagogical bragging rights, it is a struggle for moral and ethical dominance in medical institutions that affect the lives of humankind. If medical practitioners are to be the mediators of medical-ethical decision making, they must not try to eliminate value differences but, instead, to bring them into a clearer focus.

Health care is in a growing state of crisis as communities throughout the world experience too many health needs and too few resources, both medical and monetary. The problems are numerous. Specialization has estranged patients from health professionals. In the United States, inadequate private insurance and Medicare reimbursement are creating an adversarial relationship between patients and caregivers and caregivers and insurance carriers. Technology has made giant strides in medication, equipment, and procedures, but adequate care is now becoming contingent upon the patient's ability to pay. Adding fuel to this human relations fire are new technologies that proliferate the jargon practitioners use to communicate with their patients. Because of this, communication continues to deteriorate between health care professionals and their patients, especially in situations where little time is available to become acquainted before life and death procedures are undertaken. New doctors are needed. Mendelsohn (1980) described the new doctor:

> The new doctor will be conversant not only in the language of science, but in the language of *people* as well. He or she is going to be constantly *informing* patients: informing them of how certain activities and circumstances affect health. The doctor-patient relationship is democratic in the sense that both doctor and patient share information equally. But that "democracy" must necessarily break down when the doctor has to exercise his or her authority. The doctor must inform the patient of how the patient's choices will affect him, but he or she must not shrink from making a judgment based on his or her knowledge and talents. That's what the patient is paying for. (p. 23)

Too often, health care providers do not know that values are internalized beliefs that are prioritized to determine an individual's action and reaction to people, situations, and ideas. A patient's values may differ from the care provider. And value differences result in different perceptions of what is right or wrong, good or bad. In the application of values and ethics to medicine and allied health, there are only ambiguous guidelines. As we noted, many of the circumscriptions imposed on health care providers in the past were derived from philosophical and religious precepts which no longer have meaningful application in the modern world. The task is not to discard all of the existing values but to discard dysfunctional ones and add functional ones.

Medical organizations continually try to formulate new codes, but these have been basically in-house efforts without significant input from other professions or even patients who are affected by the codes. This often results in medical value guidelines that are unpremised, written in language that is difficult to understand, and built on a vision that is socially sterile. Currently, legalists and religionists are attempting to legislate ethical decisions that medical personnel must abide by. But so long as individuals exist who hold unique values, we will not be able to create an instrument profound enough to measure all the contingencies and extenuations. Still we must try to reduce the magnitude of moral uncertainty and ambiguity.

We must examine those who make and enforce medical rules. The ideal would be to eliminate at the outset medical personnel who are without sufficient character and integrity. Competence and competitiveness alone will no longer suffice. The extent of physicians' scientific knowledge and technical resources provide them with the upper limits of what can be done for patients. In many instances, it is not socially and medically acceptable to do whatever is technically possible; but most practitioners agree that it is immoral to aggravate a patient's condition when it could have been avoided. Efforts should be made to include value discernment and ethical decision making in medical and allied health curricula. Perhaps master practitioners could be trained in these disciplines to assist and oversee the beginning practice of newly graduated health care professionals.

The code of silence among the medical and allied health professions that discourages criticism of colleagues adds to the suspicions of those seeking to redress legitimate medical wrongs. There is no integrity in silence when it camouflages violations of the human care ethic. These are some of the problems that beset us, and we must not wait until we are overwhelmed by them to seek solutions. We who have inherited the earth must hurry if we are to preserve the earth and humankind's dominion over it. Medical efforts to do so will require courage, compromise, and compassion across cultures.

REFERENCES

Abram, M. B. (1983). Ethics and the new medicine. *New York Times Magazine,* June 5. 68 ff.

Almond, B. (1988). Philosophy, medicine and its technologies. *Journal of Medical Ethics, 14:* 173–178.

Beauchamp, T. L. & Childress, J. F. (1979). *Principles of biomedical ethics.* New York: Oxford University Press.

Berensen, R. A. (1989). A physician's reflections. *Hastings Center Report, 19:* 12–15.

Blendon, R. J., Aiken, L. H., Freeman, H. E. & Corey, C. R. (1989). Access to medical care for black and white Americans: A matter of concern. *JAMA, 261:* 278–281.

Boxill, B. (1985). Medical decision making under uncertainty, pp. 97–108. In J. M. Humber & R. F. Almeder (Eds.) *Biomedical ethics review.* Clifton, NJ: Humana Press.

Braverman, E. R. (1987). The religious model: Holy medicine and the Spiritual Behavior Inventory. *Southern Medical Journal, 80:* 415–420, 425.

Bronowski, J. (1965). *Science and human values.* New York: Harper & Row.

Butler, J. A., Rosenbaum, S. & Palfrey, J. (1987). Ensuring access to health care for children with disabilities. *New England Journal of Medicine, 317:* 162–164.

Chapman, C. B. (1984). *Physicians, law, and ethics.* New York: New York University Press.

Churchill, L. R. (1987). *Rationing health care in America.* Notre Dame, IN: University of Notre Dame Press.

Duff, R. & Campbell, A. G. M. (1980). Moral and ethical dilemmas: Seven years into the debate about human ambiguity. *Annals of the American Academy of Political and Social Science, 447:* 19–28.

Edwards, C. P. (1985). Rationality, culture and the construction of "ethical discourse." *Ethos, 13:* 318–339.

Eliopoulos, C. (1988). Ethics and the health care supervisor. *Health Care Supervisor, 6:* 27–37.

Engelhardt, T. H. (1986). *The foundations of bioethics.* New York: Oxford University Press.

Ginzberg, E. (1988). Medical care for the poor: No magic bullets. *JAMA, 259:* 3309–3311.

Heschel, A. J. (1975). *The prophets.* Vol. 2. New York: Harper & Row.

Howell, E. M. (1988). Low-income persons' access to health care: NMEEUS Medicaid data. *Public Health Reports, 103:* 507–514.

Jennings, B., Callahan, D. & Caplan, A. L. (1988). Ethical challenges of chronic illness. *Hastings Center Report, 18:* 1–16.

Long, K. H. (1987). The ethics of medicine. *Tampa Tribune,* November 22, pp. 11 ff.

Mendelsohn, R. (1980). I no longer believe in modern medicine. *New Physician, 2:* 18–26.

Moody, H. R. (1989). Age-based entitlements to health care: What are the limits? *Mount Sinai Journal of Medicine, 56:* 168–175.

Myers, J. M. (1969). The linneth on the leaf, pp. 59–65. In W. C. Kvaraceus & E. N. Hayes (Eds.), *If your child is handicapped.* Boston: Porter Sargent.

Neki, J. S. (1979). Medical ethics: A viewpoint from the developing world. *World Health, 2:* 18–29.

Newsweek. (1987). Should medicine use the unborn? *14:* 63.

Pinkus, R. (1981). Medical foundations of various approaches to medical ethical decision-making. *Journal of Medicine and Philosophy, 6:* 295–307.

Roemer, R. (1988). The right to health care: Gains and gaps. *American Journal of Public Health, 78:* 241–247.

Ruddick, W. (1989). Why not a general right to health care? *Mount Sinai Journal of Medicine, 56:* 161–163.

Scott, C. E. (1987). The power of medicine, the power of ethics. *Journal of Medicine and Philosophy, 12:* 335–350.

Self, D. J. (1979). Philosophical foundations of various approaches to ethical decision-making. *Journal of Medicine and Philosophy, 1:* 21–31.

Taylor, R. M. (1989). Ethical aspects of medical economics. *Neurologic Clinics, 7:* 883–900.

Veatch, R. M. (1989). *Medical ethics.* Boston: Jones & Bartlett.

Weiss, R. (1990). Drug reduces paralysis after spinal injury. *Science News, 137:* 212.

SUGGESTED READINGS

Ackerman, T. F. et al. (1987). *Clinical medical ethics: Exploration and assessment.* Lantham, MA: University Presses of America.

Anderson, G. R. & Glesnes-Anderson, V. A. (1987). *Health care ethics: A guide for decision makers.* London: Faber & Faber.

Arras, J. D. & Rhoden, N. R. (1989). *Ethical issues in modern medicine.* Mountain View, CA: Mayfield.

Baird, R. M. & Rosenbaum, S. E. (1989). *Euthanasia: The moral issues.* Buffalo, NY: Prometheus.

Bandman, E. L. & Bandman, B. (1986). *Bioethics and human rights: A reader for health professionals.* Lantham, MD: University Presses of America.

Benjamin, M. & Curtis, J. (1986). *Ethics in nursing.* New York: Oxford University Press.

Callahan, D. (1988). *Setting limits: Medical goals in an aging society.* New York: Simon & Shuster.

Calman, K. C. (1987). *Healthy respect: Ethics in health care.* London: Faber & Faber.

Christie, R. & Hoffmaster, B. (1986). *Ethical issues in family medicine.* New York: Oxford University Press.

Drane, J. F. (1988). *Becoming a good doctor: The place of virtue and character in medical ethics.* Kansas City, MO: Sheed & Ward.

Freeman, J. & McDonnell, K. (1987). *Tough decisions: A casebook in medical ethics.* New York: Oxford University Press.

Frohock, F. M. (1986). *Special care: Medical decisions at the beginning of life.* Chicago: University of Chicago Press.

Glover, J. et al. (1989). *Ethics of new reproductive technologies.* Dekalb: Northern Illinois University Press.

Graber, G. C. & Thomasma, D. C. (1989). *Theory and practice of medical ethics.* New York: Continuum.

Hull, R. T. (1990). *Ethical issues in the new reproductive technologies.* Belmont, CA: Wadsworth.

Kantor, J. E. (1989). *Medical ethics for physicians-in-training.* New York: Plenum.

Kelly, E. (1989). *Professional ethics in health care services.* Lantham, MD: University Presses of America.

Lamb, D. (1988). *Down the slippery slope: Arguing in applied ethics.* New York: Routledge Chapman & Hall.

Lammers, S. E. & Verhey, A. (1987). *On moral medicine: Theological perspectives in medical ethics.* Grand Rapids, MI: Eerdmans.

Leither, E. (1988). *The second international congress on ethics in medicine.* New York: BIMC.

Levine, R. J. (1987). *Ethics and regulations of clinical research.* New Haven: Yale University Press.

Lockwood, M. (1986). *Moral dilemmas in modern medicine.* New York: Oxford University Press.

Loewy, E. H. (1989). *Ethical dilemmas in modern medicine: A physician's viewpoint.* New York: Plenum.

Mason, J. K. (1988). *Human life and medical practice.* New York: Columbia University Press.

Menzel, P. T. (1989). *Strong medicine: The ethical rationing of health care.* New York: Oxford University Press.

Momeyer, R. W. (1988). *Confronting death.* Bloomington: Indiana University Press.

Munson, R. C. (1988). *Intervention and reflection: Basic issues in medical ethics.* Belmont, CA: Wadsworth.

Napodano, R. J. (1986). *Values in medical practice: A statement of philosophy for physicians and model for teaching a healing science.* New York: Human Sciences Press.

Palmer, L. I. (1989). *Law, medicine and social justice.* Louisville, KY: Westminister Press.

Smith, H. L. & Churchill, L. R. (1986). *Professional ethics and primary care medicine: Beyond dilemmas and decorum.* Durham, NC: Duke University Press.

VanDeVeer, D. & Regan, T. (1987). *Health care ethics: An introduction.* Philadelphia: Temple University Press.

Vaux, K. (1986). *Powers that make us human: The foundations of medical ethics.* Urbana: University of Illinois Press.

Veatch, R. (1989). *Cross-cultural perspectives in medical ethics: Readings.* Boston: Jones & Bartlett.

Weinstein, B. D. (1986). *Ethics in the hospital setting.* Morgantown: West Virginia University Press.

Wennberg, R. N. (1989). *Terminal choices: Euthanasia, suicide, and the right to die.* Grand Rapids, MI: Eerdmans.

Younger, S. J. (1986). *Human values in critical care medicine.* New York: Praeger.

Chapter 2

HEALTH AS A VALUE

There's a lot more to health than not being sick.

Bruce Larson, 1981

We do not become fully ethical beings until we are clear about our values.

E.D. Pellegrino, 1981

Goldstein (1959) said, "health is not an objective condition which can be understood by the methods of natural science alone. It is rather, a condition, related to a mental attitude by which the individual has to value what is essential for his life." Goldstein considers health the primary determinant of self-realization. " 'Health' is therefore, a value; its value consists in the individual's capacity to actualize his nature to the degree that for him is essential." Health is a significant positive value because it provides the means by which persons can achieve what is essential and meaningful to them. Something negative is usually not valued, unless, of course, someone obtains a great deal of satisfaction from malingering, or an illness is permitted to overshadow all other priorities in a person's life, or a person purposefully engages in life-threatening risks. These negative behaviors can become valued if they provide some degree of gratification or satisfaction to a person and consume a great deal of time and energy in comparison to other activities.

Values guide our conduct. A *value* is an enduring belief that a specific mode of conduct is preferable to an opposite mode of conduct. A *value system* is an enduring organization of beliefs. Gradually, through the experience of maturation, we learn to integrate isolated, absolute values, such as health. How high or low health ranks among all of our personal values influences how we conduct ourselves with respect to matters that affect our health (Rokeach, 1973).

All people everywhere possess the same values, but to different degrees. The antecedents of human values can be traced to culture, society and its institutions, and personality (Fig. 2-1). We learn what to value, and to what degree, as we grow and develop. Some values have enduring

33

importance throughout our lifetime while others change in priority. Health is an example of a value that is likely to change as we age. Health is often most valued by individuals after the loss of good health. Generally, health as a value has not been taught to children in our culture, as are such other values as independence or getting along with others. However, there are an increasing number of advocates for teaching and promoting health among school-age children, most noteworthy is the Health For All Program of the World Health Organization (Gezairy, 1990; Trichopoulos & Petridou, 1988). Personal health maintenance for children is vital for four reasons (Richmond & Kotelchuck, 1984). First, engaging in preventive behaviors such as wearing seat belts, refraining from alcohol intake, and receiving immunizations is conducive to a healthier childhood. Second, the probability of a healthier childhood is enhanced, since many of the behavioral risk factors associated with chronic disease are avoided or delayed. Third, positive health values are shaped and personal responsibility for health is assumed with an emphasis on personal health maintenance. Fourth, since adult patterns of health service utilization appear to be shaped during childhood, encouraging the development of decision-making skills regarding the appropriate use of health services may have long-term benefits.

In order for health professionals to most effectively promote health and prevent disease among school-aged populations, a knowledge of children's cognitive development is essential. An excellent overview of the literature concerning children's understanding of health and illness has been written by Mickalide (1986).

We learn about health from the media, by observing the health behavior of adults, and by determining which values are given the highest priority by the persons we respect, and which values seem to carry the greatest rewards. In general, prevention is not among the most highly rated values in our society. Only when health is lost does conversation usually turn to what caused the illness and what the individual might have done to prevent it. Although health is a personal responsibility, the tasks it requires are determined by the larger society. If society does not support health promotion, it will be difficult for most individuals to maintain the proper motivation to do so on their own (Bruhn et al., 1977).

Researchers have frequently assumed that all people uniformly place a very high value on health. Rokeach (1973) concluded that health as a value is too important to measure. Indeed, in the context of a life-

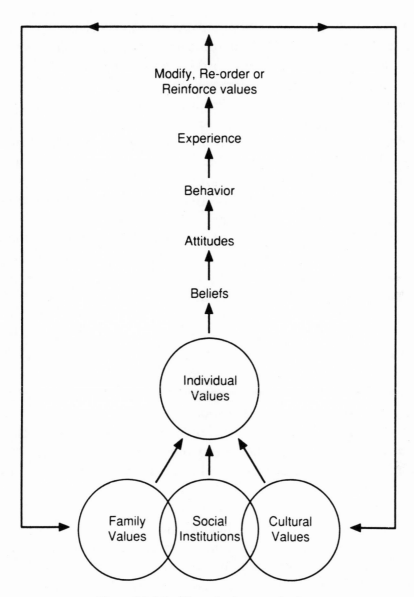

Figure 2-1. The life cycle of personal values.

threatening disease it is probably a safe assumption that the salience of health and the value placed upon it is high. However, in the domain of preventive health behavior where health actions for the purpose of remaining healthy are taken when a person is symptom free, the value placed on health may not be so high (Lau, Hartman & Ware, 1986). Ware et al., (1974) and Ware & Young (1979) studied the health perceptions of

American adults in five general population surveys. The generally healthy respondents ranked "health" in addition to 17 of Rokeach's "terminal" values, for example, happiness, wisdom, and true friendship. Although health was, on the average, the most highly ranked of the 18 values, from 20 percent to 40 percent of the respondents in the five samples did not rank health among their five highest values.

Unfortunately, there is no widely accepted method of measuring health values. The most frequent method used is some variant of Rokeach's (1973) ranking of terminal values (Kristiansen, 1985; Ware & Young, 1979). With this task, respondents are asked to rank, in order of importance to them, a series of terminal values that includes health, e.g., a comfortable life, an exciting life, friendship, salvation. Since the list of values is fairly encompassing, the relative ranking of health is assumed to measure how highly health is valued. Readers may wish to rank their personal values by completing the value survey shown in Appendix B.

One method of measuring health value was used by Fabrega and Roberts (1972). A measure they called "health salience" was constructed by asking respondents how they would spend a hypothetical $500, and then asking them to rank a series of potential uses of the $500; two of the uses involved health. Another common method is to measure health "worry" or "concern." Subjects' responses to simple statements, such as "I worry a lot about my child's health" or "Do you watch your health pretty carefully or do you take things pretty much as they come?", are taken as indicators of their concern with health. Less direct methods ask respondents how frequently they view health programs on television or score health content on projective tests. The reliability and validity of these various methods for measuring health value have not been established.

Lau and his colleagues (1986) were interested in how people learned to value health. They suggested that the value placed on health might change with health status. For example, the elderly, who typically experience more illness than younger people, might value health more highly than younger people. However, no evidence was found to support this hypothesis.

Kristiansen (1985), in a postal survey in Exeter, England, found that the value of health was related to preventive health behavior. Respondents who reported good preventive health behavior valued health more than did those who reported poor preventive health behavior. Thus, it would seem that any effort to get people to change their health beliefs and health behaviors will be most successful among people who value their health highly.

Wallston et al. (1974) used an abbreviated form of the Rokeach Value Survey in an attempt to determine the influence of values and beliefs on information-seeking behavior. Nine of the ten values used in the study were values from the Rokeach Value Survey. The remaining value included was "a healthy life." Wallston found a significantly greater amount of information-seeking behavior among those individuals who placed a greater value on a healthy life and also believed that they could control their own health.

Learning About Values

Rogers (1964) has pointed out that infants have a clear approach to values. From studying infants' behavior, we can infer that they prefer those experiences which maintain, enhance, or actualize their organism, and reject those which do not serve this end. Infants place a positive value on food, security, and new experiences and a negative value on hunger and pain, loud noises, and bitter tastes. But infants' value systems are constantly changing. The process of valuing is not fixed. Rogers also points out that the origin of the infant's approach to values is clearly within itself. Infants know what they like and dislike. At this point, parents and others are not a significant influence. As infants mature, they learn that in order to hold or gain love and approval from others, they must relinquish some values. Children learn from the behavior of others and adopt or modify the values of others as their own. Rogers believes that adults' approaches to values have several common characteristics:

1. The majority of values are introjected from significant individuals or groups, but are regarded as one's own values.
2. The source of evaluation, on most matters, lies outside of oneself.
3. The criterion by which values are set is the degree to which they will cause a person to be loved, accepted, or esteemed.
4. These preferences either are not related at all, or are not clearly related, to one's own process of experiencing.

Rogers states that the characteristic picture of a person's values are that they are fixed and rarely tested or examined. For this reason, we lose contact with our experiences and, indeed, ourselves. Rogers notes that evidence from therapy indicates that both personal and social values emerge as natural, and experienced, when individuals are close to their own valuing process. The valuing process in mature individuals is open to the acknowledgment of errors, and to feedback. Such individuals can continually correct their course toward goal fulfillment.

Learning About Health

Understanding the process by which we learn about health values is important because it relates to the practice, in health care, of including patients as agents in their own health maintenance or recovery. If patients are to be encouraged to take an active, self-initiated role in their own health maintenance, it is essential to discover what values they bring to the situation. It is equally important to discover the genesis of those values.

From early childhood, learning about health is an ongoing process. The young child's experience provides a vast source of sensory impressions and feelings, both self-initiated and derived from social stimulation, which help to shape later health attitudes and behavior. The mother, by the quality of her physical and affective response to the needs of her child, and by her verbal and nonverbal behavior as it reflects her own body image, her knowledge of health, and the health values that she has adopted from her culture, contributes to the meaning of health for her child. Society, initially through parents and by formal and informal training, orients the child to its practices, beliefs, and values regarding health (Bruhn & Cordova, 1977 & 1978).

In one of the first studies of children's understanding of health, Rashkis (1965) talked with boys and girls attending kindergarten through the third grade about the meaning of health, responsibility for health, and the prevalence of health. Rashkis found that the children could not ascribe a positive feeling tone to being well, and their tendency was to describe being well in terms of the absence of illness. They had no concept of health as a positive state. The reports of the children revealed an early and sustained awareness of many restrictions upon health. The children recognized the limitations of their ability to keep themselves well and that there are no exemptions from illness.

Eating activities were mentioned most frequently in response to the question "What do we do to be well?" Hygiene was the second most popular category. It is noteworthy that the children gave eating precedence over all other self-care activities, including prophylactic measures, in their explanation of how they keep themselves well. They ally their self-interest with a biologic drive, the economics of which they can appreciate and the satisfaction of which they can largely control.

Natapoff (1978) asked 264 first, fourth, and seventh grade children to define health, state what it felt like to be healthy and not healthy, and to give criteria they would use to judge another person's health status. She found that children saw health as a positive attribute which enabled them to participate in desired activities, that persons were healthy if they could do what they wanted to do, and that health and illness were two different concepts rather than on a continuum as is often cited in the literature. Mental health was not considered as part of being healthy except by a few of the oldest children. There were both qualitative and quantitative changes in children's views about health as they aged.

Natapoff (1978) found that children view health more positively than most definitions proposed by health professionals. Rather than seeing health as the absence of symptoms or the ability to perform minimally, they see health as feeling good and being able to participate in desired activities. Children as young as age six have ideas about health, can talk about health matters and express those ideas positively.

Children's health beliefs have been investigated by several researchers. In several studies, Gochman (1972), Gochman et al. (1972), Gochman & Sheiman (1978) found that children are consistent in their perceptions of vulnerability to health problems. These beliefs of susceptibility stabilize at approximately 9 to 11 years of age. Children's beliefs about vulnerability are more important to future behavior than perceived beliefs. Later, Gochman studied the relationship of perceived vulnerability to self-concept in children from 8–17 years of age (Gochman, 1977). A negative relationship was found in all but the youngest subjects, perhaps because they had yet to integrate the various parts of a belief system. Children's concepts of health were found to change with age (Natapoff, 1982; Palmer & Lewis, 1976).

A Piagetian framework has been used to analyze children's ideas about health (Natapoff, 1982). Using this approach, it is possible to describe the formation of health beliefs as they change over time. There is considerable evidence that children's health beliefs begin to differentiate into a coherent belief system at approximately nine years of age, a period which corresponds to Piaget's concrete operational period. Health behavior seems to change around this age as well. Eight and nine year olds are able to become active health consumers and can make their own health decisions. Abstract qualities like mental health enter into the concept of health as the child approaches adolescence.

However, children's concepts of health are influenced by variables other than just age-related cognitive development. These variables include personality, family, and the children's own state of health (Kalnis & Love, 1982). Kohlberg (1969) has noted that social development and cognitive development are interrelated. Kohlberg notes that his six stages of moral development represent successive forms of reciprocity, each more differentiated and universalized than the preceding stage. Moral development is fundamentally a process of restructuring modes of role-taking. The more individuals are responsible for the group and for their own actions, the more they must take the roles of others in the group. Values develop in the course of sharing social relationships.

Learning to Value Health

The value placed on health and the level of knowledge about health among family members represent important sources of family influences over health behavior. When mothers and fathers were asked to rate fifty-five values concerning childrearing, safety was ranked twenty-first and health thirty-eighth by mothers, while safety was ranked tenth and health twenty-fifth by fathers. The values receiving the highest scores among both mothers and fathers were independence, family unity, obedience, religion, getting along with others, responsibility, and morality (Stolz, 1967). A national survey of high school students' values found that being healthy ranked fifth in a list of twelve personal values. Being healthy was outranked by being dependable, courteous, friendly, religious, and ambitious (Remmers, 1965).

In a study of the health values of seventh grade girls and boys, McKinney and his colleagues (1985) found that the content of the children's health values were different from the values of their parents. Good health for the children amounted to avoiding concrete dangers, such as smoking, taking drugs, and eating the wrong foods. Good health to the parents consisted of more abstract prescriptions of maintaining good hygiene and a good attitude. A second difference was that the seventh graders emphasized *proscriptive* behaviors such as smoking, drug taking, etc., while parents emphasized *prescriptions* such as getting enough sleep, getting medical checkups, etc. The values were found to differ in a third way. The behaviors which the children emphasized more than the parents pertained almost exclusively to oral habits: eating, drinking, smoking, alcohol abuse, and drug taking. All of these behaviors deal with the need to be nurtured. Children apparently link health maintenance with the ability to keep oneself nurtured.

The value individuals place on their health is reflected in their health behavior. Pratt (1976) studied the health behavior of the members of 510 families to ascertain the relationships between family structure, level of health, and effectiveness of health behavior within families. Personal health behavior reflects the competence with which family members care for their health. Pratt found that encouragement and autonomy were more likely to produce in children the self-management capacities needed for caring for their own health than punishment and control. A second feature of the family form which fostered members' personal health practices was the tendency to actively and energetically attempt to cope with life's problems and issues. An egalitarian distribution of power and a flexible division of tasks and activities among family members also was found to contribute to members' personal health practices. A fourth element that fostered personal health practices of family members was a pattern of regular, frequent, and varied forms of interaction among all the members. Finally, an essential feature of the family model found to be most effective were the dynamic ties that the family maintained with the broader community through participation by all family members in external groups and activities that bear on the family's needs. Pratt called the family model, which was found to be the most effective and positive in its influence on family members' health practices, the "energized family." This implies that families that are most proactive, resilient, and which foster and encourage personal development provide the best environment for valuing health and practicing healthy behaviors.

It is interesting that *attitudes* toward prevention do not show developmental progressions (Gochman, 1985); rather, the influence of parents appears to be stable and enduring, as found in the work of Lau and his associates (1990). They explored the sources of stability and change in college students' health beliefs and behavior concerning drinking, diet, exercise, and wearing seat belts. There was substantial change in the performance of health behaviors during the first three years of college, and peers did have a strong impact on the magnitude of that change. In total, however, parents were more important than peers as sources of influence over those beliefs and behaviors. Of the various types of social influences considered, the direct modeling of behavior appears to be the most important avenue of influence for both parents and peers.

Kaplan (1987) has suggested that the family serves as a context for communicating the symbolic significance of substance abuse, and the nature of family communications influences each person to engage in or refrain from substance abuse. He notes that family members who endorse the intrinsic value of substance abuse, who view it as compatible with other values, who define situations as appropriate for the practice of substance abuse by providing the substances themselves or other opportunities to engage in it, and who teach family members in the techniques of substance abuse by modeling and/or instruction, are more likely to be substance abusers than family members who learn mutually exclusive conditions regarding substance abuse. Bush & Iannotti (1985) found that the strongest support for the modeling effect of families on their children's behaviors comes from the relationship between parental smoking and children's intentions to smoke, experimentation with smoking, and frequency of smoking. Apparently, the modeling effect is strongest in preschool and early school years, but weakens somewhat as children move through elementary school where wider social attitudes become important. Similar results have been found with other abusable substances, such as alcohol and marijuana (Bush & Iannotti, 1985).

Murray and his colleagues (1985) surveyed a cohort of about 6,000 adolescents annually for four years about their smoking behavior and attitudes. The children's parents were asked to complete similar questionnaires. The researchers found that parental smoking behavior was more important than parental attitudes in the development of smoking among children. Boys without a father and girls without a mother were most likely to smoke. This suggests that many adolescents take up smoking as part of the process of becoming an adult as modelled by the same sex parent. Even among the older adolescents, this influence of parental smoking was still apparent. Further, when the parents changed their smoking behavior, the risk of their children smoking altered accordingly.

Gillette, Wyoming has a law prohibiting anyone under age 17 from smoking in public. Recently police have enforced this law. The local judge has sentenced offenders to several hours of community service for smoking. Ninety-five percent of the youth arrested for smoking have parents who smoke.

Biglan and his colleagues (1990) studied risky sexual behaviors, other problem behaviors, and the family and peer context in two samples of adolescents. The results showed evidence that adolescents were more likely to engage in high-risk sexual behavior when they are engaging in other forms of problem behavior, including antisocial behavior, cigarette smoking, alcohol and illicit drug use. The results also implied that peer and family context influence adolescents' engagement in high-risk sexual behavior. Families in which parents were less available were strongly associated with more sexual risk-taking and, among sexually active adolescents, with less condom use. Low levels of parent availability were also associated with more antisocial behavior, more smoking, alcohol and illicit drug use, and having more friends who also engage in problem behaviors. Most current studies of adolescent problem behaviors focus on a single problem. This study indicates that prevention strategies must address a broad range of problems. Parenting and peer factors are interrelated with the influence of the broader social environment.

Umberson (1987) postulated that family ties involve social control which in turn influences to what degree family members practice health behaviors. The simple existence of family ties may facilitate health behaviors or deter risk-taking. In a national sample of 2,246 respondents Umberson found that parenting reduces the inclination to engage in negative health behaviors more when children and parents live in the same residence. The deterrent effect of parenting on negative health behaviors is most apparent for those involving substance abuse. The strongest effects are noted for marijuana use, drinking problems, and drinking and driving. Umberson also found that marital status was negatively associated with health behavior; the married had the lowest rates of negative health behaviors, and the divorced the highest rates. Marital status is somewhat more important to health behaviors than is parenting status. Parenting status, however, also has an effect on health-compromising behaviors. The deterrent value depends more on the presence of children in the home than simply on having had children. Although the effects of parenting status appear to be similar for men and women, the effects of marital status on health behaviors sometimes differ by sex; the unmarried state is more detrimental to men's health behaviors than to women's.

Learning to Value Total Health

When we discuss health in our daily lives we usually discuss physical health. Mental health is too abstract to evaluate and too personal to discuss openly. We openly value our physical health assuming mental health does not need more maintenance than an annual restful vacation. It is difficult for us to value total health because we are not taught health as a unitary concept.

Many people think of psychological health as a state of well-being, happiness, or contentment. Jahoda (1954) has suggested that there are six dimensions to a concept of positive mental health; attitudes of an individual toward oneself; an individual's style and degree of growth, development, or self-actualization; integration; autonomy; perception of reality; and environmental mastery. But what is important is that all of these aspects become part of a unifying philosophy of life which results in the individual's feeling that there is a purpose and meaning to one's life. Similar ideas occur in Maslow (1950) who speaks of people who are self-actualizers as "being the most ethical of people." There is a clear implication that healthy persons possess a unifying outlook on life. Many persons regard an individual's relation to the world as mentally healthy if it shows what is referred to as autonomy, self-determination, or independence. Most often these terms connote a relation between the individual and environment with regard to decision-making, both the process of decision-making and the outcome of decision-making in terms of independent actions.

It is interesting that when we teach children to become independent, autonomous decision-makers we do not think of it with respect to developing the child's mental health or providing him/her with the tools to formulate a life philosophy. There is no standard format for teaching children to value their total health because there are different types of health. We do not all agree on what total health is, so it is difficult to teach health as a total concept.

The discussion of mental health often makes the assumption that a mentally healthy person is one who is "good" in terms of desirable values. But as Jahoda cautions, mental health, or indeed health, is one goal among many. She notes that one value which strikes her as being compatible with almost all mental health concepts is: an individual should be able to stand on his own feet without making undue demands or impositions on others. Such a value underlies Ginsburg's (1955) idea that mental health consists of being able to hold a job, have a family, keep out of trouble with the law, and enjoy the usual opportunities for pleasure. This value seems to be somewhat outdated for the 1990s. Yet, positive mental health stems from the fact that individuals should be able to adjust their behaviors in response to changes in situations, institutions, and environment. The most practically useful behavior for children to learn to maintain their total health is adaptability. Good health is a continual struggle to maintain some semblance of harmony or balance between internal (physical and mental) and external (environment) forces. One has to learn to value the importance of "staying on top of one's life," i.e., control, in order to actively help oneself stay healthy.

Finally, total health consists of a third element in addition to mind and body. We could call this element attitude or spirit. Healthy people remember success better than failure. Healthy people assume their ability to influence events is much greater than it is. Healthy people also view the future optimistically. The mind makes up its own story about reality from the information received through our senses. These beliefs have adaptive value. People can learn to be hopeful when they are hopeless. A sense of self-control even affects our immune function. A key difference in the management of pain has appeared to be patients' perceptions of their ability to control or change their symptoms. The optimistic belief that we are in control, capable and competent to make changes, is critical to health (Ornstein & Sobel, 1989).

There is a biology of self-confidence. When it comes to health promotion, a confident attitude may contribute more to health than specific health behaviors. People who rate their health poorly die earlier and have more disease than their counterparts who view themselves as healthy. Even people suffering from illness seem to do better when they believe themselves to be healthy than when they believe themselves weak (Ornstein & Sobel, 1989).

Values Change

Health professionals intervene in clients' value systems to get them to value health more through education efforts before they become sick or by rehabilitation after an illness has occurred. The latter is easier to do than the former. In either case, it is hoped that clients will not only claim to value their health more than in the past, but demonstrate this commitment by changing their behavior to be more conducive to good health, thereby, preventing the occurrence or recurrence of a preventable illness. It is often thought that it is easier to change a person's unhealthy behaviors if there is the support of family members who assist in making health behavior changes. However, there is no conclusive evidence to indicate that interventions to change health behaviors which involve the entire family are more effective than dealing with an individual family member who exhibits unhealthy behaviors. Helping individuals and families to make changes in their lives is extremely difficult (Baranowski & Nader, 1985).

Change is difficult because behavior is tied to what a person values. The more something is valued, the more difficult it is for a person to change those behaviors most closely associated with that value. What we value is a part of our self-concept. Changing what we value means changing how we see ourselves. Unless there is a crisis which forces us to confront how we see ourselves and what we value, such as a crippling stroke or the loss of a limb in an accident, it is difficult to motivate people to change their habits or their values. Unless there is a deep-seated readiness to change, change is next to impossible.

Perhaps one of the more important aspects that dissuade people from changing their lifestyle or health behaviors is the benefit they derive from the lifestyle and behaviors with which they have become comfortable. It is difficult to persuade persons to give up a behavior or make major changes in the way they live when the benefits of these changes are unknown. Such substitutions are often viewed as a punishment or sacrifice. The trade-off between behaviors or lifestyles is not seen as an equal one (Bruhn, 1988).

Another aspect of value change involves the source of values. Values are obtained from our culture, science, religion, and personal experience. Sometimes, information about values differs between these sources, requiring that individuals make choices to guide their behavior. Indeed, individuals may make behavioral choices that appear inconsistent with respect to their value of health; for example, an individual may exercise regularly, but not wear seat belts, or adhere to dietary restrictions, but smoke cigarettes. These inconsistencies may reflect conflicts in information between sources of values and, hence, the individual's ambivalence about how total health is valued.

A third aspect of value change is related to how individuals learned their values about health, i.e., through modeling, change, or "moralizing."

Attempts to change values using the same approach in which the values were learned may have an opposite effect, especially if the conditions that surrounded the initial learning are now different. Pratt (1976) suggested that it is not simply a number of separate factors that affect how health is valued, but the overall pattern of values, of which health is one part, that is important. To cause individuals to change how they value health taps a complex, deeply embedded belief system that is not easily modifiable, at least not with simple, solitary means of intervention or modification.

Fiske & Chiriboga (1990) point out, in a study of change in the goals and values of persons over twelve years, that personal goals and values are changed to match one's current life circumstances. The priority given to goals and values does change with age. Peter Marris (1975 p. 46), who has studied how people react to change, explains the need for continuity: "Change appears as fulfillment or loss to different people, and to the same person at different times. Hence, the value placed on health can be reinterpreted and reorganized as the need arises."

Valuing Health and Value Judgments

Health professionals as a group can be assumed to value health more than nonhealth professionals. Restoring health is their business. Yet, all health professionals do not give health a high priority in their personal value systems, e.g., those who smoke cigarettes, are overweight, don't use seat belts, etc. To state that a person who smokes cigarettes does not value his/her health is a value judgment—the judgment rendered may be wrong. We make assumptions about people's values by observing their behavior. What one health professional determines to be healthy behaviors for a client may be unrealistic given the client's life situation. The client's behavior which is judged to be unhealthy might be the result of trade-offs among a series of unhealthy alternatives. Indeed, adopting new behaviors may be more stressful and destructive to a person than continuing with current unhealthy behaviors. The individual must decide on the personal benefits of change. Too often health professionals label patients who do not or will not change their behavior to what the health professional expects or wants as "uncooperative." The reluctance of patients to change is really their assertion of their value systems. The patient's priority for health may differ from that of the health professional.

Pressuring or threatening patients about their values to effect changes in their health behavior is more likely to assure that the patients will not return for future appointments than it is to get the patients to change behaviors they value and feel comfortable with.

It is difficult to assess the personal benefits of healthy lifestyles as what is considered beneficial will differ among individuals. Oster and Epstein (1986) suggested that cholesterol-lowering interventions, no matter what their cost, are unlikely to result in substantial direct savings to the health care system. However, the indirect benefits of intervention are quite high for young and middle-aged adults, as well as for those with severe elevations of cholesterol or with additional coronary risk factors. Often individuals assume that they will add years to their life. A recent follow-up of Harvard graduates showed that by the age of 80, the amount of additional life attributable to adequate exercise, as compared with sedentariness, was from 1 to more than 2 years (Paffenbarger et al., 1986). Most often, however, the personal benefits of health behavior are physiological, cognitive, and/or behavioral (Dubbert, Martin, & Epstein, 1986). Sime (1984), for example, described research showing reductions in anxiety and depression and increases in body attitude and self-confidence due to exercise.

An individual's choices and decisions about changing life style and health behaviors will also be influenced by life events and stage of development. The death of a family member from a heart attack is likely to have a greater influence in motivating a middle-aged family member than an adolescent to change his/her life style. On the other hand, wearing seat belts could be seen to have a positive benefit to all members of a family, irrespective of age, if they have lost a family member in an automobile accident where wearing a seat belt may have meant survival. Everyone, seemingly, has "times" or "teachable moments" in their life when they are more receptive to health information and perhaps more motivated to change. To capture and sustain these positive times is a continual challenge to health professionals.

Health Beliefs and Practices of Health Professionals

How well do health professionals take care of their health? Are they good role models for the clients they care for? One would assume that, since health is their business, health professionals would be good teachers of preventive medicine.

Dowling (1955) points out that physicians pay more attention to the health of their patients than to their own. Sharpe and Smith (1962), in the periodic examination of a group of middle-aged "well" physicians, found that 45.5 percent had significant, unknown diseases, the great majority of which were asymptomatic and required treatment. Kahn and her colleagues (1988) surveyed the health maintenance activities of physicians and nonphysicians in two universities regarding their personal health care. In general, physicians were less likely to have a personal physician, to perceive the need for regular health maintenance, to visit their physician, and to have clinical procedures performed.

Although there is increasing evidence that physicians are demonstrating a leadership role in nonsmoking behaviors, much less is known about physician behaviors related to the use of alcohol, weight control, dietary practices, exercise, psychological problems, and seat belt use. There appears to be a trend toward more health promoting behaviors among younger physicians, but the evidence is based on small geographic areas. Several studies have compared physicians' health behaviors among medical specialties and between professional groups, such as physicians and lawyers. According to the results of a study of health behavior among physicians and lawyers (Wyshak et al., 1980), physicians do more to guard their health than lawyers, especially with respect to wearing seat belts, not smoking, and consuming less alcohol. Studies report lower rates of cigarette smoking among internists and family physicians than among any surgical specialists (McAlister et al., 1985). Cigarette smoking in the general population has decreased during the past 25 years, but the rate is still higher than that reported for physicians (U.S. Dept. of Health, Education & Welfare, 1977).

When Glanz et al. (1982) surveyed 296 physicians' personal health attitudes and health practices at Temple University Health Sciences Center and compared the results with health practices among American adults from the National Health Interview Survey, he found that physicians do not engage in less health prevention activity than the general population.

Young (1988) also used the results from the National Health Interview Survey to compare the health promoting behaviors of family medicine residents with those of the general population. Young mailed a survey questionnaire to 781 family medicine residents who were receiving their training in a university affiliated or university administered residency program in the six-state south central region of the U.S. The results suggest that residents are modeling health promoting behaviors at a significantly higher rate than the lay public with respect to not smoking, moderate use of alcohol, low cholesterol and sodium diets, and consistent use of seat belts. Residents' behavior with respect to regular exercise and weight control was similar to that of the general population. The only negative comparison was that residents reported a significantly higher incidence of perceived personal or emotional problems than did the general population.

It is frequently suggested that dentists can motivate patients to take good care of their teeth because they believe in preventive care and practice good oral hygiene themselves. Weiss and Diserens (1980) tested this assumption by comparing the health behavior of practicing dentists to several groups, their patients, dental educators, dental hygienists, and dental students. There was no difference among the five groups in the frequency of smoking or in the frequency of physical exercise. However, dental hygienists showed significantly higher compliance in four of the five preventive health areas. Other dental professional groups were not consistently more compliant than the patients in general or in areas specifically related to oral health. Dentists, dental educators, and dental students do not excel in taking care of their oral health, but dental hygienists do.

Holcomb et al. (1985) surveyed the health beliefs and behaviors of dental hygienists, dietitians, certified nurse midwives, and physician assistants in Texas (Mullen & Holcomb, 1990; Holcomb & Mullen, 1986). The surveys were designed to elicit information regarding the health professionals' personal health behaviors, beliefs about the importance of health behaviors and screening procedures, and the significance of prevention-oriented practices in general. With respect to cigarette smoking, the numbers of smokers in each discipline was less than the national average for the general population (33%). The four disciplines also had fewer smokers than has been reported for physicians (15%) and nurses in general (23%). The proportion of respondents who reported that they always wear seat belts was greater than for the public at large (22%). Overall, the respondents were more physically active than the general public.

With respect to beliefs, there was virtual unanimity on the importance of not smoking cigarettes. Controlling weight was most important to the dietitians, moderate use of alcohol was rated highest by the midwives, there were variations among the groups with respect to avoiding stress and engaging in aerobic exercise. Ratings of importance by individual respondents, however, did not correlate with the individuals' own behavior except in the case of seat belt use. The respondents generally agreed that health promotion was a part of their role and that they should be active in community health promotion. While most of the practitioners in the four disciplines were generally good role models, many needed to change their own health behaviors.

Wilt and her colleagues (1990) studied a stratified, random sample of registered nurses at a major medical center in New York City to elicit their personal health behaviors and the influence of these behaviors on their treatment practices with cardiovascular disease. Virtually all of the sample of nurses were convinced of the importance of diet in lowering heart disease risk and most agreed that nutrition counseling should be their responsibility. Nurses who were more likely to counsel were working in general medicine, were certified nurse practitioners, knew their own blood cholesterol level, and had higher knowledge scores. The level of overall knowledge of cardiovascular disease was associated with the practice of counseling, an attitude that counseling should be a nurse's responsibility, and personal health behavior, regardless of age or degree status.

Glazer-Waldman et al. (1989) studied the health beliefs and health behaviors of a random sample of licensed physical therapists in Texas. The physical therapists reported less cigarette smoking and less alcohol consumption than reported from the National Health Interview Survey for the general population. Twice as many physical therapists (64.5%) reported a high level of physical activity than was reported in the national survey for the general population (21.9%). Only 2.6 percent of the physical therapists reported the use of drugs that affect mood or help them to relax. Somewhat surprising was that only two health behaviors examined in this study had a statistically significant relationship to health beliefs. Tobacco use and alcohol use were not related to health beliefs. The use of drugs or medications and physical activity did show significant positive correlations with health beliefs. The relatively central role of health beliefs for physical therapists is perhaps explained in part by the type of individual who selects physical therapy as a profession, the nature of their professional preparation, and the environment in which they work, all of which focus on illness and sick-role behavior as being undesirable end points which can be modified so that the patient can lead an active, meaningful life.

Disincentives to Valuing Health

Shangold (1979) said "Teaching by example is the most fundamental educational technique. Many professionals are guided into career choices by inspiring role models. No greater flattery exists than the initiation of another's life style. It is somewhat surprising, then, that those who prescribe health care for others set such poor examples themselves." Basically, no health professional is against health promotion and health education. It would be like being against motherhood and apple pie. There are two essential questions which permeate the literature with respect to our ambivalence as health professionals in putting health promotion into practice. One question is "Health education takes time. What are the incentives to incorporate health education into my care of patients?" A second question is "Will health education make a difference?"

Relman (1982) discusses the first question. He notes that there are many reasons why physicians and most patients are not very interested in primary preventive medicine. From the physician's point of view, the most obvious of these reasons is that third parties reimburse little or nothing for counseling, screening examinations, checkups, and other forms of preventive activity. The result is that practitioners neglect these activities which are not reimbursed. Relman suggests that if we are to make preventive medicine and health promotion more attractive to physicians and patients, we will have to give them both more incentives. Physicians will have to be paid more for the time they spend in prevention activities. Patients will have to be persuaded that they stand to benefit in the long run from prevention and promotion activities.

An even more compelling barrier to getting physicians and other health professionals to teach and model preventive health behavior to their clients (the well and the sick) is the suspicion that it won't make any difference, that is, people aren't really motivated to be more healthy.

A national sample of family practice physicians reported on the treatments and referrals they provide for each of three behavioral health risks—cigarette smoking, obesity, and insufficient exercise—and obstacles to effective office-based health promotion (Orleans et al., 1985). Most of the physicians reported giving regular education and advice, but infrequent treatment or referral for the substantial numbers of their patients who smoke cigarettes, are obese, or get too little exercise. The results confirmed impressions that primary-care physicians are reluctant to treat such problems and underutilize behavioral or psychological treatments in their practice or referral to other specialists. Physicians' pessimism about their patients' abilities to change life styles, a lack of confidence in their own and outside treatments, and perceived patient rejection, along with financial and time disincentives, appear the major contributors to this underutilization.

A survey sent to physicians in Monterey County, California to assess their attitudes and practices regarding hypertension and cigarette smoking showed that only half of the physicians advised patients to quit smoking. Physicians who doubted the effectiveness of their antismoking advice or who did not know what to say to smoking patients were less likely to provide advice. Most physicians felt that their smoking patients lacked sufficient motivation to quit (Fortmann et al., 1985).

Several studies have shown that physicians perceive that they have little success in getting patients to adopt more healthy life styles (Valente et al., 1986; Rosen et al., 1984). In addition, there is not full agreement among physicians on the importance of some types of health-promoting behavior such as aerobic exercise, nutrition, and moderate alcohol use (Wechsler et al., 1983). While physicians feel obligated to endorse the rhetoric of prevention, they also agree that prevention is not interesting to them (Rosen et al., 1984).

Certainly, a great deal of the variation that has been observed in physicians' preventive practices are related to factors such as age; sex; specialty; organizational factors, such as mode of payment and practice setting; as well as individual attitudes (Maheux et al., 1989). Physicians' personal health behaviors affect their level of reducing certain risk factors among their patients (McAlister et al., 1985). It has been found that physicians with good personal health habits counsel their patients significantly more about all habits, regardless of their clinical specialty. Physicians with poor habits are unlikely to counsel their patients (Wells et al., 1984). These authors suggest that physicians may operate on a self-referential principle such as "As long as your patient drinks, smokes, and exercises less than you do, he's okay."

Making Health Promotion Clinically Relevant and Practical

The similarity between senior medical students' and practicing physicians' beliefs about health promotion suggests that attitudes on this topic are fairly well fixed by the time of medical school graduation (Rubin et al., 1990). These findings indicate that the most important barrier to clinical preventive practices is not the lack of knowledge about risk factors, but rather the difficulty in translating knowledge into practice. The goal of health professional education should not be to change students' attitudes about prevention, but instead provide students with appropriate skills to assist them in implementing changes in health behaviors. Philips et al. (1989) have developed the behavioral prescription as a practical, familiar, and efficient method for achieving smoking cessation. The behavioral prescription involves writing prescriptions based on a plan that leads the patient through five successive weeks of behavioral modification, culminating in complete cessation of cigarette use. Physician time is minimal, since the approach requires only two face-to-face meetings. Physician advice to a smoker has been shown to be effective, especially when a patient's health has already been affected by smoking.

Lewis (1988) notes that there are more data on smoking counseling than on that for any other risk factor. Exercise counseling, counseling about the excessive use of alcohol, diet counseling, and the use of seat belts are next in frequency. Lewis notes that at the time of his literature review no studies of the sexual counseling activities of physicians had been published. The absence of such studies prior to the AIDS epidemic reflects both the apathy and discomfort surrounding this topic. The increasing incidence of AIDS and the vulnerability of all persons in the population to AIDS make the physician a key contact in providing safe sex information. This can range from literature in the office to referral to a community agency or another professional. Indeed, if the physician's responsibility is to provide information to increase risk sensitivity among all his/her patients, it should be provided in a variety of ways so that it is palatable to the majority of patients.

A Clinical Model of Behavioral Risk Reduction

The American life and health insurance industry planned the INSURE Project to study how age-related preventive services—including patient education for health risk reduction—could be implemented in private physicians' offices, what would be the cost of such a program, and whether or not these services would have any impact on medical care cost containment (Rosen et al., 1984); Rosen & Logsdon, 1985). The INSURE Project began in 1982 as a feasibility study and in 1984 was extended to evaluate long-term behavioral risk reduction among adult patients in primary medical care. At baseline, seventy-four primary care physicians were surveyed regarding their attitudes toward and practices of preventive medicine. Physicians reported that they were conscientious about educating their patients about health risks, but they spent little time doing so and had doubts about their efficacy in patient education. The preventive interventions and patient surveys were continued over the next five years to determine the long-term effectiveness and costs of preventive services (Karson, 1990).

The effects of preventive medical services involving behavioral risk reduction and counseling were demonstrated over a 12-month period in this feasibility study (Logsdon et al., 1989). Primary care physicians at group practice study sites brought about greater improvements in self-reported, health-related behavior among their adult study patients than the changes reported by control patients at reference sites. These short-term results indicate the potential benefits of a medical model for reducing five important behavioral risks associated with morbidity and mortality among adults: lack of regular exercise, nonuse of auto seat belts, overweight, misuse of alcohol, and irregular or no breast self-exam among women. A trend toward increased smoking cessation was noted.

Implementation of the protocols for preventive medical services included a continuing medical education module with training for physicians in patient communication skills and the epidemiologic evidence for disease prevention. This study showed that the initial costs for the medical model for preventive services in primary care are controllable and that patient utilization patterns are definable. Thus, the implementation of preventive medical services appears feasible if medical training is provided and financial barriers for patients and physicians are removed.

The press to help more people stay healthy is tempered by the words of Lewis Thomas (1979, pp. 49–50), who wrote: "As a people, we have become obsessed with health . . . We are, in real life, a reasonably healthy people . . . The new danger to our well-being, if we continue to listen to all the talk, is in becoming a nation of healthy hypochondriacs, living gingerly, worrying ourselves half to death." Yet, as Knowles (1977 pp.

6–7) points out, physician-educators "are not at all satisfied with the way things seem to be moving...we feel dis-eased. We find intolerable the levels of deprivation and ill health suffered by significant numbers of the American people." Callahan (1977) asks, "How much health do people need?" He suggests that a theory of medical limits will evolve—a new balance between public needs and private desires and between responsibility and duty. Callahan (1990, p. 1813) states, "Whether we like modifying our values or not it seems impossible to achieve equity and efficiency without doing so. We need to restrain our demands for unlimited medical progress, maximal choice, perfect health, and profits and income."

In Retrospect

The requirements for health include: adequate nutrition, protection from environmental hazards, and common sense in avoiding excesses in personal behaviors such as smoking, drinking alcohol, overeating, sedentariness, etc. The responsibility for the prevention of disease and disability through healthier life styles and a cleaner environment extends to all levels of society, the individual, family, community, and government. But in seeking changes in societal values and attitudes toward health there are trade-offs between these values and individual values and freedoms. Kass (1975) has warned that health, while good, cannot be the greatest good for the individual or society. Politically, excessive preoccupation with health can conflict with other important social and economic goals. While there is no such thing as being too healthy, there is the possibility of being too concerned about health. Kass (1975, p. 42) states, "To be preoccupied with the body is to neglect the soul, for which we should indeed care 'first and foremost,' and more than we now do."

REFERENCES

Baranowski, T. & Nader, P.R. (1985). Family health behavior. In D.C. Turk & R.D. Kerns (Eds.), *Health, illness, and families: A life-span perspective* (pp. 51–80). New York: Wiley.

Biglan, A., Metzler, C.W., Wirt, R., Ary, D., Noell, Jr., Ochs, L., French, C. & Hood, D. (1990). Social and behavioral factors associated with high-risk sexual behavior among adolescents. *Journal of Behavioral Medicine, 13,* 245–261.

Bruhn, J.G. & Cordova, F.D. (1977). A developmental approach to learning wellness behavior. Part I. Infancy to early adolescence. *Health Values, 1,* 246–254.

Bruhn, J.G. & Cordova, F.D. (1978). A developmental approach to learning wellness behavior. Part II. Adolescence to maturity. *Health Values, 2,* 16–21.

Bruhn, J.G., Cordova, F.D., Williams, J.A. & Fuentes, R.G. (1977). The wellness process. *Journal of Community Health, 2,* 209–221.

Bruhn, J.G. (1988). Life-style and health behavior. In D.S. Gochman (Ed.), *Health behavior: Emerging research perspectives* (pp. 71–86). New York: Plenum.

Bush, P.J. & Iannotti, R. (1985). The development of children's health orientations and behaviors: Lessons for substance abuse prevention. In C.L. Jones & R.J. Battjes (Eds.), *Etiology of drug use, implications for prevention* (NIDA Research Monograph 56). Washington, DC: U.S. Department of Health and Human Services.

Callahan, D. (1977). Health and society: Some ethical imperatives. In J.H. Knowles (Ed.), *Doing better and feeling worse: Health in the United States* (pp. 23–33). New York: W.W. Norton.

Callahan, D. (1990). Rationing medical progress: The way to affordable health care. *The New England Journal of Medicine, 322* 1810–1813.

Dowling, H.F. (1955). Physician heal thyself. *GP, 11,* 69–73.

Dubbert, P.M., Martin, J.E., & Epstein, L.H. (1986). Exercise. In K.A. Holroyd & T.L. Creer (Eds.), *Self-management of chronic disease: Handbook of clinical interventions and research* (pp. 127–161). New York: Academic Press.

Fabrega, H. Jr. & Roberts, R.E. (1972). Social psychological correlates of physician use by economically disadvantaged Negro urban students. *Medical Care, 10,* 215–223.

Fiske, M. & Chiriboga, D.A. (1990). *Change and continuity in adult life.* San Francisco, CA: Jossey-Bass.

Fortmann, S.P., Sallis, J.F., Magnus, P.M., & Farquhar, J.W. (1985). Attitudes and practices of physicians regarding hypertension and smoking: The Stanford Five City Project. *Preventive Medicine, 14,* 70–80.

Gezairy, H.A. (1990). Health education: Begin with children. *Hygie, 9,* 29–32.

Ginsburg, S.W. (1955). The mental health movement and its theoretical assumptions. In R. Kotinsky & H. Witmer (Eds.), *Community programs for mental health* (pp. 7, 21). Cambridge, MA: Harvard University Press.

Glanz, K., Fiel, S.B., Walker, L.R. & Levy, M.R. (1982). Preventive health behavior of physicians. *Journal of Medical Education, 57,* 637–639.

Glazer-Waldman, H.R., Hart, J.P. & LeVeau, B.F. (1989). Health beliefs and health behaviors of physical therapists. *Physical Therapy, 69,* 204–210.

Gochman, D.S., Bagramian, R. & Sheiham, A. (1972). Consistency in children's perceptions of vulnerability to health problems. *Health Services Report 87,* 282–287.

Gochman, D.S. (1972). The organizing role of motivation in health beliefs and intentions. *Journal of Health & Social Behavior, 13,* 285–293.

Gochman, D.S. & Sheiman, J.A. (1978). Cross-national consistency in children's beliefs about vulnerability. *International Journal of Health Education, 21,* 189–193.

Gochman, D.S. (1977). Perceived vulnerability and its psychosocial context. *Social Science & Medicine, 11,* 115–120.

Gochman, D.S. (1985). Family determinants of children's concepts of health and illness. In D.C. Turk & R.D. Kerns (Eds.), *Health, illness, and families: A life-span perspective* (pp. 23–50). New York: John Wiley.

Goldstein, K. (1959). Health as value. In A.H. Maslow (Ed.), *New knowledge in human values* (pp. 178–188). New York: Harper and Brothers.

Holcomb, J.D. & Mullen, P.D. (1986). Certified nurse-midwives and health promotion and disease prevention. *Journal of Nursing-Midwifery, 31,* 141–148.

Holcomb, J.D., Mullen, P.D., Fasser, C.E., Smith, Q., Martin, J.B., Parks, L.A. & Wente, S.M. (1985). Health behaviors and beliefs of four allied health professions regarding health promotion and disease prevention. *Journal of Allied Health, 14,* 373–384.

Jahoda, M. (1954). *Current concepts of positive mental health.* New York: Basic Books.

Kahn, K.L., Goldberg, R.J., DeCosimo, D. & Dalen, J.E. (1988). Health maintenance activities of physicians and non-physicians. *Archives of Internal Medicine, 148,* 2433–2436.

Kalnins, I. & Love, R. (1982). Children's concepts of health and illness—and implications for health education: An overview. *Health Education Quarterly, 9,* 8–18.

Kaplan, H.B. (1987). Substance abuse patterns and their relationship to family attitudes and values. *Health Values, 11,* 40–46.

Karson, S.G. (1990). INSURE Project Report. In C.B. Arnold (Ed.), *Transactions of the Association of Life Insurance Medical Directors of America,* (pp. 202–207). Tampa, FL: Joe B. Klay & Sons.

Kass, L.R. (1975). Regarding the end of medicine and the pursuit of health. *The Public Interest, 40,* 11–42.

Knowles, J.H. (Ed.). (1977). *Doing better and feeling worse: Health in the United States.* New York: W.W. Norton.

Kohlberg, L. (1969). Stage and sequence: The cognitive-developmental approach to socialization. In G.A. Goslin (Ed.) *Handbook of socialization theory and research* (pp. 347–380). Chicago: Rand McNally.

Kristiansen, C.M. (1985). Value correlates of preventive health behavior *Journal of Personality and Social Psychology, 49,* 748–758.

Lau, R.R., Hartman, K.A. & Ware, J.E., Jr. (1986). Health as a value: Methodological and theoretical considerations. *Health Psychology, 5,* 25–43.

Lau, R.R., Quadrel, M.J. & Hartman, K.A. (1990). Development and change of young adults' preventive health beliefs and behavior: Influence from parents and peers. *Journal of Health & Social Behavior, 31,* 240–259.

Lewis, C.E. (1988). Disease prevention and health promotion practices of primary care physicians in the United States. *American Journal of Preventive Medicine, 4,* 9–16.

Logsdon, D.N., Lazaro, C.M. & Meier, R.V. (1989). The feasibility of behavioral risk reduction in primary medical care. *American Journal of Preventive Medicine, 5,* 249–256.

Maheux, B., Pineault, R., Lambert, J., Beland, F. & Berthiaume, M. (1989). Factors influencing physicians preventive practices. *American Journal of Preventive Medicine, 5,* 201–206.

Marris, P. (1975). *Loss and change.* Garden City, NY: Anchor Press.

Maslow, A.H. (1950). Self-actualizing people: A study of psychological health. *Personality Symposia, 1,* 16.

McAlister, A., Mullen, P.D., Nixon, S.A., Dickson, C., Gottlieb, N., McCuan, R. & Green, L. (1985). Health promotion among primary care physicians in Texas. *Texas Medicine, 81,* 55–58.

McKinney, J.P., Chin, R.J. & Reinhart, M.A. (1985). Health values in early adolescence. *Journal of Clinical Child Psychology, 14,* 315–319.

Mickalide, A.D. (1986). Children's understanding of health and illness: Implications for health promotion. *Health Values, 10,* 5–21.

Mullen, P.D. & Holcomb, J.D. (1990). Selected predictors of health promotion counseling by three groups of allied health professionals. *American Journal of Preventive Medicine, 6,* 153–160.

Murray, M., Kiryluk, S. & Swan, A.V. (1985). Relation between parents' and children's smoking behavior and attitudes. *Journal of Epidemiology & Community Health, 39,* 169–174.

Natapoff, J.N. (1982). A developmental analysis of children's ideas of health. *Health Education Quarterly, 9,* 34–44.

Natapoff, J.N. (1978). Children's view of health: A developmental study. *American Journal of Public Health, 68,* 995–1000.

Orleans, C.T., George, L.K., Houpt, J.L. & Brodie, K.H. (1985). Health promotion in primary care: A survey of U.S. family practitioners. *Preventive Medicine, 14,* 636–647.

Ornstein, R. & Sobel, D. (1989). *Healthy pleasures.* Reading, MA: Addison-Wesley.

Oster, G., & Epstein, A.M. (1986). Primary prevention and coronary heart disease: The economic benefits of lowering serum cholesterol. *American Journal of Public Health, 76,* 647–656.

Paffenbarger, R.S., Hyde, R.T., Wing, A.L. & Hsieh, C.C. (1986). Physical activity, all-cause mortality, and longevity of college alumni. *New England Journal of Medicine, 314,* 605–613.

Palmer, B.B. & Lewis, C.E. (1976). Development of health attitudes and behaviors. *Journal of School Health, 46,* 401–402.

Philips, B.U., Longoria, J.M., Calhoun, K.H. & Bates, D.F. (1989). Behavioral prescription writing in smoking cessation counseling: A new use for a familiar tool. *Southern Medical Journal, 82,* 946–953.

Pratt, L. (1976). *Family structure and effective health behavior: The energized family.* Boston: Houghton Mifflin.

Rashkis, S.R. (1965). Child's understanding of health. *Archives of General Psychiatry, 12,* 10–17.

Relman, A.S. (1982). Encouraging the practice of preventive medicine and health promotion. *Public Health Reports, 97,* 216–219.

Remmers, H.H. (1965). *Report of Poll 74: The Purdue Opinion Panel.* West Lafayette, IN: Purdue University, Purdue Research Foundation.

Richmond, J.G. & Kotelchuck, M. (1984). Personal health maintenance for children. *Western Journal of Medicine, 141,* 816–823.

Rogers, C.R. (1964). Toward a modern approach to values: The valuing process in the mature person. *Journal of Abnormal & Social Psychology 68,* 160–167.

Rokeach, M. (1973). *The nature of human values.* New York: Free Press.

Rosen, M.A., Logsdon, D.N. & Demak, M.M. (1984). Prevention and health promotion in primary care: Baseline results on physicians from the INSURE Project on lifecycle preventive health services. *Preventive Medicine, 13,* 535–548.

Rosen, M.A. & Logsdon, D.N. (1985). The INSURE Project on preventive health services. *Statistical Bulletin,* January–March, 25–27.

Rubin, J.D., Sobal, J. & Moran, M.T. (1990). Health promotion beliefs and practices of fourth-year medical students. *American Journal of Preventive Medicine, 6,* 106–111.

Shangold, M.M. (1979). The health care of physicians: 'Do as I say and not as I do'. *Journal of Medical Education, 54,* 668.

Sharpe, J.C. & Smith, W.W. (1962). Physician, heal thyself. *Journal of the American Medical Association, 182,* 234–237.

Sime, W.E. (1984). Psychological benefits of exercise training in the healthy individual. In J.D. Matarazzo, S.M., Weiss, J.A., Herd, N.E. Miller, & S.M. Weiss (Eds.), *Behavioral health: A handbook of health enhancement and disease prevention* (pp. 488–508). New York: John Wiley.

Stolz, L.M. (1967). *Influences on parent behavior.* Stanford, CA: Stanford University Press.

Thomas, L. (1979). *The medusa and the snail: More notes of a biology watcher.* New York: Viking Press.

Trichopoulos, D. & Petridou, E. (1988). Promoting health among school age children. *Scandinavian Journal of Social Medicine, 16,* 251–255.

Umberson, D. (1987). Family status and health behaviors: Social control as a dimension of social integration. *Journal of Health & Social Behavior, 28,* 306–319.

United States Department of Health, Education, and Welfare, Public Health Service, National Institutes of Health. (1977). *The smoking digest: Progress report on a nation kicking the habit.* Bethesda, MD.

Valente, C.M., Sobal, J., Muncie, H.L., Jr., Levine, D.M. & Antlitz, A.M. (1986). Health promotion: Physicians' beliefs, attitudes, and practices. *American Journal of Preventive Medicine, 2,* 82–88.

Wallston, K.A., Maides, S.A. & Wallston, A.A. (1974). *Health care information seeking as a function of health locus of control and health values* (Mimeographed paper). Nashville, TN: Vanderbilt University.

Ware, J.E., Jr., & Young, J. (1979). Issues in the conceptualization and measurement of value placed on health. In S.J. Mushkin & D.W. Dunlap (Eds.), *Health: What is it worth?* (pp. 141–166). New York: Pergamon.

Ware, J.E., Jr., Young, J.A., Snyder, M.K. & Wright, W.R. (1974). *The measurement of health as a value: Preliminary findings regarding scale reliability, validity and administration procedures.* (Tech. Rep. No. MHC 74-11). Washington, DC: National Technical Information Service, U.S. Department of Commerce.

Wechsler, H., Levine, S., Idelson, R.K., Rohman, M. & Taylor, J.O. (1983). The physician's role in health promotion—A survey of primary care practitioners. *The New England Journal of Medicine, 308,* 97–100.

Weiss, J. & Diserens, D. (1980). Health behavior of dental professionals. *Clinical Preventive Dentistry, 2,* 5–8.

Wells, K.B., Lewis, C.E., Leake, B. & Ware, J.E., Jr. (1984). Do physicians preach what they practice? A study of physicians' health habits and counseling practices. *Journal of the American Medical Association, 252,* 2846–2648.

Wilt, S., Hubbard, A. & Thomas, A. (1990). Knowledge, attitudes, treatment practices and health behaviors of nurses regarding blood cholesterol and cardiovascular disease. *Preventive Medicine, 19,* 466–475.

Wyshak, G., Lamb, G.A., Lawrence, R.S. & Curran, W.J. (1980). A profile of the health-promoting behaviors of physicians and lawyers. *The New England Journal of Medicine, 303,* 104–107.

Young, E.H. (1988). Health promoting behaviors of family practice residents: Do they compare with the general public? *Family Medicine, 20,* 437–442.

SUGGESTED READINGS

Abeles, R.P. (Ed.) (1987). *Life-span perspectives and social psychology.* Hillsdale, NJ: Lawrence Erlbaum.

Baltes, P.B., & Schaie, K.W. (Eds.). (1973). *Life-span developmental psychology: Personality and socialization.* New York: Academic Press.

Eurich, A.C. (Ed.). (1981). *Major transitions in the human life cycle.* Lexington, MA: D.C. Heath.

Gould, S.J. (1990). Health consciousness and health behavior: The application of a new health consciousness scale. *American Journal of Preventive Medicine, 6,* 228–238.

Kaluger, G. & Kaluger, M.F. (1974). *Human development: The span of life.* St. Louis: C.V. Mosby.

Nemcek, M.A. (1990). Health beliefs and preventive behavior. *AAOHN Journal, 38,* 127–138.

Chapter 3

PREVENTION AS A VALUE

Prevention is so much better than healing because it saves the labor of being sick.

Thomas Adams (d.1653), Works
"The Happinesse of the Church"

Illness is the night-side of life, a more onerous citizenship. Everyone who is born holds dual citizenship, in the Kingdom of the well and in the Kingdom of the sick. Although we all prefer to use only the good passport, sooner or later each of us is obliged, at least for a spell, to identify ourselves as citizens of that other place.

Susan Sontag
Illness as a Metaphor (1978)

Concepts of healthful living have an ancient lineage. However, as long as infectious disease was prevalent and society was preoccupied with the spread of disease, prevention was directed toward such maladies. Much of the practice of preventive medicine has been effective without a basic knowledge of why it worked. Jenner introduced a vaccination for smallpox without a knowledge of virology. Cholera was controlled by implementing findings from a simple epidemiologic study by John Snow. The decline of the mortality rate in the second half of the 19th Century was influenced by the reduction of exposure to infection which resulted directly from improved hygiene affecting the quality of water and food (Saward & Sorensen, 1978). All of the elements that historically have been associated with preventive medicine—environmental sanitation, proper nutrition, physical fitness, and moderation in the common vices— are still with us, but the spectrum of health issues has broadened. Now we are concerned about gun control, seat belts, violence on television, drug use and abuse, human abuse, and the right to die. The conquest of infectious disease has brought into focus a different set of methods to improve health. The most effective means of disease prevention and improved health lie outside the medical care process and are related to reducing hazards in the environment, improving nutrition, and adopting appropriate personal habits. McKeown (1976) has expressed the challenge to improve health stating that, "Those fortunate enough to be born free of significant congenital disease or disability will remain well if three basic needs are met: they must be adequately fed; they must be protected from a wide range of hazards in the environment; and they must not depart radically from the pattern of personal behavior under which man evolved, for example, by smoking, overeating, or sedentary living."

The purposes of this chapter are to: (1) examine our societal values about health and prevention; (2) review the concept of risk as it relates to attitudes, behaviors, and lifestyles which promote good health; (3) describe the burden of illness and the benefits of preventive behavior; (4) discuss the relationship of values to health behavior; and (5) point out ethical issues associated with the promotion of health.

Definitions and Perspectives:
Disease Prevention and Health Promotion

The importance of the prevention of disease has gained wide acceptance among professionals and the public. As with crime, prevention generally is reiterated to be better than cure. Prevention requires that medicine shift its focus from treating the ill to maintaining the healthy. Since the aim of prevention is to stop illness before it starts, or before it becomes apparent, it is necessary to intervene in the lives of people who regard themselves as healthy (Miles, 1978). Disease prevention begins by recognizing a threat to health—a disease or environmental hazard—and seeks to protect as many people as possible from the harmful consequences of that threat. Health promotion begins with people who basically are healthy and seeks to develop community and individual life style measures to help them maintain and enhance their state of well-being (Becker & Rosenstock, 1989). Health promotion is based on a broad understanding of "health" as the extent to which an individual or group is able to realize aspirations, satisfy needs, and change or cope with the environment. This reaffirms the World Health Organization's definition of health, reiterating that health goes beyond the absence of disease, but adding a dynamic and process-based dimension. Health, as defined by WHO, is based on the understanding of public health that encompasses the notion of social responsibility for health: the components of physical and mental well-being need a foundation in a secure society. Kickbusch (1988) proposes that we adopt an ecological and social understanding of health as the conceptual basis of health promotion and suggests the following eight characteristics for this model:

1. concern for the "whole person" which considers the interaction between the individual, family, community, society, and culture, and emphasizes well-being, fulfillment, independence, and functioning in social roles;
2. concern with the social distribution of health and with how life styles reflect life changes;
3. attempts to understand the cultural and personal meaning of health and its ranking in people's hierarchy of values;
4. takes into account the perceptions and emotions related to health;
5. aims to understand health actions in the context of everyday life;
6. views health as a resource;
7. views self-reliance (self-care) as an expression of human dignity;
8. considers more than one form of caring, curing, and healing.

Blum (1983) also takes an ecologic or systems approach to health, stating that causes of ill-health are not thrust singly upon individuals, but are the result of perturbations in a system. He notes that a person's well-being is determined by the interrelationships between three levels: somatic, psychic, and social. Prevention efforts should be aimed at maintaining some semblance of harmony or balance between these levels. Figure 3-1 shows the complex interrelationships of factors influencing the individual practice of preventive health behaviors.

The biomedical model focuses on three types of prevention, primary, secondary, and tertiary. Primary prevention encompasses all actions and technology to prevent disease prior to its occurrence. Secondary prevention is concerned with the detection of early signs of disease prior to the occurrence of the disease and the elimination of the disease process. Tertiary prevention involves treating and halting the development of disease to limit damage and restore normal functioning. There is a need for developing a model for teaching prevention if we expect people to initiate and sustain complex sets of health behaviors and be supported by their immediate social environment, as well as by the culture in which they live (Leventhal & Hirschman, 1982). The basic foundation for teaching prevention revolves around our perceptions of risk in general, how we personalize and select risk, how risk relates to our values and

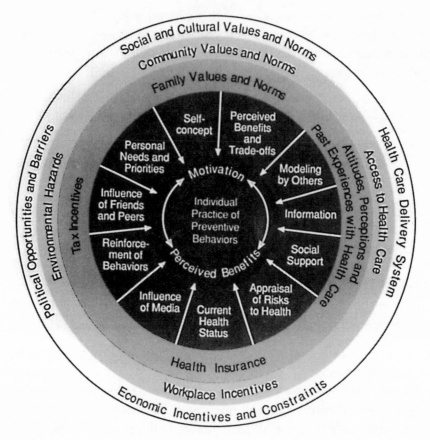

Figure 3-1. Interrelationships of factors influencing the individual practice of preventive health behaviors.

their priorities, and how we assess the short- and long-term consequences of taking or not taking certain risks.

Good Health Is a Choice

Most individuals do not worry about their health until they lose it (Knowles, 1977). Prevention means forsaking the bad habits which many people enjoy and doing things which require special effort. We take pride in the freedom we have to make personal choices in our lives. There is a repugnance to being told one cannot do something, especially if it is a behavior one has chosen and one enjoys. As children, we were not taught that health was an individual responsibility and that we could make choices about the level of health we wished to experience. Health, in schools, was usually taught by coaches and was limited to first aid and emergency procedures. Health was learned in the home by observing parental health behavior. Traditionally, health has been viewed as what it is *not.* Just as peace has been defined as the absence of war, and sanity as the absence of insanity, health has been defined as the absence of illness (Ng et al., 1981). In household surveys, Americans say that what health means to them is their ability to do what they need to do. Their judgment of their physical capacity depends on how many health problems they have. The more health problems curtail their freedom to do for themselves, the less they enjoy living. People's sense of their own health is tied to more than the restrictions imposed by health problems. The types of problems make a difference. Specific diagnoses also evoke different judgments about the loss of health Americans feel. Health means more than the absence of symptoms or restricted activity; it also means freedom from the constraints of medical treatment and freedom to use one's time as he/she chooses (Milio, 1983).

Lay conceptions of health vary culturally and socioeconomically, tend to focus on the present, and involve a feeling state. Conceptions also are formed by an individual's assessment of his/her ability to function in roles that the individual considers important, and by the individual's assessment of change in his/her biology (Levine & Sorenson, 1984). Most laymen's conceptions of health are passive; that is, health is considered an attribute much like personality that one can do little about. Until the last decade, there was no conception that one could actively do things to improve his/her health or well-being. All the talk of "health" was about care for the sick. We have learned a clear-cut process for taking care of our health. When symptoms appear, a person can seek medical help, receive treatment, and regain his/her health. As Ornstein & Sobel (1987) point out, providing more and more medical care does not necessarily produce healthier people. Access to medical care has definite value in the prevention of disease and promotion of health. However, medical care should not be counterposed to prevention, but rather should be integrated with it (Roemer, 1984). Only in the last 10 to 15 years, has prevention been rediscovered by health professionals. This is primarily because seven of the ten leading causes of death and disability today could be substantially reduced if people chose to eat properly, exercise more, refrain from smoking or abusing alcohol and other drugs, drive safely, and reduce stress. In contradistinction to illness, prevention views health, aggressively and affirmatively, as a continual process of learning, growth, and development throughout life. Good health, or wellness, is a choice.

Good health is not only an individual, but a social choice. While we espouse health as a right, this right usually refers to the access to and availability of health services. The realization of that right is always incomplete because some of the resources that could be used for health are allocated to other purposes. As Fuchs (1974) notes, "No country is as healthy as it could be." Many deaths could be prevented if we were to devote more resources to that end. Every nation chooses its own death rate by its evaluation of health compared with other goals. One of the most important choices every individual and every society has to make is between using existing resources to satisfy current desires or applying them to activities in anticipation of future needs. As a society, we do not have a history of planning for future needs. As individuals, our planning often has been limited to protecting ourselves economically in the event that a catastrophic event will no longer permit us to work at our usual job. Unfortunately, good health often is not a choice we make consciously, individually, or collectively as a society. Too often, we wait for a crisis to elicit our choice when time and options are limited. Even then we may default and let circumstances make the choice for us.

The Illusion of Immortality

Prevention is not more highly valued by some in our society because they avoid confrontation with their own mortality believing that they cannot affect the number of years they will live. Others do not wish to take responsibility and relegate it to God. Still others, in varying degrees, incorporate health promoting behaviors and activities into their daily lives. It is not a question of the length of life, but rather the quality of life. Some individuals do not want to assume responsibility for the quality of their lives. The illusion of personal invulnerability is reinforced in societies where life is comparatively easy, affluent, longevity is extended, and the miracles of medical technology are extolled in the daily media (Montagu, 1976).

Our feelings of immortality are somewhat paradoxical; we easily buy into the current "quick fixes" to prevent disease or extend our lives, e.g., oat bran for colon cancer, drugs for lowering cholesterol, aspirin to prevent strokes. Prevention is not an effective "single bullet." Perhaps one reason that we do not have a more comprehensive and continuous view of prevention is that prevention is not "natural" to us. Only recently have we come to learn about prevention as a series of unrelated actions with unknown long-term effects in which we are encouraged to engage to remedy or prevent health problems. Prevention has been marketed as the responsibility of industry, technology, and medicine to develop better products to forestall disease. Individual actions to change one's health status seem impotent, especially when the effects may not be immediately measurable or perceptible. Thus, despite their cost, "quick fixes" are readily accepted by consumers who continue to feel invulnerable.

It should be pointed out that no matter how purely we eat and drink, no matter how carefully we guard the air we breathe, no matter how much we become involved with our doctors, the mortality rate will still be 100 percent. Not all diseases and decay are self-induced. The process of living wears us down as much as we wear ourselves down. We must guard against the notion that, if we can only control enough, be disciplined enough, and be powerful enough, we can prevent all that is potentially bad in our lives (Shapiro & Shapiro, 1979).

Risk and Prevention

Accepting risks has become second nature to us. Not many of us insist on a zero risk society. But acceptability is subjective, danger is a matter of degree (Imperato & Mitchell, 1985). We choose or embrace many risks ourselves, from smoking to speeding. One person's chosen risk is another person's imposed risk, e.g., drunken drivers. We choose some risks freely because of our lack of information or our misinformation. Other risks, such as radiation, air and water pollution, and food additives are imposed upon us. It is difficult not to concede that people do have the moral right to take personal risks (Amartya, 1986). The importance of the right to take risks varies with the nature of the activity involved. It also varies from person to person. Risk-taking rarely has consequences for only one individual. The effects of one person's risk-taking impact on others, i.e., physical, psychological, economic, and social. For example, the family of a race car driver may worry about the family member's physical safety each time he enters a race, but the family will have to deal with the physical and economic consequences should the person become injured or disabled. Social costs involve possible limitations or changes in one's

ORCHESTRA CONDUCTORS' LONGEVITY:
A CLUE FOR PREVENTIVE MEDICINE*

Hans H. Neumann, M.D.

Medical Director of the Department of Health, New Haven, Conn.

Why do so many orchestra conductors remain intensely active and energetic well into their late 80s or longer? Leading an orchestra seems to be a prescription for longevity and this phenomenon has led to lofty theories to explain it, such as the possession of unusual talents, endowment with genius or driving motivation. Another hypothesis credits it to a sense of fulfillment and happiness this activity produces.

From a physician's viewpoint, one may advance a more prosaic interpretation. Conducting requires long, sustained, aerobic action of the upper extremities. There is evidence that exercise of the upper extremities is more beneficial for the cardiovascular system than training and use of the lower half of the body. While the weight carried by the conductor is no heavier than a baton, and his work is not overly taxing in any short unit of time, the activity is protracted and does not allow one to give in to fatigue. Compared with a runner's effort, it does not approach the hazards of functioning close to the endurance limit.

When those undergoing training of the arms only are retested after such a program, they show a decrease in the resting heart rate and of the systolic blood pressure, more so than after training with leg work. Perhaps the major favorable impact of sustained, submaximal arm exercises is the lesser increase in the heart rate under physical stress, and the smaller rise in the systolic blood pressure. Their daily work makes orchestra conductors function further away from the threshold of ischemia.

Add to this the general benefits of exercising large muscle groups, not just the upper extremities. Among these benefits are a lowering of the triglyceride levels and an increase in the high-density lipoproteins. Moderate muscle action over prolonged periods increases endurance and contributes to improved well-being. Psychological standard tests show that such types of training reduce leanings to depression and anxiety and those who exercise are less likely to be affected by the emotional complications of aging.

The list of conductors who stayed on their jobs well into their eighties, even into their 90s, is strikingly long. Arthur Fiedler, Richard Strauss, and Ernest Ansermer till 86, Walter Damrosch to 88, Arturo Toscanini was active as a conductor to the age of 90. Leopold Stokowski died at the age of 96. Karl Boehm, the director of the Vienna Opera, made repeated guest appearances at the Metropolitan Opera in New York in his mid-80s. He died last year at the age of 87. These are but a few examples.

If conducting an orchestra is an exercise of optimal duration and intensity, it is difficult for lesser mortals to come up with similar types of physical activity. One cannot advise hiring an orchestra for physical training purposes. But there are practical alternatives. Among them are piano or violin playing on a regular basis, not just dabbling. The pianist Arthur Rubinstein died recently at the age of 94, Eubie Blake celebrated his 100 birthday playing the piano as usual, and Vladimir Horowitz is no youngster either.

Other activities are swimming and rowing. Instead of the stationary bicycle, one should recommend the stationary rowboat. Training should be done without trying to hike up the resistance of the oars to a high level. The effort should be moderate and for prolonged periods. To reduce boredom, one can play on the hi-fi one's favorite symphony while rowing that boat in synchrony.

These alternatives may not offer the fun, exhilaration, and excitement of conducting an orchestra, but they can provide acceptable alternatives for those whose genius lies in fields other than music.

*Reprinted from *Medical News*, Monday, October 17, 1983, with permission from the author and Medical Tribune US, Inc., New York, NY.

job, leisure activities, and friends should one become disabled or disfigured while racing.

Research has confirmed that some behaviors are risk factors of disease. That means that people who engage in such behaviors are more likely to develop certain types of illnesses than are people who do not. Perhaps the most widely known association of this type is that of cigarette smoking as a risk factor for lung cancer. To be a risk factor, the behavior must be present before the disease begins; it cannot be an early symptom of the disease, as coughing, for example, is an early indication of lung disease. However, a risk factor need not cause the disorder. It may merely be closely associated with some underlying process that eventually produces the disease state. As a result, once a type of behavior is identified as a risk factor, additional studies are needed to determine whether changes in behavior are of value in preventing or treating the disease. Known behavioral risk factors include cigarette smoking, excessive consumption of alcoholic beverages, use of illicit drugs, certain dietary habits, insufficient exercise, reckless driving, nonadherence with

sound medication regimens, and maladaptive responses to social pressures (Hamburg et al., 1982).

If our society is to be more successful in getting people to assume more
responsibility for their health and to make healthy choices in the risks
they take, we need to consider what risk-taking means in the context of a
person's life style and provide health risk information that will be within
"learning range" for that individual. Too often, the media and health
experts present health risk information for the public that is not heard
by most, heard and dismissed by some, seriously considered by a few,
and used by very few (Bruhn, 1988b).

Risk-taking as Normal Behavior

Risk behavior helps to establish an identity and test the control an
individual has over the environment and self; this aspect of risk behavior is important when trying to understand why young people adopt
patterns of behavior that involve risks to their health. Risk behavior can
compensate for conflicts that arise in everyday life and help one regain
the physical and psychological ability to face up to them again (Health
Education Unit, 1986). Escape from conflicts is promoted by the mass
media advertising: "Have a cigarette," "Take a pill," and "Enjoy Happy
Hour." Attempts to influence individuals to adopt healthy forms of
behavior must allow for the fact that their present behavior is not merely
a matter of free choice; it may often be a way of coping with conflict that
has been learned, and with which the individual has come to feel
comfortable. Positive health behavior and risk behavior are part of a
wider life-orientation, including a sense of well-being and confidence in
coping with one's environment.

A study of risk-taking behaviors in children in grades 5–8 found that
peer pressure was especially prevalent among eighth graders. About 50
percent of the dares encouraged problem behaviors that placed the
children or others at risk for personal injury, or the potential development of habits hazardous to their health. With increasing age/grade,
dares from peers occurred more often and more frequently within the
school environment; the junior high school was almost twice as common
a site for such challenges as the elementary school. The dared behaviors
were said to be performed more frequently by those in the eighth grade,
who also reported they were responding to urges or requests. Among 8th

graders, the content of dares changed. More young people were challenged to smoke marijuana, vandalize, and commit acts of violence to others. More challenges for sexual experimentation were presented, especially to girls (Lewis & Lewis, 1984).

In another study, ninth grade students were asked to make a decision on a hypothetical dilemma scenario. Based upon their choice, they were classified either as health-promoting decision makers or as health-risk decision makers. They were subsequently asked a series of questions dealing with future health choices, degrees of reflection, the effect of stress upon choice selection, and type of cognition during decision-making. Results indicated that health-promoting decision makers intended not to engage in future, risky sexual behavior, drinking, or driving. Health-risk decision makers were, however, more reflective in making their initial choice (Duryea & Okwumabua, 1985). Radius et al. (1980) found that youths, aged 6–17, who reported doing things that they considered bad for their health also tended not to accept personal responsibility for poor health outcomes.

Risk-taking is an aspect of our culture that is learned and changeable throughout an individual's life cycle. Our attitudes toward risk vary according to what has happened to us, what we expect, what we feel, what we know, and what we care about. We ignore some risks and overestimate others. Our perceptions are selective and change as our social life changes (Teuber, 1990). Experience with risk also modifies our perceptions of new risks and our evaluation of the trade-offs to taking a risk. Figure 3-2 shows a series of hypothetical curves to illustrate the different kinds of risks that may be predominate at different points along the lifecycle. In recent years, the government and the health professions have begun to set limits for risk-taking behavior that has an effect on health, e.g., warnings about smoking cigarettes, labels on food products indicating the percentage of cholesterol and saturated fat, and safe sex information. As we learn more about healthy persons, we find some of their characteristics to be: more control of their environment, personal involvement and commitment to a task, choice of a life style that augments an ability to cope with life events, and the availability and use of a social support network to help manage life stress (Flannery, 1987).

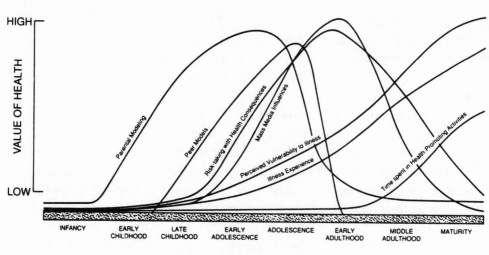

Figure 3-2. Factors affecting the personal value of health at various stages of the life cycle.

Decisions to Risk

While risk-taking decisions do not always occur in an orderly predictable manner, the ingredients of probability, contingencies, acceptability of the risk, alternatives, and outcome are usually present in deciding whether or not to take a risk. (Weinstein, 1989). Consciously or unconsciously, we continually make decisions about whether or not to put ourselves at risk with respect to our health. According to Baric (1969), the "at risk" role is a commitment we make toward becoming more sick or more well. For example, we make choices about whether or not to increase our risk of sickness by continuing to smoke tobacco and whether to enhance our wellness by beginning an exercise program. Many of our decisions about risking are based on uncertainty or incomplete knowledge, e.g., whether pregnant women should jog, while other decisions are made with full awareness of the possible consequences (Cohen, 1972), e.g., a diabetic patient who has a casual attitude about taking his insulin.

Health professionals play a key role in an individual's decision-making process about taking health risks. This does not mean that health professionals are consulted about all health risk-taking or that their advice is always taken. Nonetheless, health professionals are often consulted and their reaction to the behaviors engaged in does influence some individuals some of the time. Too often, we emphasize the hazards of engaging in a certain behavior rather than the benefits of not engaging in that behavior. Clarke and Parcel (1975) pointed out that emphasizing specific behaviors, such as observing safety precautions, exercising, or eating low fat foods, make specific behaviors the goal rather than the means to the goal of good health. Our strategies in getting individuals and patients to become more healthy, or to regain their health, often emphasize specific behaviors as goals. Reducing risks to our health, therefore, is not so that we can live longer, but so that we can live better.

We do not take risks without a reason. The reason is closely associated with what we value. If status or prestige is valued more than health, it is likely the individual will not be dissuaded from taking a high-prestige job because of the possible effects of increased stress on his health. If, on the other hand, health is valued more than status or prestige, an individual may pass up a promotion in order not to sacrifice time with his family or to accept the pressure of additional job responsibility.

We seldom take health risks impulsively or purposefully. Those individuals who seek out or create stress for excitement, or who are masochistic, or suicidal, are exceptions (Bruhn, 1987a). Most individuals live lives of routine and are not aware of health risks on a daily basis, except, for example, people living near petrochemical or nuclear plants. In this case, health risks often appear to be of less concern than the risk of not finding a job should the person or family relocate; hence, concerns about health consequences may be superceded by a more immediate need, namely income. There is usually planning time in deciding to take a risk. During this interval, many factors, such as peer pressure, cultural values, personal expectations, and so forth influence a person's weighing of whether or not to accept the risk. Often, a person may not consider his health in these deliberations because of a lack of information, and/or health may be perceived to be of lesser importance and have fewer consequences than the immediate choice. Even when a person has the appropriate knowledge or experience about a health risk, other factors or needs may seem more important than changing health-threatening behavior (e.g., a pathologist who smokes cigarettes or an obese obstetrician who advises pregnant mothers to watch their weight). While individuals are free to make choices about their own health, public pressure to take steps to reduce hazards to its collective health is increasing, e.g., the prohibition of smoking in public places, such as airplanes, the call for widespread voluntary HIV testing of sexually active adults, and the development of standards for safe sex (Goedert, 1987). In order to affect decisions in risk-taking regarding health, we need to consider individual values (Kristiansen, 1985). Risk-taking regarding health will not be changed unless health is highly valued by the individual and society.

The Unnecessary Burden of Illness

The heaviest burdens of illness in the United States, today, are related to aspects of individual behavior, especially long-term patterns of behaviors referred to as life style. The Centers for Disease Control of the United States Public Health Service have estimated that 50 percent of mortality from the ten leading causes of death in the United States can be traced to life style (Hamburg et al., 1982). Life styles are the patterns of choices we learn from early childhood and vary according to socioeconomic and cultural circumstances (Bruhn, 1988a; Health Education Unit, 1986; Hetzel & McMichael, 1988). Table 3-1 shows some of the personal behaviors that are associated with increased risk for certain diseases (Office of Disease Prevention and Health Promotion, 1988; Hetzel and McMichael, 1988; Hamburg et al., 1982).

Belloc & Breslow (1972) examined the relationship between common health practices, including hours of sleep, regularity of meals, physical activity, smoking and drinking, and physical health status. They found that good health practices were associated with positive health and the relationship of these activities was cumulative; those who followed all of the good health practices being in better health, even though older, than those who failed to do so. Belloc (1973) also found that the number of health practices showed an inverse relationship with mortality rates, especially for men. This relationship was independent of income level and physical health status. The average life expectancy of men, age 45, who reported six or seven good health practices was more than 11 years more than that of men reporting fewer than four. For women, the relationship between health practices and mortality was less strong, and the difference between life expectancy at age 45 for those who reported six or seven good health practices, and those who reported fewer than four, was 7 years.

The major causes of the almost two million deaths each year in the United States are cardiovascular diseases, including heart disease, stroke, hypertension, and the various manifestations of atherosclerosis; cancers, accidents; violence, including homicide and suicide; diabetes mellitus;

Table 3-1. Major causes of mortality and morbidity in western society and their associated risk factors

Cause	Risk factors
Bowel Disorders	Diet
Breast Cancer	Reproductive history, body weight, diet
Cancers of digestive system	Diet, alcohol and smoking
Chronic lung disease (bronchitis, emphysema, etc.	Smoking, occupational exposure to dust, fumes, etc.
Cirrhosis of liver	Alcohol consumption
Coronary heart disease	Smoking, hypertension, blood lipid levels, diet, exercise, weight
Dental caries	Diet
Diabetes mellitus (adult-onset)	Diet, relative weight, exercise
Drug abuse	Overuse of or dependence upon pre-scribed drugs including alcohol, use of illicit drugs (cocaine, heroine, LSD, etc.), social and psychological factors
Gallstones	Diet, reproductive history, oral contraceptive usage
Human abuse	Social and psychological factors
Lung cancer	Smoking, occupational exposures
Malignant melanoma and other skin cancers	Exposure to sunlight
Motor vehicle accidents	Alcohol and other drugs, driver's skill, vehicle safety, road conditions
Obesity and other eating disorders	Diet
Occupational injuries and diseases	Chemicals, fumes, dust, noise, stress, unsafe work conditions
Other accidents, poisoning and violence	Alcohol, social and psychological factors, environmental conditions at home and work
Sexually transmitted diseases diseases and cancer of the cervix	Semen, blood and blood products, multiple sex partners, unprotected sex
Stroke	Hypertension, diet, smoking, oral contraceptives plus smoking (young women)
Suicide	Social and psychological factors

cirrhosis of the liver; and lung disease. Many of the leading causes of death are chronic and progressively disabling diseases. Years of limitation in function and associated health care costs may precede death.

Premature mortality is an important aspect of the burden of illness. The term refers to deaths that occur prior to the age of average longevity. More sensitive measures of the relative burden of several types of illness include days in hospitals or long-term care facilities, number of visits to physicians, days of restricted activity, direct costs of treatment, indirect costs, such as work days lost, and costs of home health care. Causes of death for which life style factors are especially significant continue to predominate, e.g., heart disease, cancer, accidents, and violence. The impact of behavior on the burden of illness is reflected in the observation that alcohol abuse, cigarette smoking, and obesity are disproportionately present among the 20 percent of patients with the highest hospitalization costs (Milio, 1981).

The government of Canada has made a very strong effort to change individual attitudes about safety, smoking, and drinking. The purpose is to change habits. In a pioneering 1974 report, the Canadian government noted that making health services available to all Canadians had little impact on morbidity and mortality rates. An analysis of the principal causes of mortality and morbidity revealed that environmental factors and life style were the keys to effective disease control (LaLonde, 1974). The Canadian study focused on four components: environment, life style, health care organization, and human biology. In this way, program planners could focus their attention on the most important contributing factors. For example, the underlying causes of death from traffic accidents were found to be mainly due to risks taken by individuals, not to roads or the design of cars.

Blum (1982) and Mechanic (1989) suggest there is a need for a mixture of micro (individual) and macro (societal) approaches to reduce risks for disease. The most powerful interventions are macro interventions, such as taxing or general prohibitions, which focus on the socioeconomic environment. There is little doubt that how society views major problems will be critical to how society acts on the problems.

Values as Predictors of Health Behavior

One reason for the difficulty in getting people to change their health behaviors is that preserving health is not our society's highest value. It competes with many other values, including wealth, power, security, knowledge, and social acceptance (Mechanic & Cleary, 1980 Mechanic, 1982).

Many studies have reported that people's knowledge of health and health risks has increased, and beliefs have changed as the result of interventions. Efforts to mold or change values and influence behavior have been less successful. Health beliefs vary from disease to disease, person to person, and even in the same person over time (Kristiansen, 1985). Thus, singular appeals to change health behavior or life style have to be meaningful to an individual at a particular point in time. In other words, individuals have to be "ready" to change. Times when fewer pressing or compelling priorities compete for an individual's personal resources might be most appropriate for change.

Perhaps one of the more predominent aspects that dissuade people from changing their life styles or health behaviors is the *benefit* they derive from the life styles and behaviors with which they have become comfortable. It is difficult to persuade persons to give up a behavior or make major changes in the way they live when the benefits of these changes are unknown. Such substitutions are often viewed as punishment or sacrifice. The trade-off between behaviors or life styles is not seen as an equal one.

Another aspect of value change involves the *source* of values. Values are derived from our culture, science, religion, and personal experience. Sometimes, these sources present conflicting values, requiring that individuals make choices to guide their behavior. Indeed, individuals may make behavioral choices that appear inconsistent with their values of health; for example, an individual may exercise regularly, but not wear seat belts, adhere to dietary restrictions, but smoke cigarettes. These inconsistencies may reflect conflicting values derived from various sources and, hence, the individual's ambivalence about how total health is valued.

A third aspect of value change relates to *how individuals obtained* their values about health, i.e., through modeling, chance, or "moralizing." Attempts to change values using the same approach in which the values were learned may have the opposite effect, especially if the conditions that surrounded the initial learning are now different. Pratt (1976) suggested that it is not simply a number of separate factors that affect how health is valued, but the overall pattern of values, of which health is one part, that is important. To cause individuals to change the way in which they value health taps a complex, deeply embedded belief system that is not easily modifiable, at least with simple, solitary means of intervention or modification (Richards, 1975).

Value change is one of the most formidable tasks in health education.

Indeed, it would seem more prudent with respect to time, effort, and cost to begin in early childhood to teach and model healthy life styles and health behaviors than to attempt to change deeply entrenched values in adulthood.

Lifestyle and Health Behavior

It is difficult to assess the personal benefits of healthy life styles; what is considered beneficial will differ among individuals. Oster and Epstein (1986) suggested that cholesterol-lowering interventions, no matter what their cost, are unlikely to result in substantial direct savings to the health care system. However, the indirect benefits of intervention are quite high for young and middle-aged adults, as well as for those with severe elevations of cholesterol or with additional coronary risk factors. Often individuals assume that they will add years to their life. A recent follow-up of Harvard graduates showed that by the age of 80, the amount of additional life attributable to adequate exercise, as compared with sedentariness, was from 1 to more than 2 years (Paffenbarger et al., 1986). Most often, the personal benefits of health behavior are physiological, cognitive, and/or behavioral (Dubbert et al., 1986). Sime (1984), for example, described research showing reductions in anxiety and depression and increases in body attitude and self-confidence due to exercise.

An individual's choices and decisions about life style and health behaviors will also be influenced by life events and stage of development. The death of a family member from a heart attack is likely to have a greater influence in motivating a middle-aged family member than an adolescent to change his/her life style. On the other hand, wearing seat belts could be seen to have a positive benefit to all members of a family, irrespective of age, if they have lost a family member in an automobile accident in which wearing a seat belt might have meant survival. Everyone, seemingly, has "times" or "points" in their life when they are more receptive to health information and perhaps more motivated to change. To capture and sustain these positive times is a continual challenge to health professionals. Pill and Stott (1987) have developed an index to measure the extent to which people perceive their daily decisions regarding diet, exercise, smoking, drinking, and so on as choices that determine future health. This index has the potential for identifying those segments of a population most ready to alter their life style.

It is important to note that people who participate in one form of health behavior may not participate in other health-related behaviors. This suggests that each behavior or type of behavior may have its own unique determinants and situational reinforcers, and, thus, must be analyzed separately (Mechanic, 1979). There does not appear to be a general or common "preventive health personality," or type of person who is likely to engage in a broad variety of preventive health behaviors. There are, however, characteristics that seem to distinguish between individuals who follow a wellness versus an illness lifestyle (Table 3-2).

Harris and Guten (1979) propose that all individuals engage in some behaviors intended to protect their health. These researchers set out to identify the activities an individual performs in the belief that they protect his/her health. They also wanted to find out if there were any patterns among these activities. Over 70 percent of the 1,250 randomly chosen respondents reported health behaviors related to general nutrition. The next most frequently related behaviors concerned how, when, how long, and how frequently the respondents slept, rested, and relaxed. About one-third of the respondents reported behavior related to physical activity and recreation. Preventive health care behaviors were affected by sex, race, income, education, satisfaction with health, perceived vulnerability, and health condition. While this study was exploratory and limited in time and depth, it did indicate what laymen consider health behaviors, rather than what health professionals recommend.

Even if an individual recognizes health behaviors and practices one or more preventive health behaviors, there must be a payoff to motivate the person to continue to act over time. Many characteristics or factors that have been uncovered by researchers comprise a rough profile of a wellness versus an illness life style (Table 3-2). Individuals persist in living life styles they feel satisfying and comfortable. In order to ascertain the degree to which a life style is healthy or unhealthy a "behavioral diagnosis" is needed (Jenkins, 1979). The individual should participate with the health professional in making this diagnosis and in discussing any changes or trade-offs in behaviors. Individuals will not give up or trade behaviors they find satisfying unless the consequences directly threaten their most highly held values (Bruhn, 1988b).

Table 3-2. Some characteristics of illness and wellness lifestyles

Illness Lifestyle	Wellness Lifestyle
Use of limited coping skills	Learns new or modifies old coping skills
Socially withdrawn, shy, minimal interaction	Open and receptive to others
Sees change as barrier, obstacle	Initiates and directs change
Perceives few choices and options in problem-solving	Perceives and exercises choices and options in problem-solving
No clear-cut goals or purpose to life	Has purpose to life and goals
Limited use of resources in adapting	Makes use of resources of all kinds in adapting
Relies on already acquired skills, limited skills	Enhances personal, social and other skills
Black-white view of issues and problems	Integrating approach to issues and problems
Crisis-oriented approach to problems	Problem-solving/preventive attitude
Passive/reactive behavior	Active/initiating behavior
Minimal self-care activities	Maximal self-care activities
Socially isolated or weak social ties	Strong social ties
Risk-seeking health behavior	Risk-conscious health behavior
Pessimistic/fatalistic attitude	Optimistic/hopeful attitude
Stress producing behavior	Stress reducing behavior
External locus of control	Internal locus of control
Anger/depression common emotions	Frustration, anxiety and compulsive behavior common
Negative self-image, low self-esteem	Positive self-image, high self-esteem

The Many Sides of Health Promotion

Health promotion does not only apply to physical health. Eisenberg (1981) discusses the need to promote mental health and prevent mental illness. Epidemiologic studies have documented increased rates of psychiatric disorder and of general morbidity and mortality among persons who are socially isolated. There is also general agreement on the deleterious health consequences of bereavement and of racism on mental health. Eisenberg notes that programs for mental hygiene all too often imply the prevention of all mental illness. There is no single entity of "mental illness," but rather a variety of disorders. The task is to devise methods to prevent particular disorders. Perhaps less interest and emphasis has been given to the prevention of mental illness than to physical illness because many of the root causes and mechanisms of mental disorders are deeply embedded in the fabric of society, e.g., poverty, unemployment, "social malnutrition," abandonment, and abuse. It is often assumed that if physical health is improved, improvement in mental health will follow and vice versa.

Health professionals often regard prevention and rehabilitation as opposite poles on a continuum of care, viewing the former as avoiding illness, injury, or disability, and the latter as restoring lost function. This view of rehabilitation is unnecessarily restrictive. Rehabilitation should be concerned with restoration and prevention. The rehabilitation process generally unfolds over a substantially longer period of time than does that of acute care. This creates many opportunities for members of the rehabilitation team to become familiar with their patients, to assess their life styles, to determine their physical and emotional responses to their illnesses or injuries, to determine factors placing patients at risk for additional adverse outcomes, and to assess those risks that are potentially correctable (DeVellis & Sauter, 1985). A characteristic that facilitates prevention is the multidisciplinary nature of rehabilitation teams. Each member has a special awareness and sensitivity to a particular set of concerns. A physical therapist, for example, may be particularly attentive to the potential problems of body mechanics and the risk of falling, while a social worker may concentrate on the long-term handicap of a low self-image. Incorporating prevention into rehabilitation services could lead to more efficient and effective patient management strategies, which will benefit all parties.

Examples of Prevention: The Case of AIDS

The strategy of prevention of HIV transmission through education and the modification of behaviors is the most realistic approach to the prevention of AIDS. Educating persons with information that leads to changed behaviors that reduce or eliminate high-risk, unprotected sexual encounters constitutes effective prevention. Safer sexual practices reduce the likelihood of transmission. Educating intravenous drug users about the use of clean needles and techniques for sterilizing needles and the related paraphernalia can reduce the transmission of AIDS (Mays et al., 1989). Transmission of the virus can occur during high-risk activities with any HIV-infected person, regardless of that person's clinical health; the majority of transmission episodes occur between people who appear to be in good health. Because HIV-infected individuals do not show visable manifestations of their viral carrier status, a person's healthful appearance provides no information concerning HIV infection. The most appropriate prevention objective is to encourage and assist persons to refrain from engaging in high-risk practices with any partner who might carry the HIV virus (Kelly & St. Lawrence, 1988).

There is considerable public policy debate concerning the focus of AIDS prevention efforts. Some persons stress that the only means of avoiding sexually-transmitted HIV exposure is the maintenance of either celibacy or a completely monogamous relationship with one other person when both are HIV-unexposed. Proponents of this viewpoint suggest that programs to prevent the spread of AIDS should stress the values of chastity until marriage, the maintenance of a lifelong marital relationship with the same person, and strict monogamy. Others note that it is naive to assume that most people, now or in the future, will successfully adopt such life styles, and that prevention efforts should teach individuals to minimize their likelihood of HIV exposure, regardless of their sexual preference and relationship fidelity (Kelly & St. Lawrence, 1988).

Printed materials and education through the mass media are necessary to educate persons about ways to reduce exposure risks. Personal communication and community education with efforts aimed at specific age, ethnic, socioeconomic, and cultural groups is also needed (Bruhn, 1990). Government decisions to emphasize moral education for AIDS prevention have been enacted against a background of public opinion that has become, in general, more tolerant of nonmarital heterosexual intercourse. The climate of increasing social tolerance for nonmarital sex can be observed most reliably during 1972–1988, for which there are reliable national indicators of public attitudes. Some of the federal guidelines regarding AIDS education in schools require that programs be consistent with the moral values of parents and the community; others require that the values presented in the programs correspond to those of monogamous marriage. However, given the pluralistic nature of the United States, such guidelines are sure to offend some group. One way to avoid such problems is to leave out the moral dimension of AIDS messages and allow individuals and families to supply their own value judgments. This approach embodies a respect for private beliefs (Turner et al., 1989).

The uphill battle to inform the public, especially adolescents, about AIDS is evident in the study and literature review conducted by Sunenblick (1988). She investigated the knowledge about AIDS and attitudes toward personal susceptibility among 90 freshmen (ages 17–23) enrolled at a university in Maine. The major finding revealed that the level of knowledge and perception of susceptibility was not significantly associated with safe sexual behaviors. The students had a high level of knowledge about the cause, transmission, and treatment of AIDS and the more knowledge they had, the less they were concerned about personal susceptibility. However, their awareness did not always result in safe sexual behavior. The literature suggests that even the most healthy adolescents are governed by the push toward impulse gratification and may have difficulty with the kinds of behavioral change required to prevent the transmission of AIDS. The major lesson for AIDS prevention efforts is that cognitive efforts to instruct adolescents about safe sex practices will be unsuccessful unless the emotional aspects of adolescent development are addressed. Adolescents are asked to face their mortality at a time when their feelings of immortality and invincibility are at their highest. Public health educators and clinicians should deal with the denial against the painful realities of AIDS. They can work toward creating environments in which adolescents can talk safely about mortality, sex, safe practices, homosexuality, drug use, and AIDS. Reluctance to address the value issues that are related to AIDS contributes to the highly emotional and often irrational responses to the AIDS epidemic (Sunenblick, 1988).

Examples of Prevention: The Healthy Workplace

Growing evidence suggests that workplace health promotion programs can be effective in reducing smoking, controlling hypertension, reducing obesity, and increasing exercise levels, possibly more effective than similar programs outside of work (House & Cottington, 1986). Studies have shown a higher degree of voluntary employee participation in health services offered at the worksite than anywhere else. Multiphasic screening programs in industry regularly achieve 90 percent to 95 percent participation, whereas identical programs, offered without cost after extensive community publicity, rarely get more than 30 percent participation (Bruhn & Cordova, 1987b).

Health services at the worksite are convenient, free and, employees often assume, of good quality. For the employer who pays a sizable portion of the costs of health care and of disability and death, the economic return of health services at the worksite is important. Changing societal attitudes and regulatory pressures also encourage the development of the work setting as a site for health promotion for much of the population. The worksite offers a management structure and relationships with employees that can facilitate health promotion programs. Finally, the workplace offers technical advantages that help to ensure change in health behavior (such as the ability to apply long-term interventions) and to acquire health-related data easily, which make it possible to follow individuals and groups over time and thus provide communication, information, and social support for health promotion endeavors (McGill, 1979).

Several investigators have reported the effects of corporate health and fitness programs on physiological and psychological parameters (Baun et al., 1986). In most studies, significant improvements were found in psychological parameters such as self-concept, trait anxiety, and job satisfaction, as well as improvement in physiological parameters such as resting heart rate and blood pressure, concentrations of triglycerides and total concentration of cholesterol in blood. The psychological benefits of exercise are apparent in the mentally well as well as in those with psychological disorders.

The four reasons given for the establishment of health and fitness programs by the Washington Business Group for Health are as follows: (1) improve human relations through improving morale; (2) improve productivity; (3) lower health care costs; and (4) improve the company image with the community. Corporate fitness programs are generally found in larger organizations, and the current trend is to provide services to all employees, emphasizing preventive health practices other than just exercise.

Wellness in the Workplace: Some Prototypes

In 1977, the Kimberly-Clark Corporation initiated a health maintenance effort called the Health Management Program. The program includes a medical history and health risk profile, multiphasic screening, a physical examination, exercise-testing by treadmill or bicycle ergometer, a health review and recommendations by a physician or nurse practitioner, an aerobic exercise program that uses the company's 32,000 square foot exercise facility, health education classes, and an employee-assistance program for chemical dependency and other special health problems. The program aims to achieve a higher level of wellness and productivity in employees and to reduce absenteeism and the rate of escalation in health care costs (Dedmon et al., 1980).

About 300 of the 1,800 eligible hourly employees and 2,400 (90%) of the 2,700 eligible salaried employees in the Fox Valley Wisconsin Kimberly-Clark mills have had multiphasic screening and exercise tests. The highest monthly participation rate is 7.5 per employee; about 25 percent of eligible employees currently participate in a regular exercise program. About 1,500 employees and family members have registered for health education classes, which include training in cardiopulmonary respiratory training (Dedman et al., 1979).

In the developing stages, employees were not required to participate. Years of observation will be necessary before any estimate can be made of the effect of the program on morbidity or mortality rates. It will be difficult to evaluate individual components of the program and to distinguish a cause-and-effect relationship between them and disease episodes. Also, since the employees who participate in these programs are self-selected, the results may be biased.

A different approach is provided by Honeywell, Inc. (1981). Employees and their dependents are eligible to enroll in any one of six Health Maintenance Organizations (HMOs) or Blue Cross/Blue Shield Insurance plans at Honeywell's cost. When an employee retires, HMO coverage continues until the employee is 65. The six plans vary somewhat according to the site at which health care is provided and the kind of services offered.

The Kaiser-Permanente Medical Care Program, which was initiated in 1933, is one of the oldest industrial health plans in the United States (Newman, 1981). The purpose of the program is to provide quality care at a reasonable cost to subscriber-members on a prepaid basis. The program operates in six geographic regions and consists of several separate but cooperating organizations that provide health-care services to about 3.5 million health plan members. It is the largest prepaid group practice in the nation and is a prototype of all HMOs. As part of this program, preventive medicine measures, such as periodic tests, are recommended by each physician, although the process may be initiated by either the physician or the patient. Considerable evidence shows that if a program of prevention is to be cost-effective, it should be based on the individual patient's age, sex, and specific risk factors. Risk factors should be identified and a cost-effective set of tests performed, with reexamination at time intervals appropriate for each individual's risk category.

A multiphasic health check-up system based on 25 years of experience classifies individuals by health status. Then, appropriate recommendations are made, which are based on each person's needs. The process selects out high-risk persons and those who have early asymptomatic illness. Sick people are referred to "sick-care services" and well people to health-education and health-counseling services to further improve their health status. The approach provides for an efficient entry into the health care system, an appropriate use of the health professional's time, and an education of patients regarding the proper use of health services.

Does Health Promotion Pay?

A survey of the literature (Rogers et al., 1981) on the cost-effectiveness of health promotion programs showed that we know little about the effectiveness of health promotion for several reasons: little if any evaluation of programs is built into them at their onset, so available data must be collected after interventions have begun; few programs seek to change health behavior because it would take a long commitment of time, money, and manpower, and government, business, and industry are often reluctant to wait that long for answers; no general agreement on how to measure costs exists, and practically no comparable measures or standards for deciding whether costs are high or low are available; it is usually assumed that health education and health promotion are justified only if they prove to be cost-effective; and, since few organizations share information about the type, extent, and results of their health programs, assessment of those programs is difficult.

The findings with respect to the cost-effectiveness of health promotion activities are contradictory. Higgins (1988) concludes that health promotion may have been oversold as a cost containment strategy. Prevention is not always cheaper than cure, and judging health promotion solely on the basis of savings in health care costs overlooks other important benefits. For example, Spilman et al., (1986) reports that the health promotion program at A, T, & T was found to lower health risks and improve health-related and job-related attitudes among the study group.

Recently, a report by the Health Insurance Association of America (HIAA) offered persuasive evidence that a company profits when it keeps its employees healthy. Dr. Loring Wood, medical director for research at New York Telephone Company, reported that nine disease-prevention programs for some 80,000 employees at his company resulted in annual savings of $2.7 million. The HIAA report also noted that a colon and rectal cancer screening program at the Campbell Soup Company saved that company $245,000 over 10 years. The extensive health promotion program at Kimberly-Clark, described earlier, may take as long as 10 years to be cost-effective.

In a comprehensive review of the economics of fitness and sport with particular reference to the worksite, Shepherd (1989) found that costs vary greatly with the scale of facilities and the level of program supervision that is offered. Beyond a certain ceiling, further expenditures do not seem to enhance program effectiveness. Likely benefits to a company include an improved corporate image, recruitment of premium employees, gains in the quality and quantity of production, a decrease in absenteeism and turnover, lower medical costs, an improvement in personal life styles, and a reduced incidence of industrial injuries. While current evidence has many limitations, it does suggest that exercise, in the context of more general health promotion, is both cost-effective and cost-beneficial: the immediate return may be as much as $2 to $5 per dollar invested.

There is a widespread perception that prevention programs will save money. The Centers for Disease Control calculated that the first five years of the measles immunization program led to the avoidance of almost 10 million cases, averted more than 3,000 cases of mental retardation, and saved about 1,000 lives. The cost of the program was just over $100 million. The net direct economic savings from averted doctor visits, hospitalization, and long-term care of those who would have been permanently disabled exceeded $275 million. Almost as great were the indirect savings due to loss of time from work, lifetime earnings, etc. Immunization against other childhood diseases including rubella and whooping cough, has also been shown to be cost-saving. Fluoridation of the water supply saves large sums of money. Testing for and removing lead paint in urban neighborhoods where lead poisoning is prevalent among children is cost-saving. Yet, these cases are exceptional. Most prevention programs do not save money; for example, intensive care units for newborns, periodic stool exams for traces of blood to detect cancer of the bowel, vaccinations of the elderly against pneumococcal pneumonia, high blood pressure screening, and mandatory air bags in automobiles (Hiatt, 1987). Evidence also shows that, even allowing for savings in treatment, prevention usually adds to medical expenditures. Prevention cannot be assumed to be a less expensive choice than cure in every case.

The Ethics of Disease Prevention/Health Promotion

Prevention is neither costless nor riskless. Every preventive measure involves some degree of risk (Russell, 1986). For example, taking the flu vaccine does not ensure that you will not get the flu; the cholesterol-lowering drug, Mevacor®, carries the risk of possible kidney damage. Prevention aimed at correcting or enhancing one aspect of health may have adverse affects on other aspects of one's health. The aim of prevention, therefore, is to "normalize or equalize risk," not eliminate it completely. The effects and limitations of preventive measures should be realistically and honestly presented. Prevention cannot ensure a longer life, but it can affect the quality of life.

Some preventive options may not be available to all persons because of cost. For example, not everyone can afford to join a health club, or afford preventive drugs, or afford to buy foods at health stores. This raises the ethical question of whether it is right for some persons to have access to options to improve their health and well-being while others cannot experience these options. Prevention should be as much a part of the "right to health care" as treatment is.

Prevention also raises the issue of personal autonomy and freedom of choice (Eisenberg, 1987). Some community preventive efforts such as the fluoridation of water are voted on by the public. Other preventive efforts, such as prohibiting smoking in public buildings and on airlines, give no choice to the individual except alternative means of transportation. Most preventive health behaviors are a matter of individual choice, for example, to quit smoking, to exercise, to lose weight, to use seat belts, etc.

The self-care movement, whereby a layperson functions on his/her own behalf in health maintenance, disease prevention, self-diagnosis, self-medication, and self-treatment, is perhaps the extreme example of personal autonomy and freedom of choice (Levin et al., 1976). Self-care has generated many ethical, legal, and philosophical issues among medical practitioners. Perhaps a more currently acceptable means of patient participation is a voice in decision-making about their treatment and the freedom to seek other opinions. This would apply to preventive measures as well as corrective interventions.

One might raise the question of whether it is ethical for a physician and other health professionals not to routinely offer information about how they can enhance their health to clients as a part of medical treatment. Some clients may be unaware of sources of preventive health measures and self-help groups. There are preventive measures that have mixed endorsements in medicine, such as routine chest x-rays, mammographies, Pap smears, and routine physical examinations. The physician one chooses for health care influences greatly the preventive attitudes of his/her patients.

The success of efforts to prevent disease and enhance health rests with the individual. Individuals who feel helpless to change the course of their health will become consumers of health services sooner or later and will place their lives in the hands of the latest medical technology. Technology may provide them with longer lives, but not necessarily enjoyable ones. When individuals who take the initiative to become more aware of their health and engage in activities thought to enhance their general physical and/or mental well-being do become consumers of health services, they will also be more likely to take initiatives to return to an active, independent state. Preventive medicine cannot expect to win all to its side. We are all the products of a complex upbringing, laden with attitudes, values, and role models who influence our lives. To decide to give a higher rank to our health than we had previously means making significant changes in our lifestyles and behavior. Each individual gives a rank of importance to his/her health either by choice or by default. Unfortunately, after the symptoms of chronic disease have become overt it is too late to change the value one places on his/her health. We need to value our health before we lose it.

In Retrospect

An appraisal of influences in the past suggests that the contribution of modern medicine to the increase of life expectancy has been much smaller than most people believe. Health improved because people became ill less often. We remain well because of immunization, a high standard of nutrition, a healthier environment, and we have fewer children (McKeown, 1978). Today's problems are mainly with noncommunicable diseases. Most diseases are associated with influences that might be controlled. Among such influences are those that the individual determines by his/her own behavior. Both behavioral and environmental influences are more important than medical care. Few people, however, see themselves as having the major responsibility for their own health. The public believes that health depends primarily on intervention by the doctor and that the essential requirement for health is the early discovery of disease.

The failure to recognize personal vulnerability has long been a barrier to the adoption of precautions. People tend to be unrealistically optimistic about their own susceptibility to harm. This has been a major challenge in the primary prevention of AIDS (Weinstein, 1989). Prevention involves personal risk assessment and choice. If health is not as high a priority to an individual as other values, preventive activities are not likely to be of interest to him/her, even when the consequences are known, and the fact that they will eventually be disabling and painful. It is difficult for a health professional to accept the fact that not everyone values health to the same extent, resulting in patients choosing to live in ways that will eventually result in pain, disability and death, which may have been avoided, or at least postponed, e.g., cigarette smoking with the risk of developing emphysema. Illness behavior is as much a choice as health behavior. In the health professions, we prefer to work with "good patients," that is, patients who have similar values, follow directions, and come back to see us. Patients who do not conform to our ways, we label as "unmotivated," "crocks," or "gomers." As Golin (1979) noted, there is no such thing as an unmotivated patient, since any patient who is alive — eating, breathing, sleeping — is obviously motivated. The label generally refers to a patient who is not motivated to the degree expected, or in the direction expected by the health professional. As health professionals, we need to validate individuals and not their values.

REFERENCES

Amartya, S. (1986). The right to take personal risks. In D. MacLean (Ed.), *Values at risk.* (pp. 155–169). Totowa, NJ: Rowman & Allenheld.

Baric, L. (1969). Recognition of the "at-risk" role. *International Journal of Health Education, 12,* 24–34.

Baun, W.B., Bernacki, E.J., & Herd, J.A. (1986). Corporate health and fitness programs and the prevention of work stress. In J.C. Quick, R.S. Bhagat, J.E. Dalton & J.D. Quick (Eds.), *Work stress: Health care systems in the work place* (pp. 217–234). New York: Praeger.

Becker, M.H. & Rosenstock, I.M. (1989). Health promotion, disease prevention, and program retention. In H.E. Freeman & L. Levine (Eds.), *Handbook of medical sociology,* 4th ed. (pp. 284–305). Englewood Cliffs, N.J.: Prentice Hall.

Belloc, N.B. (1973). Relationship of health practices and mortality. *Preventive Medicine, 2,* 67–81.

Belloc, N.B. & Breslow, L. (1972). Relationship of physical health status and health practices. *Preventive Medicine, 1,* 409–421.

Blum, H.L. (1983). *Expanding health care horizons.* 2nd ed. Oakland, CA: Third Party Publishing.

Blum, H.L. (1982). Social perspective on risk reduction. In M.M. Faber & A.M. Reinhardt (Eds.), *Promoting health through risk reduction* (pp. 19–36). New York: Macmillan.

Bruhn, J.G. (1987a). The novelty of stress. *Southern Medical Journal, 80,* 1398–1406.

Bruhn, J.G. & Cordova, F.D. (1987b). Promoting healthy behavior in the workplace. *Health Values, 11,* 39–48.

Bruhn, J.G. (1988a). Life-style and health behavior. In D.S. Gochman (Ed.). *Health behavior* (pp. 71–86). New York: Plenum.

Bruhn, J.G. (1988b). Creating risk-sensitive persons: The roles of choice and chance in staying healthy. *Southern Medical Journal, 81,* 624–629.

Bruhn, J.G. (1990). A community model for the prevention of AIDS. *Family and Community Health, 12,* 65–77.

Clarke, K.S., Parcel, G.S. (1975). Values and risk-taking behavior: The concept of calculated risk. *Health Education, 6,* 26–28.

Cohen, J. (1972). *Psychological probability or the art of doubt.* London: George Allen and Unwin.

Dedmon, R.E., Gander, J.W., & O'Conner, M.P., et al. (1979). An industry health management program. *The Physician and Sports Medicine, 7,* 56–57.

Dedmon, R.E., Kubiak, M.K., & Konkol, P.O., et al. (1980). Employees as health educators: A reality at Kimberly-Clark. *Occupational Health and Safety, 49,* 18–24.

DeVellis, R.F. & Sauter, S.V.H. (1985). Recognizing the challenges of prevention in rehabilitation. *Archives of Physical Medicine and Rehabilitation, 66,* 52–54.

Dubbert, P.M., Martin, J.E., & Epstein, L.H. (1986). Exercise. In K.A. Holroyd & T.L. Creer (Eds.), *Self-management of chronic disease: Handbook of clinical interventions and research* (pp. 127–161). New York: Academic Press.

Ducanis, A.J. & Golin, A. (1979). The sick role. In N. Abrams & M.D. Buckner (Eds.), *Medical ethics.* (pp. 169–171). Cambridge, MA: The MIT Press.

Duryea, E.J., Okwumabua, J. (1985). An explanatory study of the health decision-making variables of New York and Montana ninth-graders. *Adolescence, 20,* 899–908.

Eisenberg, L. (1981). A research framework for evaluating the promotion of mental health and the prevention of mental illness. *Public Health Reports, 96,* 3–19.

Eisenberg, L. (1987). Value conflicts in social policies for promoting health. In S. Doxiadis (Ed.), *Ethical dilemmas in health promotion* pp. 99–116. New York: John Wiley.

Flannery, R.B. (1987). Towards stress-resistant persons: A stress management approach to the treatment of anxiety. *American Journal of Preventive Medicine, 25,* 25–30.

Fuchs, V.R. (1974). *Who shall live? Health, economics, and social choice.* New York: Basic Books.

Goedert, J.J. (1987). What is safe sex? Suggested standards linked to testing for human immunodeficiency virus. *New England Journal of Medicine, 316,* 1339–1341.

Golin, S. (1979). Illusion of control among depressed patients. *Journal of Abnormal Psychology 88:* 454–457.

Hamburg, D.A., Elliott, G.R., & Parron, D.L. (1982). *Health behavior. Frontiers of research in the biobehavioral sciences.* Washington, D.C.: National Academy Press.

Harris, D.M. and Guten, S. (1979). Health-protective behavior: An exploratory study. *Journal of Health and Human Behavior, 20,* 17–29.

Health Education Unit, WHO Regional Office for Europe. (1986). Life-styles and health. *Social Science and Medicine, 22,* 117–124.

Hetzel, B. & McMichael, T. (1988). *The LS factor.* Auckland, Australia: Penguin Books.

Hiatt, H.H. (1987). *America's health in the balance.* New York: Harper & Row.

Higgins, C.W. (1988). The economics of health promotion. *Health Values, 12,* 39–45.

Honeywell Health Maintenance Organization. (1981). Pub. No. 59-7354. Minneapolis, Honeywell, Inc.

House, J.S. & Cottington, E.M. (1986). Health and the workplace. In L.H. Aiken & D. Mechanic (Eds.), *Applications of social science to clinical medicine and health policy.* (pp. 392–416). New Brunswick, NJ: Rutgers University Press.

Imperato, P.J. & Mitchell, G. (1985). *Acceptable risks.* New York: Viking.

Jenkins, C.D. (1979). An approach to the diagnosis and treatment of problems of health related behavior. *International Journal of Health Education, 22,* 1–24.

Kelly, J.A., & St. Lawrence, J.S. (1988). *The AIDS health crisis: Psychological and social interventions.* New York: Plenum.

Kickbusch, I. (1988). Introduction. In R. Anderson, J.K. Davies, I. Kickbusch, D.V. McQueen, & J. Turner (Eds.), *Health behavior research and health promotion* (pp. 1–3). New York: Oxford University Press.

Knowles, J.H. (1977). The responsibility of the individual. In J.H. Knowles (Ed.) *Doing better and feeling worse: Health in the United States* (pp. 57–80). New York: W.W. Norton.

Kristiansen, C.M. (1985). Value correlates of preventive health behavior. *Journal of Personality and Social Psychology, 49,* 748–758.

LaLonde, M. (1974). *A new perspective on the health of Canadians: A working document.* Ottawa: Ministry of Health and Welfare.

Leventhal, H. & Hirschman, R.S. (1982). Social psychology and prevention. In G.S. Sanders & J. Suls (Eds.), *Social psychology of health and illness* (pp. 183–226). Hillsdale, NJ: Lawrence Erlbaum.

Levin, L.S., Katz, A.H., & Holst, E. (1976). *Self-care: Lay initiatives in health.* New York: Prodist.

Levine, S. & Sorenson, J.R. (1984). Social and cultural factors in health promotion. In J.D. Matarazzo, S.M. Weiss, J.A. Herd, N.E. Miller, & S.M. Weiss (Eds.), *Behavioral health: A handbook of health enhancement and disease prevention* (pp. 222–229). New York: John Wiley.

Lewis, C.E. & Lewis, M.A. (1984). Peer pressure and risk-taking behaviors in children. *American Journal of Public Health, 74,* 580–584.

Mays, V.M., Albee, G.W., & Schneider, S.F. (1989). *Primary prevention of AIDS: Psychological approaches.* Newbury Park, CA: Sage.

McGill, A.M. (Ed.) (1979). *Proceedings of the national conference on health promotion programs in occupational settings.* January 17–19. Washington, D.C.: Government Printing Office.

McKeown, T. (1978). Determinants of health. *Human Nature.* April: 60–67.

McKeown, T. (1976). *The role of medicine: Dream, mirage, or nemesis?* London: Nuffield Provencial Hospitals Trust.

Mechanic, D. (1982). Disease, mortality, and the promotion of health. *Health Affairs, 1,* 28–38.

Mechanic, D. (1989). *Painful choices: Research and essays on health care.* New Brunswick, NJ: Transaction Publishers.

Mechanic, D. (1979). The stability of health and illness behavior: Results from a 16-year follow-up. *American Journal of Public Health, 69,* 1142–1145.

Mechanic, D. & Cleary, P.D. (1980). Factors associated with the maintenance of positive health behavior. *Preventive Medicine, 9,* 805–814.

Miles, A. (1978). The social content of health. In P. Brearley, J. Gibbons, A. Miles, E. Topliss, & G. Woods, *The social context of health care* (pp. 7–37). London: Martin Robertson.

Milio, N. (1983). *Primary care and the public's health.* Lexington, Mass: D.C. Heath and Co.

Milio, N. (1981). *Promoting health through public policy.* Philadelphia, PA: F.A. Davis.

Montagu, A. (1976). The illusion of immortality and health. *Preventive Medicine, 5,* 496–507.

Ng, L.K.Y., Davis, D.L., Manderscheid, R.W., & Elkes, J. (1981). Toward a conceptual formulation of health and well-being. In L.K.Y. Ng, & D.L. Davis, (Eds.), *Strategies for public health: Promoting health and preventing disease* (pp. 44–58). New York: Van Nostrand Reinhold.

Newman, H.F. (1981). Kaiser-Permanente: Preventive medicine and health promotion.

In Lorenz, L.Y., & Davis, D.L. (Eds.) *Strategies for public health: Promoting health and preventing disease.* (pp. 388–396) New York: Van Nostrand Reinhold.

Office of Disease Prevention and Health Promotion, U.S. Public Health Service, U.S. Department of Health and Human Services. (1988). *Disease prevention/health promotion. The facts.* Palo Alto, CA: Bull.

Ornstein, R. & Sobel, D. (1987). *The healing brain.* New York: Simon and Schuster.

Oster, G. & Epstein, A.M. (1986). Primary prevention and coronary heart disease: The economic benefits of lowering serum cholesterol. *American Journal of Public Health, 76,* 647–656.

Paffenbarger, R.S., Hyde, R.T., Wing, A.L., & Hsieh, C.C. (1986). Physical activity, all-cause mortality, and longevity of college alumni. *New England Journal of Medicine, 314,* 605–613.

Pill, R. & Stott, N.C.H. (1987). Development of a measure of potential health behavior. A salience of lifestyle. *Social Science and Medicine, 24,* 125–134.

Pratt, L. (1976). Child rearing methods and children's health behavior. *Journal of Health and Social Behavior, 14,* 61–69.

Radius, S.M., Dielman, T.E., Becker, M.H., et al. (1980). Health beliefs of the school-aged child and their relationship to risk-taking behaviors. *International Journal of Health Education, 23,* 227–235.

Richards, N.D. (1975). Methods and effectiveness of health education: The past, present, and future of social scientific involvement. *Social Science and Medicine, 9,* 141–156.

Rogers, P.J., Eaton, E.K., & Bruhn, J.G. (1981). Is health promotion cost effective? *Preventive Medicine, 10,* 324–339.

Roemer, M.I. (1984). The value of medical care for health promotion. *American Journal of Public Health, 74,* 243–248.

Russell, L.B. (1986). *Is prevention better than cure?* Washington, D.C.: The Brookings Institution.

Saward, E. & Sorensen, A. (1978). The current emphasis on preventive medicine. *Science, 200,* 26 May, 889–894.

Shapiro, J. & Shapiro, D.H., Jr. (1979). The psychology of responsibility: Some second thoughts on holistic medicine. *The New England Journal of Medicine, 301,* 26 July, 211–212.

Shepherd, R.J. (1989). Current perspectives on the economics of fitness and sport with particular reference to work. *Sports Medicine, 7,* 286–309.

Sime, W.E. (1984). Psychological benefits of exercise training in the healthy individual. In J.D. Matarazzo, S.M. Weiss, J.A. Herd, N.E. Miller, & S.M. Weiss, (Eds.), *Behavioral health: A handbook of health enhancement and disease prevention* (pp. 488–508). New York: Wiley.

Spilman, M.A., Goetz, A., Schultz, J., Bellingham, R., & Johnson, D. (1986). Effects of a corporate health promotion program. *Journal of Occupational Medicine, 28,* 285–289.

Sunenblick, M.B. (1988). The AIDS epidemic: Sexual behaviors of adolescents. *Smith College Studies in Social Work, 59,* 21–37.

Teuber, A. (1990). Justifying risk. *Daedalus 119:*235–254.

Turner, C.F., Miller, H.G., & Moses, L.E. (Eds.) (1989). *AIDS: Sexual behavior and intravenous drug use.* Washington, D.C.: National Academy Press.

Weinstein, N.D. (1989). Perceptions of personal susceptibility to harm. In V.M. Mays, G.W. Albee & S.F. Schneider (Eds.), *Primary prevention of AIDS: Psychological approaches,* (pp. 142–167). Newbury Park, California:Sage.

SUGGESTED READINGS

Amler, R.W. & Dull, H.B. (Eds.). (1987). *Closing the gap: The burden of unnecessary illness.* New York, Oxford University Press.

Cousins, N. (1989). *Headfirst: The biology of hope.* New York: Dutton.

Doxiadis, S. (Ed.). (1987). *Ethical dilemmas in health promotion.* New York: Wiley.

Felner, R.D., Jason, L.A., Moritsugu, J.N. & Farber, S.S. (Eds.). (1983). *Preventive psychology: Theory, research & practice.* New York: Pergamon Press.

Justice, B. (1987). *Who gets sick.* Houston, Texas: Peak Press.

Kar, S.B. (Ed.). (1989). *Health promotion indicators and actions.* New York: Springer.

Karasek, R. & Theonell, T. (1990). *Healthy work: Stress, productivity, and the reconstruction of working life.* New York: Basic Books.

Ornstein, R. & Sobel, D. (1989). *Healthy pleasures.* Reading, MA: Addison-Wesley.

Pellegrino, E.D. (1981). Health promotion as public policy: The need for moral groundings. *Preventive Medicine, 10,* 371–378.

Preventive Medicine. (1972). Vol. 1. Entire issue.

Somers, A.R. (Ed.) (1976). *Promoting health.* Germantown, MD: Aspen.

Wikler, D. (1978). Persuasion and coercion for health. *Health and Society, 56,* 303–338.

Chapter 4

NORMALITY AS A VALUE

Health is only a word; there wouldn't be any inconvenience if it were taken from our vocabulary. For my part, I only know people who are more or less sick with a larger or smaller number of diseases which are developing more or less rapidly.

Dr. Knock, or the Triumph of Medicine,
Jules Romains, A play first performed in 1923.

What does it mean to be "normal"? Does being "normal" mean the same as being "average"? Is normality the absence of disease? Or does normality convey the capacity of a person to adapt or adjust to life circumstances? We do not possess any general definition of normality, yet laymen and professionals make judgments every day about what is normal behavior or what is a normal condition. We cannot avoid making value judgments, but we need to be aware that we are making them and to understand how our judgments affect the ways in which we see and act toward other people. The purpose of this chapter is to examine the meanings and dimensions of normality and to make health professionals in particular, more aware of how judgments about normality affect the ways in which they relate to patients.

Normality as a Value

To be normal, in lay terms, means that a person looks, acts, and thinks within a certain boundary. To be normal means that a person's behavior is "not too different" from what is tolerated by society. While society and professionals do not generally agree about what is "normal," there is reasonable agreement about extreme abnormality, e.g., hallucinations. Even in evaluating abnormality, we use value judgments, e.g., severely abnormal (or "way out") or mildly abnormal ("he's just expressing his individuality"). Some severe illnesses and abnormalities may be camou-

99

flaged by a seemingly normal surface; the degree of sickness or abnormality may not be detectable by all persons and at all times. Therefore, judgments about normality may be based on incomplete information.

In our society, we place a high value on being normal. There is social pressure to conform to the way of life of the majority, and we reward those who do conform. We regard having a job and being independent as normal, and unemployment and dependence as abnormal. We value people who are physically attractive, active, and youthful, and we make heroes of people who possess these characteristics in our advertisements, television, and movies. As people age and increasingly deviate from youthfulness, they may begin to withdraw from others and others to withdraw from them, resulting in social isolation. Similarly, the handicapped are treated differently—they deviate from the standard way of life of the "normal" person. Health professionals are not free from making judgments about the patients they treat, they tend to catagorize their patients as "good" or "bad" according to how well they conform to expectations. We all judge other people according to how well they agree with our individual beliefs, life styles, and expectations. This can lead to categorization, stereotyping, and a preference for treating certain types of patients.

The concept of normality encourages taking extreme positions such as positive or negative, right or wrong, sick or well, good or bad. Contrary to what we may think, normality does not imply an ideal or harmonious condition. The concept of normality is relative. What is normal under one set of circumstances may be abnormal under other circumstances. We know when a car is "normal" or "abnormal" because we generally agree on what cars are used for and we know something about their limits, but we do not all agree on how life should be lived and how we should treat our bodies. It is for this reason that we must look at the relationship of society to the individual when assessing normality. Iron does not react to sulfur, iron and sulfur react together. In the same way, the adjustment of the individual to society is a mutual one. Normality is a dynamic process. Just as every organ and tissue has a natural range of variability in respect to its structure and function, variations exist in the ways in which humans adapt to their environment. As Bateson (1979) has said, "The world partly. . . . comes to be how it is imagined."

The Relationship of Normality to Health

When we speak of health or disease, we use implicit values. Health is something good and desirable, while disease implies something bad (Eaton, 1951). "Health" and "normality" are generally considered positive concepts that are defined in terms of the absence of observable negative manifestations of abnormality and disease (Lewis, 1953). Popular belief asserts that individuals who see physicians are sick and those who do not are "well." Illness or abnormality cannot be defined, however, solely as that which physicians treat (Ryle, 1947). The following vignette humorously portrays the expectations of some health professionals when individuals appear in a health facility.

> "What's your name and address, child? What are your symptoms?" A woman in a white uniform shook Alice to wake her.
> "My name is Alice. I haven't any symptoms. I'm not sick. I just don't know where I am."
> "No symptoms?" the woman exclaimed in annoyance.
> "You must have. Everyone has. We'll send you to the multiphasic screening unit immediately.
> The computer will find some symptoms. This is Mediland. Everyone here is either a consumer of medical care, or a provider, or a third party. You've got to be one or the other." (Somers, 1972).

Assessing normality is implicit in the diagnostic process practiced by every physician; however, in the absence of a medical nosology for normality, physicians routinely assess the nature and degree to which patients deviate from agreed-upon clinical "norms" for bodily structures and functions. Those "norms" have been established, in turn, on the basis of clinical observation and experience, e.g., height and weight tables help to determine obesity; clinical experience influences what is considered a normal pulse and normal respiration. Each person has his/her own range of variations (Engel, 1960). Therefore, in assessing a patient's degree of normality, the physician must weigh the patient's current functioning against established clinical "norms" and the patient's past functioning against that of the present. This assessment process is influenced by the physician's clinical experience and by his/her sensitivity to individual and temporal variations. Past experience with patients experiencing similar symptoms, in turn, influences the physician's definition of "health" or "normality," his/her judgments about the nature of the therapeutic regimen, i.e., what has worked best in treating previous patients with the same condition, and the degree of normality the patient can be expected to achieve following treatment, i.e., the patient's motivation to get well and the recovery patients treated previously have achieved.

Customarily, medicine emphasizes phenomena that can be measured objectively and uses diagnostic labels that have statistical and predictive value (King, 1954). While more easily measured than health, disease is not a discrete and discontinuous state, nor is its assessment a completely objective process (Fabrega, 1972; Sabshin, 1967). The determination of etiology requires the physician to learn not only "what" the abnormality is, but also "how" and "why" it exists. These all involve value judgments about the patient's normal physical and mental functioning as well as about his/her life style and deviations from them. In assessing abnormality, the physician makes a series of deductions regarding various types of deviations from normality, e.g., physiological, psychological, social. These deductions are based on the patient's own assessment of his/her normal functioning (what "normal" is for him/her), the physician's interpretations of the patient's behavior and condition, what the patient tells and does not tell the physician, the physician's interpretations of laboratory results, and objective signs in the clinical examination (Redlich, 1952). Several visits may be necessary before the physician can assess the full extent of the patient's deviations from normality. Even then, many ills may be perceived by the patient as a sense of "not feeling his/her typical self," and cannot be assessed objectively by the physician or classified according to disease nosology. The complexity of this process of diagnosing departures from normality accounts, in part, for the need for specialists who are trained to assess deviations in specific bodily parts or organ systems. Multiple problems involving several parts or organ systems require that specialists consult one another in order to weigh the extent of deviation of various structures and functions before they can arrive at a total assessment of the degree of normality or abnormality present.

The process of assessing patients with psychiatric or psychosomatic complaints is even more complex (Carstairs, 1959; Glover, 1932; Grinker, 1967; Hacker, 1945; King, 1945; Kubie, 1954; Reider, 1950; Smith, 1950; Wegrocki, 1939). Psychological assessments often require that the physician depend less upon established nosology and more upon clinical experience and intuition to determine what is a "normal" mind. Psychiatry and psychosomatic medicine have no absolute clinical norms for variations in feeling and mood; hence, judgments of normality cannot be based solely on objective signs and symptoms. The criteria of normality are intimately tied to the psychological and social needs of each patient and to the culture and community in which he/she lives (Cantor, 1941; Lafave et al., 1967; Zusman, 1966). Individual needs, life styles, societal values, and norms change. Ultimately, the physician must translate psychosocial, ethical, and/or legal deviations into established clinical nosology (Opler, 1963). Clinical nosologies can also change. What constitutes a "normal" range for serum cholesterol is much lower today than it was a decade ago (Wynder & Hill, 1972). The American Psychiatric Association removed homosexuality from the third version of the Diagnostic and Statistical Manual, stating that it was no longer a disease, but included tobacco use as a new psychiatric disorder (Rakoff, Stancer & Kedward, 1977).

Eaton (1951) pointed out that mental health is a conceptual abstraction, that we know mental health only through its manifestations. Therefore, mental health is a value judgment. In a classic study, Rosenhan (1973) described an experiment in which eight sane people gained admission to psychiatric hospitals with a diagnosis of schizophrenia. Despite their "show" of sanity, the pseudopatients were never detected. They were all discharged with a diagnosis of "schizophrenia in remission." Beyond the tendency to call the healthy sick, the study addressed the issues of psychiatric labeling. Having once been labeled, there is little that one can do to overcome the label, which profoundly colors others' perceptions and expectations of a person. Indeed, a history of psychiatric treatment will introduce the question in some people's minds, "Is he/she normal now?"

The process of diagnosing abnormality involves the patient and the physician, but may also include the family, community agencies, or the court. Individuals who seek medical treatment have already gone through some type of assessment of their normality by themselves and/or with others. Basic decisions usually are not made first by professional personnel, but rather by an individual, his family, and/or community members who differ in their kinds and degrees of tolerance for various behaviors. The size and form of the social structure of a community can affect the visibility, definition, and consequences of symptomatology (Mechanic, 1962). In some instances, community or family pressures may be such that the patient is obliged to remain sick (Bursten & D'Esopo, 1965), e.g., a physically and/or mentally handicapped person; in others, behavior that would be regarded as clinically aberrant might be socially acceptable, e.g., bulemia and anorexia among adolescents; and, in still others, socially unacceptable behavior might be regarded as clinically normal, e.g., biting fingernails, picking one's nose, or purposefully burping at the dinner table. A patient's assessment of his own normality or deviations may depend upon a social rather than a clinical definition. A patient's expectations regarding treatment and prognosis may encompass the return to his former state of normality, a new level of normality with the alleviation of present abnormalities, or a more ideal state of enhanced well-being and functioning. When the physician and patient cannot agree upon their respective definitions of normality-abnormality or prognosis, the patient may search for another health professional in closer agreement with his definition and expectations. Furthermore, both physicians and patients may alter their definitions as the diagnosed deviation changes. Patients with chronic illnesses, for example, continually redefine normality as their perceptions of their illnesses, along with those of their physicians, change, e.g., persons who have strokes, heart attacks, or cancer.

Physicians base their diagnosis of deviations from normality on anatomical and clinical classifications, while patients describe health complaints, problems, and symptoms, not diseases, when they appear for medical help (Scarlett, 1962). If these "health problems" translate into established disease categories, the patient learns to view his situation as one of "disease" rather than a problem of "health." In essence, the patient is obliged to act in concert with the physician to reestablish a state or stage of "health," i.e., where his bodily structure and functioning will once again fall within established clinical "norms" for health. Because they are oriented toward looking for deviations from established clinical norms, physicians often have only a biological view of man's ailments based upon their clinical experience (Lafave et al., 1967). Our complex system of specialized medical care has also encouraged patients to translate their "health problems" into disease nosology, and accordingly, seek out those specialists who are experts in diagnosing deviations from normality with respect to a specific bodily part or organ system. Accordingly, our system of medical care has taught potential consumers to narrow their conceptions of "health" in order to obtain expeditious help when they experience deviations from their usual states of health. However, this encourages consumers to act on symptoms they can see or recognize as needing attention. Many of the early signs and symptoms of heart disease or cancer, for example, may be missed or dismissed by the layman. As chronic degenerative diseases have rapidly come to dominate the causes of death and disability, and as environment and life style play a larger role in influencing the health of individuals, the presence or absence of "health" can no longer be assessed solely on the basis of whether or not "health complaints" or "problems" fit an established clinical nosology of disease (Scarlett, 1962; Strauss, 1967; Wolff, 1962).

Normality as Balance

The principle that all organisms react to changing conditions in a manner that maintains a relatively constant "internal environment," as Claude Bernard (1927) called it, or a "steady state," a term which von Bertalanffy (1950) prefers, was introduced into physiology from chemistry by Claude Bernard (1927). It was most clearly and convincingly presented by Walter Cannon (1939) in his book, *The Wisdom of the Body*, in which he wrote, "the constant conditions which are maintained in the body might be termed *equilibria.*" That word, however, has come to have a fairly exact meaning as applied to relatively simple physiochemical states in closed systems where known forces are balanced. The coordinated physiological processes which maintain most of the steady states in the organism are very complex and peculiar to living beings, involving the brain, nerves, heart, lungs, kidneys, and spleen, all working cooperatively. Menninger (1963) referred to this state of balance as *homeostasis.*[1] The principle of homeostasis has been extended to higher levels of organismic behavior and emphasizes man's attempt to maintain a steady state outside, as well as inside his body. Menninger points out that a person has some vague sense of the unity and integrity of his personality. He *feels* rather than *knows* this to be a normal or ideal characteristic of his life. The awareness of an equilibrium is what Menninger calls "the vital balance" (Perkins, 1938). Scarlett (1962) sees the constant struggle of man to reach an equilibrium or balance as an unattainable goal, but, nonetheless, a lifelong process. Normality is also continually changing, modified as a consequence of man's relationships with his physical, social, psychological, and spiritual environments (see Fig. 4-1). The

---

[1]Clark (1969) has addressed the question, "What constitutes a healthy organization?" He notes that, since man is a social being, and business a group activity, the healthy organization must afford groups as well as individuals chances to fulfill their tendencies and capacities for equilibrium and growth. It must do this for small groups, for intergroup relationships and for the total organization. Clark defines the healthy organization as one in which its component parts—group and individual—somehow manage to achieve an optional resolution of their tendencies toward equilibrium (maintenance, homeostasis, or status quo) and their capacities for growth (elaboration, complication, differentiation, negative entropy).

hour glass in Figure 4-1 shows the dynamic nature of "what constitutes normality" and how man's various environments meld together to affect his unique normality.

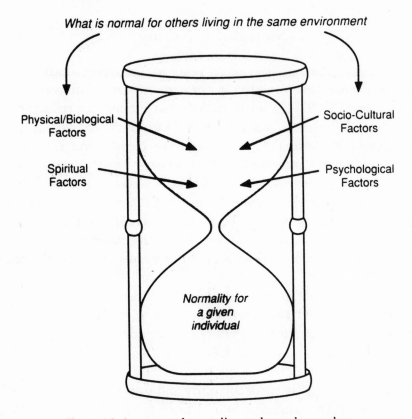

Figure 4-1. A concept of normality: an hour-glass analogy.

Perkins (1938) has attempted to define a normal, healthy person . . . "as one who can retain all of his organs and tissues in a state of efficient function and physical organization against those external and internal forces that are constantly tending to disturb him. Every function can be stressed beyond the limits of its accepted norm; when this is so, the altered function is called abnormal, and the evidence of it is pathology. In so doing, an arbitrary, indefinite line has been created between the two states, which is invariably called 'the borderline of disease,' 'the limits of safety,' the 'limit of tolerance,' or 'the normal limit,' each of which implies that the processes of change have been forced to some point that is intolerable or dangerous." Other definitions of health are provided in Table 4-1.

Table 4-1. Sample definitions of health

"Health is an activity of the living body in accordance with its specific excellences."
Leo Kass (1975)

"Mentally healthy individuals should be in touch with their own identity and their own feelings; they should be oriented toward the future and over time they should be fruitfully invested in life; their psyches should be integrated and provide them a resistance to stress; they should possess autonomy and recognize what suits their needs; they should perceive reality without distortion and yet possess empathy; they should be masters of their environment—able to work, to love, to play, and be efficient in problem-solving."
Marie Jahoda (1959)

"The condition of being sound in body, mind, and spirit."
Webster (1988)

"Health consists in the capacity of the organism to maintain a balance in which it may be reasonably free of undue pain, discomfort, disability, or limitation of action including social incapacity."
John Romano (1950)

"High level wellness for the individual is defined as an integrated method of functioning which is oriented toward maximizing the potential of which the individual is capable. It requires that the individual maintain a continuum of balance and purposeful direction within the environment where he is functioning."
Halbert L. Dunn (1961)

Using the rubber band as an analogy helps to illustrate the unique, changeable nature of normality. If one stretches a rubber band between two fingers, one can vary its degree of expansion. If one does not stretch the rubber band at all, it will lie limp on one's fingers. If one stretches the rubber band too far, it will snap or break. The degree of stretchability between these two extremes is analogous to a person's continual stretching to adapt to life. All of us reach a comfortable degree of stretchability on a day-to-day basis until a crisis arises to test us, or we feel unchallenged and lie limp waiting for an opportunity to emerge. Just as each rubber band has its unique character and durability, normality for each individual is different.

What is the "normal" person like? If "normal" is taken to mean "ideal" or "perfectly adjusted," no one meets the criteria for a "normal person." On the other hand, if "normal" is taken to mean "typical," information which permits an answer, is available. The first scientific study ever

directed to the psychological study of "normal" adults was begun in 1952
by Robert Havighurst, who studied the lives of a representative cross-
section of middle-aged men and women in Kansas City. Robert Peck
reported the results of this four-year study to answer the question, "What
is a normal person?" (Peck, 1959). The researchers found the joy of the
utter mastery of life to be rare. For most people, life meant settling for a
good deal less than they wanted, yet, for the average American, life was
not really a matter for despair. There were no completely happy people
in the study. There was no one whose life was without frustration or
sorrow. Most people lived through their daily hassles and catastrophes.
Peck says that to be normal, "is to be unreasonable with one's spouse, or
children, several times a week, yet try in a fumbling, half inept, but
sincere way to make it up. It is to spend money foolishly, then work hard
to stretch what is left until pay day. It is to work all your life wishing you
had gone into another job or career, yet proud of your 25 years of
service. . . . It is to marry in haste, divorce in haste, and marry five years
later to a person you love all the rest of your life. This is what it means to
be a typical, normal American."

According to Kubie (1954), the essential difference between what is
neurotic and what is normal is a fine line that can be expressed only in
relation to single behavioral events. Hacker (1945) proposes a reformulation
of the concept of normality. He proposes, "since the total personality and
not only one of its aspects is treated, integration of the personality is the
yardstick of normality. Integration is biologically and culturally determined and is to be understood in terms of the individual patient. This
inherent quality of the patient-doctor relationship should be consciously
realized by the physician and treatment methods should be formulated
in every case according to the basic set of values expressed by the concept
of normality in terms of the individual personality and its integration."

Normality and Change

We talk about "normal aging" and "normal adolescence," acknowledging that recognizable changes accompany the process of human growth
and development. There are different criteria for judging normality at
different phases or stages of human development. Each person is a
unique homeostatic organism. Many different factors influence what is
considered normal at different phases of the life cycle. Just as there is a

natural range of variability for our organs and tissues as they age, there is a natural range of variability for persons as they adapt to temporal variations in the life cycle. For example, premature infants are labeled "high risks," but 80 percent will be developmentally normal at three to five years of age. Therefore, the pediatrician must be aware of the self-fulfilling prophecy that if the baby is premature, the child will be abnormal. Repeated evaluations of the child for minor deviations from what is considered normal need to be avoided in order for the family to establish normal relationships (Glick, Clarkin & Kessler, 1987).

As Twaddle (1979) points out, another dimension of health is the capacity of individuals to perform roles and tasks. These may change as one ages. Health has different values and priorities in various socio-economic, ethnic, and cultural groups that may change as one progresses along the life cycle. Education, marriage, and changes in occupation or residence all can have an impact on health as a value and its priority among competing values. To prevent misjudgments of normality, we need to know more about normality at various points in the life cycle.

Heath (1983) has proposed a model to yield information about what defines the effective adult and the determinants of effectiveness that social institutions may be able to affect. He proposes the need to study the maturation of a person's cognitive skills, self-concept, values, and interpersonal relationships along five dimensions: allocentricism (allocentric growth is the humanizing, socializing influence others have in furthering our development); integration or internal consistency; stability; and autonomy. Heath believes that this model will help identify the skills, values, and interpersonal traits that are the core qualities that facilitate adaptation. Walsh and Shapiro (1983), on the other hand, believe that we need to study healthy people to learn what they are like, and how and why they got that way. Such a study would need to start with an agreement among investigators about a definition of health.

Finkel (1976), pursuing the ideas of Hollister (1967), investigated whether certain experiences strengthen the personality and contribute to the psychological growth of an individual. Hollister (1967) recounted that Margaret Mead pointed out a lack in the English language of an antonym for the word *trauma* — a word that would describe an experience that strengthens the personality. Therefore, he coined the term "stren." The 1950 White House Conference on education and curriculum took the position that "a healthy personality integration" was the goal of the American school, and that intellectual and vocational tasks were secondary to the program of producing an "integrated mature person." But how would such a goal be put into action? Finkel (1974, 1975) found that stren and trauma producing events were numerous and varied and tied closely to the age group being studied, in his case, college students. Finkel raises the point that, "if our ego and coping skills are strengthened during childhood and adolescence, we would expect fewer traumas later." Adulthood brings greater responsibilities, decisions, and events that we consider potentially stressful (marriage, divorce, childbirth, job loss, geographical moves). If the stresses multiply, so does the likelihood for more trauma. One noted commonality of stren events is their unexpected and unplanned nature (e.g., praise by a teacher), making it difficult to program strens into the school curriculum.

When project TALENT was conceived and organized in the late 1950s, it was designed as a long-range research project to determine the best methods for the identification, development, and utilization of human talents (Flanagan et al., 1962; Abeles, Steel & Wise, 1980). In 1960, a probability sample of about 5 percent of the public, private, and parochial high schools in the United States was drawn. The 400,000 students were administered tests and inventories. Follow-up studies were carried out for 1, 5, 10, and 20 years after each of the classes graduated from high school. The researchers had predicted that order, timing, and discontinuity would be important factors in influencing an individual's later occupational achievement. They predicted that those individuals who experienced role transitions in order of completion of school, start of first job, marriage, and childbirth would do better in their occupational achievements than individuals who did not follow this order. They also predicted that individuals who were "on time" would be more successful occupationally than those individuals who were "off time." Finally, the researchers expected individuals who had no educational and/or work discontinuities would have more job prestige and higher incomes than individuals with discontinuities. It is interesting that the order and timing of role transitions did not predict occupational achievement; however, job discontinuity was associated with lower job prestige and lower income. This study emphasizes that we have certain expectations about "normal" progression through life with respect to taking on certain social roles, completing certain tasks, and the relationship of this progression to later success. We believe and often reinforce for our children the importance of these "normal" progressions. The data from the TALENT study do not show that the strict patterning of educational, occupational, and familial careers leads to greater success as measured by prestige and income. However, there is some evidence that early career decisions can have far-reaching and perhaps irreversible consequences, both positive and negative.

One of the difficulties in expanding our knowledge of a normal person is that normality for each individual is continually changing as he/she grows and develops. Society's view of normality is also continually changing. Rather than attempt to search for the secrets of normality or health to apply these to others, it seems more useful to learn how individuals and families adapt to change. Moos and Tsu (1976) ask, "What is it that keeps people going?" Many theorists have ideas about what human fulfillment and growth is. Among the best known of these theorists are Carl Rogers and Abraham Maslow. Rogers (1961) hypothesizes that the core tendency of man is self-actualization. Each person attempts to actualize or develop all of his/her capacities in ways that serve to maintain and enhance life. Maslow (1954) postulates two underlying patterns of motivation: growth motivation and deficiency or deprivation motivation. Deficiency motivation aims to decrease tension arising from unfulfilled tissue needs, such as hunger and thirst. Growth motivation, on the other hand, reflects the tendency toward self-actualization and involves the urge to enrich our experience and to expand our horizons.

Growth and fulfillment theories have led to studies of normal, healthy people and their patterns of adaptation and coping. Maslow informally studied a number of outstanding historical figures whom he regarded as self-actualized, e.g., Abraham Lincoln, Albert Einstein, Jane Addams, Eleanor Roosevelt. Maslow noted several characteristics in the lives of these people that he felt facilitated their effective coping: an efficient perception of reality and comfortable relations with it, a problem-centered focus, and a broad view of life in the widest frame of reference. Maslow described these self-actualized people as spontaneous in their behavior, as having a strong social interest and a genuine desire to help others, having a small, intimate circle of friends, and being somewhat independent of their culture and environment.

Other investigators have addressed themselves to studying normal, mentally healthy people. An unusual opportunity for this kind of investigation was provided by the follow-up program of the Oakland Growth Study (Stewart, 1962). About 25 years ago, the subjects of the Oakland Growth Study were studied intensively for a period of seven years, beginning when they were in the sixth grade of school and continuing until they graduated from high school. The same subjects were studied at age 33 in order to obtain a series of follow-up records, as well as a thorough medical examination. In the course of this medical assessment, it was found that a number of the subjects had developed disorders of a probable psychosomatic nature. This finding provided the basis for an investigation in an attempt to define some factors of social and emotional adjustment in adolescence that may be associated with the subsequent development of psychosomatic disorders. Stewart reported that the results of this study supported the hypothesis that a basic depressive tendency is an important factor in the etiology of psychosomatic disorders.

Grinker (1962) studied a group of young male college students whom he labeled homoclites (people who were normal and healthy). He found that these students did reasonably well academically and were able to play well and with satisfaction. They were adequately adjusted to reality, and had a firm sense of identity, felt good, and had hope for the future. They had warm human relationships with parents, teachers, and friends, both male and female. Their aspirations were to be successful, to make some contribution, and to be liked. Grinker identified a cluster of conditions associated with this mentally healthy group, such as sound physical health, average intelligence, satisfactory relationships with both parents, parental agreement and cooperation in child rearing, definite and known limitations or boundaries placed on behavior, sound early religious training, early work history, action orientation, and so forth.

Vaillant (1974, 1975, 1977, 1978) studied 95 healthy men and followed them prospectively from age 18 until age 47. At age 47, independent raters, blind to the previous data on the men, rated the men's overall adjustment. Child environment had relatively little association with work history, ego mechanisms of defense, or psychosomatic illness. Sustained childhood stresses, but not isolated trauma, were associated with subsequent poor overall mental health. Fifty of the originally healthy men developed illness patterns sometimes called psychosomatic (ulcer, colitis, allergy, hypertension, musculoskeletal disorders). These men were compared with 45 similarly studied men who never developed such illnesses. The men who developed psychosomatic illnesses as children and adults had more physical illnesses of all kinds. They were less likely to indulge in vacations and athletics and more likely to use tranquilizers and excessive alcohol. Men with psychosomatic illnesses experienced a greater variety of somatic symptoms under stress. Twenty men who eventually developed serious irreversible physical illnesses had more psychopathology than the 45 who developed psychosomatic illnesses.

Kobasa (1985) examined how highly stressed people who remain healthy differ from those who show illness along with high stress. Her proposition was that persons who experience high degrees of stress without falling ill have a personality structure which differentiates them from persons who become sick under stress. This personality difference is called *hardiness*. From her study of 837 middle-aged adults, Kobasa gained insights into how hardy individuals evaluated stress and coped with it. She profiles a healthy, hardy, but stressed executive as follows: "The hardy executive will approach the necessary readjustments in his life with (a) a clear sense of his values, goals, and capabilities, and a belief in their importance and, (b) a strong tendency toward active involvement with his environment. Hence, the executive actively deals with the stress utilizing his inner resources. Another characteristic of the hardy executive is an unshakable sense of meaningfulness and ability to evaluate the impact of the stress in terms of a general life plan with established priorities. In contrast, the executive low in hardiness will react to the stress with less sense of personal resource, more acquiescence, more encroachments of meaninglessness, and a conviction that the stress has been externally determined with no possibility of control on his part."

Peterson and his colleagues (1988) followed 99 men, randomly chosen from a sample of 268 who participated in the Study of Adult Development, which began with mentally and physically healthy and successful members of the classes of 1942 through 1944 at Harvard University. They found that men who explained events with stable, global, or internal causes at age 25 were less healthy later in life than men who made unstable, specific and external explanations. Men who were more pessimistic tended to be at greater risk for poor health in middle and late adulthood. The investigators speculate that the pessimists were poor problem solvers and therefore accumulated more unsolved crises. Furthermore, persons who are negative tend to be more socially withdrawn and lack social resources.

There have been many studies of normal adolescent development, of the development of maturity in college students, and of outstanding individuals, such as the first astronauts and Peace Corps volunteers. These studies focused on how these individuals coped with their life situations and handled specific, relatively stressful experiences. Interest in studying normal healthy individuals and their adaptation and coping patterns has given rise to a multitude of psychological assessment techniques, such as self esteem, ego identity, novelty needs, self-actualization, stimulus-seeking motivation, self efficacy and competence. The complexity of the interaction between normality, health, coping, and the process of growth and development can be illustrated by using the slide rule as an analogy, showing homeostasis as a continually changing situation for each individual (see Fig. 4-2).

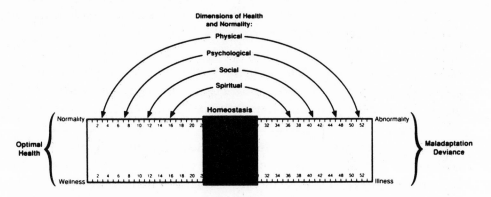

Figure 4-2. Relationship between health and normality continua and their dimensions.

Normality, Intervention, and Rehabilitation

Health professionals make judgments about normality so that they can classify, label, and intervene to return individuals and families to normality (Leifer, 1969). Rehabilitation is a facilitative process, enabling a person with a handicap to attain usefulness and satisfaction in life. The individual's handicap may result from any type of disability, i.e., physical, mental, or emotional, and from various causes, e.g., birth defects, sickness and disease, accidents, or stress. People are handicapped by cultural disadvantages, social, financial, or educational, whenever these conditions cause difficulties in life adjustment. Rehabilitation then equalizes opportunity for life attainment as a human right and societal obligation (Wright, 1980).

Comprehensive rehabilitation is a multifaceted effort. It involves evaluation of a patient's functioning, and often long-term treatment, in areas such as mobility, self-care, communication, personal and family adjustment, sexuality, vocational and avocational planning, and social integration. Specific goals in each of these areas are shaped by the needs expressed by the patient as well as by suggestions from rehabilitation specialists. Although the focus of rehabilitation is primarily on the patient, the family and extended social network also must be considered. In a family, for example, disability suffered by one person typically demands that other family members accommodate to the new circumstances and cope with the loved one's misfortune. The family's positive adjustment becomes a goal during rehabilitation, both as a worthy aim and because it can enhance the patient's progress (Greif & Matarazzo, 1982).

The "normalization principle" was formulated by Scandinavian workers in mental retardation (Wolfensberger, 1970). Reduced to its essentials, the principle states that human management practices should enable a "deviant" person to function within the acceptable norms of his/her society. Similarly, human management practices should enable a person who is not "deviant" to continue to function within the acceptable norms of his/her society. The following specifics of human management are stressed: the goal is not to impose social conformity, but to prevent or reverse involuntary or unconscious "deviancy"; by using culturally normative means, the appearance of separateness of deviant persons is minimized; and the attitudes and values of society should be shaped to be more accepting and tolerant of harmless differences, such as differences in appearance, speech, language, nationality, education, race, and dress.

Normalization means that "deviant" persons should be exposed to experiences that are likely to elicit or maintain accepted behavior. These experiences can be derived from physical activities and social interaction so that both the physical and social environments are reinforcing. Since exposure to normative experiences is a crucial aspect of normalization, every effort should be made to avoid conditions that are apt to inhibit or prohibit normal behavior. It is essential that associations and experiences be age-specific. Normalization means that a person should live a normal routine of life and that a person should be independent and empowered to make choices. Normalization suggests action on three levels: clinical, public, and societal.

Leigh and Reiser (1985) suggest that the approach to a person who is "sick," "abnormal," or in need of help should be three dimensional. In repairing an automobile, the mechanic must know the state of all of the component parts, the way the car functions as a whole, and the interaction of the car with other factors, e.g., how the owner maintains it. In approaching clients or patients, a similar conceptual approach, which includes organizing data according to three dimensions, is useful: (1) the biological dimension, the structure and function of the components including both healthy and diseased or abnormal parts; (2) the personal dimension, the behavior or functioning of the whole person; and (3) the environmental dimension, the interaction of the person with the physical environment, including work, family, and leisure activities. These three dimensions can be seen as a system with interaction between and within each level. Leigh and Reiser utilize this scheme in formulating a Patient Evaluation Grid (PEG) to assist in evaluating a patient. The three dimensions (biological, personal, and environmental) are matrixed with three longitudinal time contexts (current, recent, and background). This nine compartment grid is useful in taking a complete history, performing an examination of the patient, and planning special procedures. The PEG will show the precipitating and contributing factors to the person's condition or situation and, in most situations, will identify the strains in the biological, personal, and environmental systems. In many cases, the etiologic, precipitating, and influencing factors in the illness or condition will become clear. Rational care plans for the whole patient will emerge and be three dimensional.

The ultimate premise of the rehabilitation philosophy is an all-encompassing concern for the person to be rehabilitated. The rehabilitation process is individualized. Each person is unique in skills, limitations, resources, and desires, and the manifestations of sickness and disability have varying meanings and implications. Successful rehabilitation must identify the unmet needs of a particular client and plan a treatment program that satisfies the unique patterns of that person's needs and desires. The individual's conception of what is normal for him/her must be meshed with the therapist's conception of a possible level of normality given the person's condition, characteristics, such as age, and his/her life circumstances. A major dimension in which persons with disabilities may differ from each other is that of age group. The most immediate effect of a disabling condition is the obstruction of activities normal for a particular life stage. A further consequence of the disrupting influence on development is the failure to acquire essential qualities required for a healthy and complete ego. A developmental approach to restoration of health and normality suggests that interventions be based upon capacities that the individual might reasonably be expected to possess at his/her life stage, and that treatment demands that call for more mature capacities be avoided (Eisenberg, Sutkin, & Jansen, 1984).

Variations in the Restoration of Normality

Illness as a biological state involves changes in bone, tissues, fluids, etc. Illness as a social state involves changes in behavior. When a health professional diagnoses a human condition as illness, that person's behavior is changed by the diagnosis. Being sick is a form of deviance in that it separates a person from the well, exempts the person from normal obligations, and places the control for restoring the person to health in the hands of health professionals, specifically the physician. The proper management of deviance is "treatment" in the hands of a responsible and skilled professional.

Both the patient and health professional organize the social state of being sick, i.e., whether or not one is "really" ill and can or must adopt a sick role; whether or not one may assume a new, special social identity; whether or not one must be worked on by others; and whether or not one can ever again assume a normal identity and social status. Thus, a health professional treats a biological organism, and also organizes the social identity of the person into being a patient. In applying their knowledge, health professionals cannot avoid making social as well as medical decisions about the people they deal with (Freidson, 1970).

Health professionals also make value judgments about the potential of a person's return to normality. Their judgments are based on the clinical experience of the physician and other health professionals with the abnormality or illness and the unique personality and life situation of each patient. The judgments are also affected by the expectations of the patient and family regarding the extent of the patient's recovery, as well as the realities of the illness (Fig. 4-3). Mutual agreement between the health professional, the family, and the patient about when the patient will return "to his/her normal self" is relatively straightforward in the case of acute illness and minor accidents. The disparities between expectations and realities regarding the return to normality are greatest for chronic illness and major accidents. There are many social and biological intervening factors that influence prognosis in chronic illness, such as the patient's current physical condition and stamina, the patient's degree of hopefulness and motivation to get well, the degree of social and family support, the extent of physical and/or mental impairment or limitation, and the availability and accessibility of occupational, physical, speech, and other rehabilitation therapists.

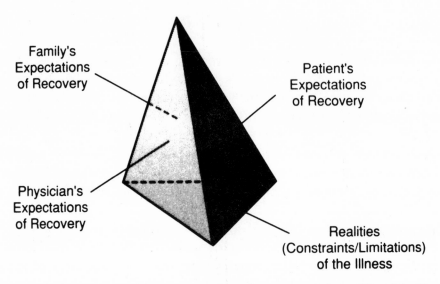

Figure 4-3. Interrelationships between expectations of recovery and the realities of the illness.

Our personal experiences tell us that illness is a potent agent of change. Chronic illness, especially, disrupts the usual ways in which family members behave toward one another and hampers their ability to overcome the effects of this disruption. The effects of chronic illness on families are more often disintegrative than integrative; indeed, they change the attitudes and behavior of both sick and well family members, as individuals and as members of a family unit. Tasks and responsibilities must often be reassigned and this creates a period of disequilibrium. The duration and outcome of family disequilibrium is influenced by the clinical manifestations and management of the illness as well as by how well the family adapts to the changes created by the illness (Bruhn, 1977).

Chronic Illness and Role Change

Short-term changes in the role structure and task allocation in families as a result of illness are similar to the permanent or long-term changes caused by loss of one parent (Roghmann, Hecht & Haggerty, 1973).

When duties and responsibilities are taken away from one family member and assumed by another, often one will feel a sense of loss and the other will feel burdened. Role change and task reallocation is, perhaps, easier to accept in short-term illness. In chronic illness, the ill person and other family members assume or hope, at first, that role change will be temporary. Indeed, if the clinical course of the illness stabilizes, or there is improvement, the ill person may regain some of his former family functions. If the clinical course of the illness declines, however, and duties and responsibilities must be removed from the ill person rather abruptly, he/she may feel a sense of personal loss. The patient, especially one with a long-term illness, is sensitive to his dependence upon others and, if his former duties and responsibilities within the family are completely removed, will feel unneeded. Roles must be changed and reallocated in ways which minimize a sense of personal loss and prevent the ill person's social and psychological withdrawal from the family. We are familiar with chronically ill persons who "gave up" living and became resigned to their illnesses and with ill persons who attempted to overcome the effects of their illness with determination, hope, and a "will to live." Members of the latter group usually retain a role within the family and feel wanted and needed.

It is possible for a person disabled by illness to achieve secondary gains for himself as well as to behave in a manner that will increase gains for others. It has been found, for example, that when some husbands lose their capacity to earn a livelihood, they attempt to compensate for this inadequacy by becoming more considerate of their wives, helping around the house, and changing their usual role behaviors in the family (Komarovsky, 1940). It may be that the value the person places on his various life activities helps to determine how disability in one role affects his performance in others. If the disability occurs in a role which is only one of several that are important and satisfying to the person, disability will be less destructive to his identity than if there are no role options.

In the clinical management of chronic illness, it is important to recognize that a sick member may become sicker in response to role changes in the family and "well" members may become "sick" to call attention to themselves or to the need to reallocate tasks, especially if they feel overshadowed or overburdened by the ill family member.

Role Expectations and Adjustment to Chronic Illness

The rate of breakdown in families with severe chronic disease is high. It has been shown that the combined effects of poor health and unfavorable family situations are cumulative over time (Pless, Roghmann & Haggerty, 1972). Diabetes mellitus, hemophilia, and epilepsy are examples of chronic illnesses with high rates of family breakdown. Family breakdown, in these instances, often results because family members would not or could not change roles and reallocate tasks.

What others expect of the ill person will influence how he adjusts to illness as well as the degree of success in the clinical management of the illness. The physician also has expectations of the ill person regarding motivation, compliance with clinical regimen, and cooperation in controlling the illness. The ill person must sometimes balance the expectations of family members with those of the physician. It is important that the physician, the family, and the patient discuss expectations jointly so that all will arrive at realistic expectations regarding adjustment.

Implications for Health Professionals

Doctor-patient and doctor-family relationships are critical ones for chronically ill patients. For some chronic illnesses, such as cancer, there is little patients can do to alter the disease once treatment has begun. For other chronic illnesses, such as diabetes, patients can control their disease through diet and medication. Whatever the degree of individual control over the illness, the physician is seen as a symbol of hope by the chronically ill person. The key to coping with chronic illness is having and maintaining hope. Although the patient and his family have to cope somehow with changes in life style and roles, few people can make these adjustments without periods of discouragement, anxiety, and resentment. The physician is in a key position to enhance the changes for successful clinical and psychosocial adjustment to chronic illness by using his knowledge of the family and its dynamics to create strong family support for the ill person. Physicians, like their patients, are not immune to feelings of discouragement in treating chronic disease. Many physicians prefer not to tell their patients and families the truth about the clinical course of a chronic illness. Direct two-way communication between the physician and the family is essential because it builds confidence and rapport. This is often the most effective treatment available for chronic illness.

In Retrospect

Each of us makes judgments about other people's behavior every day. These judgments help us to classify people into those we like and those we don't like. Our judgments affect how we behave toward others. It is not a personal fault to make value judgments as long as we are aware that our values affect the ways in which we treat others. Health professionals are bound by professional ethics to acknowledge health care as a right and to provide care to those who seek it. Value judgments come into play at the first encounter between a client and a health professional. How we "size up" potential patients influences how we behave toward them and, many times, influences the quality of care provided.

Value judgments are involved in determining whether someone is sick or well, normal or abnormal. There are societal guidelines for "normal" behavior, such as wearing clothes in public. There are specific places, such as beaches, where people can wear little or no clothing and be considered within normal bounds; there are individuals who may test the limits of these rules by wearing few clothes in other public places. Despite general societal guidelines, we make judgments about what we consider proper attire and what is prudent behavior, which may be more or less strict than the societal guidelines. A similar process of assessment is used by health professionals. Assessments lead us to prioritize individuals according to who needs emergency attention, who is sick but is not in a life-threatening situation, who is a malingerer, and who needs preventive care. We expect patients to cooperate in the treatment process so that they can return to a state of health and assume their normal roles. Health professionals, the family, and the patient all have expectations about the extent of the patient's recovery. These expectations also reflect personal values. Acceptance of the abnormality or illness by the patient and his/her family will influence the process of rehabilitation and habilitation. Health professionals are often in the position of helping the family and patient adjust their expectations of recovery according to the realities of the illness or accident.

We often hear the phrase, "I'm back to normal," following an illness, yet we never return to the same state of normality we experienced before an illness; we are continuously changing. We return to a "feeling state of normality," which is comfortable for us. Health professionals need to know their patients well enough to know what being normal means to them.

Like most other general concepts—"peace," and "freedom," "normality," and "health" pose enormous difficulties of definition. We all know what it means to be sick, yet we all do not know what it means to be healthy. People can learn to adapt to illness, and do so in different ways. Most people have a rough idea of what it means to be sick. However, the idea of being in "good health" is bland and rarely noticed. We take our individual health for granted. It is something we assume is present unless our daily routines are disrupted by uncomfortable feelings or unusual symptoms. Knowles (1977) has stated, "Most individuals do not worry about their health until they lose it." Prevention of disease means forsaking the bad habits many people enjoy. The idea of individual responsibility for one's health conflicts with the principles of individual freedom, yet the majority of chronic illness in developed countries can be directly traced to individual behaviors and lifestyles.

Health professionals must be teachers of preventive medicine to their clients, sick and well. As individuals and as a society, we need to give substance to the concept of health. Health is more than something that we need to maintain or regain. Health can be promoted and enhanced on a personal level. Individuals have the power and moral responsibility to do more than keep their health; they can enhance it. Health professionals have a responsibility to help make the concept of "health" more than an abstraction by actively teaching and modeling the principles and ethics of "good health."

REFERENCES

Abeles, R.P., Steel, L., & Wise, L.L. (1980). Patterns and implications of life-course organization: Studies from Project TALENT. In P.B. Baltes & O.G. Brim, Jr. (Eds.), *Life-span development and behavior, Vol. 3.* (pp. 307–337). New York: Academic Press.

Bateson, G. (1979). *Mind and nature: A necessary unity.* New York: Dutton.

Bernard, C. (1927). *An introduction to the study of experimental Medicine.* New York: Macmillan.

Bertalanffy, L. von. (1950). An outline of general systems theory. *British Journal of Philosophy of Science, 1,* 134–163.

Bruhn, J.G. (1977). Effects of chronic illness on the family. *The Journal of Family Practice, 4,* 1057–1060.

Bursten, B. & D'Esopo, R. (1965). The obligation to remain sick. *Archives of General Psychiatry, 12,* 402–407.

Cannon, W.B. (1939). *The wisdom of the body.* New York: Norton.

Cantor, N. (1941). What is a normal mind? *American Journal of Orthopsychiatry, 11,* 676–683.

Carstairs, G.M. (1959). The social limits of eccentricity: an English study. In M.K. Opler (Ed.), *Culture and mental health.* New York: Macmillan.

Clark, J.V. (1969). A healthy organization. In W.G. Bennis, K.O. Benne & R. Chin (Eds.), *The planning of change.* New York: Holt, Rinehart & Winston.

Dunn, H.L. (1961). *High level wellness.* (pp. 4–5). Thorofare, New Jersey: Charles Slack.

Eaton, J.W. (1951). The assessment of mental health. *American Journal of Psychiatry, 108,* 81–90.

Eisenberg, M.G., Sutkin, L.C. & Jansen, M.A. (Eds.). (1984). *Chronic illness and disability through the life span: Effects on self and family.* New York: Springer.

Engel, G.L. (1960). A unified concept of health and disease. *Perspectives in Biology and Medicine, 3,* 459–485.

Fabrega, H. (1972). Concepts of disease: Logical features and social implications. *Perspectives in Biology and Medicine, 15,* 583–616.

Finkel, N.J. (1974). Stress and traumas: An attempt at categorization. *American Journal of Community Psychology, 2,* 265–273.

Finkel, N.J. (1975). Stress, traumas, and trauma resolution. *American Journal of Community Psychology, 3,* 173–178.

Finkel, N.J. (1976). *Mental illness and health.* New York: Macmillan.

Flanagan, J.C., Dailey, J.T., Shaycoft, M.F., Gorham, W.A., Orr, D.B., & Goldberg, I. (1962). *Design for a study of American youth.* Boston: Houghton Mifflin.

Freidson, E. (1970). *Profession of medicine.* New York: Dodd, Mead & Co.

Glick, I.D., Clarkin, J.F., & Kessler, D.R. (1987). *Marital and family therapy.* 3rd edition. New York: Grune & Stratton.

Glover, E. (1932). Medico-psychological aspects of normality. *British Journal of Psychiatry, 23,* 152–166.

Greif, E. & Matarazzo, R.G. (1982). *Behavioral approaches to rehabilitation: Coping with change.* Boston: Springer.

Grinker, R.R. (1962). "Mentally healthy" young males (homoclites): A study. *Archives of General Psychology, 6,* 405–453.

Grinker, R.R. (1967). Normality viewed as a system. *Archives of General Psychiatry, 17,* 320–324.

Hacker, F.J. (1945). The concept of normality and its practical significance. *American Journal of Orthopsychiatry, 15,* 47–64.

Heath, D. (1983). The maturing person. In R. Walsh & D.H. Shapiro, Jr. (Eds.), *Beyond health and normality: Explorations of exceptional psychological well-being* (pp. 152–214). New York: Van Nostrand Reinhold.

Hollister, W.G. (1967). The concept of stress in education: A challenge to curriculum development. In E.M. Bower & W.G. Hollister (Eds.), *Behavioral science frontiers in education* (pp. 193–205). New York: Wiley.

Jahoda, M. (1959). *Current concepts of positive mental health.* New York: Basic Books.

Kass, L.R. (1975). The meaning of the measurement of ego development. *The Public Interest, 40,* 11–42, 28.

King, C.D. (1945). The meaning of normal. *Yale Journal of Biology and Medicine, 17,* 493–501.

King, L. (1954). What is disease? *Philosophy of Science, 21,* 193–203.

Knowles, J.H. (Ed.) (1977). *Doing better and feeling worse: Health in the United States.* New York: W.W. Norton.

Kobasa, S.C. (1985). Stressful life events, personality, and health: An inquiry into hardiness. In A. Monat & R.S. Lazarus (Eds.), *Stress and coping: An anthology,* 2nd ed. New York: Columbia University Press.

Komarovsky, M. (1940). *The unemployed man and his family.* New York: Dryden.

Kubie, L.S. (1954). The fundamental nature of the distinction between normality and neurosis. *Psychoanalytic Quarterly, 23,* 167–204.

Lafave, H.G., Rootman, I., Sydiaha, D., & Duckworth, R. (1967). The ethnic community and the definition of mental illness. *Psychiatric Quarterly, 41,* 211–227.

Leifer, R. (1969). *In the name of mental health.* New York: Science House.

Leigh, H. & Reiser, M.F. (1985). *The patient: Biological, psychological, and social dimensions of medical practice,* 2nd ed. New York: Plenum.

Lewis, A. (1953). Health as a social concept. *British Journal of Sociology, 4,* 109–124.

Maslow, A. (1954). *Motivation and personality.* New York: Harper.

Mechanic, D. (1962). Some factors in identifying and defining mental illness. *Mental Hygiene, 46,* 66–74.

Menninger, D. (1963). *The vital balance.* New York: Viking.

Moos, R.H. & Tsu, V.D. (1976). Human competence and coping. In R.H. Moos (Ed.), *Human adaptation: Coping with life crises.* Lexington, MA: D.C. Heath.

Opler, M.K. (1963). The need for new diagnostic categories in psychiatry. *Journal of the National Medical Association, 55,* 133–137.

Peck, R.F. (1959). Measuring the mental health of normal adults. *Genetic Psychology Monographs, 60,* 197–255.

Perkins, W.H. (1938). *Cause and prevention of disease.* Philadelphia: Lea and Febiger.

Peterson, C., Seligman, M.E.P. & Vaillant, G.E. (1988). Pessimistic explanatory style is a risk factor for physical illness: A thirty-five-year longitudinal study. *Journal of Personality and Social Psychology, 55,* 23–27.

Pless, I.B., Roghmann, K.J. & Haggerty, R.J. (1972). Chronic illness, family functioning and psychological adjustment: A model for the allocation of preventive mental health services. *International Journal of Epidemiology, 1,* 271–277.

Rakoff, V.M., Stancer, H.C. & Kedward, H.B. (Eds.). (1977). *Psychiatric diagnosis.* New York: Brunner/Mazel.

Redlich, F.C. (1952). The concept of normality. *American Journal of Psychotherapy, 6,* 551–576.

Reider, N. (1950). The concept of normality. *Psychiatric Quarterly, 19,* 43–51.

Rogers, C. (1961). *On becoming a person.* Boston: Houghton Mifflin.

Roghmann, K.J., Hecht, P.K. & Haggerty, R.J. (1973). Family coping with everyday illness: Self reports from a household survey. *Journal of Comparative Family Studies, 4,* 49–62.

Romano, J. (1950). Basic orientation and education of the medical student. *Journal of the American Medical Association, 143* (June 3), p. 411.

Rosenhan, D.L. (1973). On being sane in insane places. *Science, 179,* 250–258.

Ryle, J.A. (1947). The meaning of normal. *Lancet,* 1, 1–5.

Sabshin, M. (1967). Psychiatric perspectives on normality. *Archives of General Psychiatry, 17,* 258–264.

Scarlett, E.P. (1962). What is health? *New Physician, 11,* 28–29.

Smith, M.B. (1950). Optima of mental health: A general frame of reference. *Psychiatry, 13,* 503–510.

Somers, A.R. (1972). Who's in charge here—Alice searches for a king in Mediland. *New England Journal of Medicine, 287* (October), 849–855.

Stewart, L.H. (1962). Social and emotional adjustment during adolescence as related to the development of psychosomatic illness in adulthood. *Genetic Psychology Monographs, 65,* 175–215.

Strauss, A.L. (1967). A sociological view of normality. *Archives of General Psychiatry, 17,* 265–270.

Twaddle, A.C. (1979). The concept of health status. In E.G. Jaco (Ed.) *Patients, physicians and illness.* New York: Free Press.

Vaillant, G.E. (1974). Natural history of male psychological health. II: Some antecedents of healthy adult adjustment. *Archives of General Psychiatry, 31,* 15–22.

Vaillant, G.E. (1975). Natural history of male psychological health. III: Empirical dimensions of mental health. *Archives of General Psychiatry, 32,* 420–426.

Vaillant, G.E. (1977). *Adaptation to life.* Boston: Little, Brown.

Vaillant, G.E. (1978). Natural history of male psychological health. IV: What kinds of men do not get psychosomatic illness. *Psychosomatic Medicine, 40,* 420–431.

Walsh, R. & Shapiro, D.H., Jr. (1983). In search of a healthy person. In R. Walsh & D.H. Shapiro, Jr., (Eds.), *Beyond health and normality: Explorations of exceptional psychological well-being* (pp. 3–12). New York: Van Nostrand Reinhold.

Webster's ninth new collegiate dictionary. (1988). (p. 558). Springfield, Massachusetts: Merrian-Webster, Inc.

Wegrocki, H.J. (1939). A critique of cultural and statistical concepts of abnormality. *Journal of Abnormal and Social Psychology, 34,* 166–178.

Wolfensberger, W. (1970). The principle of normalization and its implications to psychiatric services. *American Journal of Psychiatry, 127,* 291–297.

Wolff, H.G. (1962). A concept of disease in man. *Psychosomatic Medicine, 24,* 25–30.

Wright, G.N. (1980). *Total rehabilitation.* Boston: Little, Brown.

Wynder, E.L. & Hill, P. (1972). Blood lipids: How normal is normal? *Preventive Medicine, 1,* 161–166.

Zusman, J. (1966). Sociology and mental illness. *Archives of General Psychiatry, 15,* 635–648.

SUGGESTED READINGS

Ahmed, P.J. & Coelho, G.V. (1979). *Toward a new definition of health: Psychosocial dimensions.* New York: Plenum.

Duhl, J. (1986). *Health planning and social change.* New York: Human Sciences Press.

Erde, E.L. (1979). Philosophical considerations regarding defining "health", "disease", etc., and their bearing on medical practice. *Ethics in Science and Medicine, 6,* 31–48.

Fabrega, H. (1974). *Disease and social behavior: An interdisciplinary perspective.* Cambridge, MA: MIT Press.

Fromm, E. (1955). *The sane society.* New York: Holt, Rinehart and Winston.

Jourard, S.M. (1974). *Healthy personality.* New York: Macmillan.

Mercer, J.R. (1972). Who is normal? Two perspectives on mild mental retardation. In E.G. Jaco (Ed.), *Patients, physicians, and illness,* 2nd ed., pp. 56–75. New York: Free Press.

Offer, D. & Sabshin, M. (1966). *Normality: Theoretical and clinical concepts of mental health.* New York: Basic Books.

Offer, D. & Sabshin, M. (1984). *Normality and the life cycle: A critical integration.* New York: Basic Books.

Sontag, S. (1977). *Illness as a metaphor.* New York: Farrar, Straus and Giroux.

Szasz, T.S. (1961). *The myth of mental illness.* New York: Haeber-Harper.

Wood, G. (1983). *The myth of neurosis: Overcoming the illness excuse.* New York: Harper and Row.

Chapter 5

HEALTH VALUES AND RELIGIOUS BELIEFS

Science without religion is lame, religion without science is blind.

Albert Einstein, 1955

The disparate and collective efforts of human beings to understand their existence is a classical study in frustration. This frustration notwithstanding, human beings have tried continually to understand their present by extracting significance from their past, and even by imposing upon their present a social order which is shaped by their expectation of the future. Stated another way, most of us are puzzled by the cyclic patterns of the seasons, the unerring polarities of days and nights, the conflict between reason and emotion, the glorious process of birth, and the inevitable call of death. Indeed, we are in awe when we consider the idea of infinite movement and our smallness in comparison to the magnitude of the universe. In short, human life seems to have a complexity beyond our powers of comprehension. The human race has always been concerned with the need for structuring universal reality, not only temporarily, but ultimately. In this regard, perhaps the oldest area of human activity is religion.

No other pursuit reveals more of the paradoxical nature of the human make-up than religion, which is a concern for the ultimate value of life and how to attain it, preserve it, and enjoy it (Bahm, 1964). Despite differences of opinion regarding our ultimate value, and despite elaborate and conflicting schemes for determining and systematizing values, this problem is fundamental to health care. Historically, religion is one of the foremost institutions humans have turned to in attempting to work out the meaning of illness and health. For countless persons, religion offers a philosophic border that gives at least a semblance of order to their lives. Indeed, religions offer perhaps our most comprehensive beliefs about the basic nature of human beings—beliefs that have significantly affected theories and practices of medical care. This has been borne out in numerous studies of the religious-medical practices of

127

primitive and modern peoples. The word "primitive" is used here in the sense of "lineally ancestral," not with the negative or culturally prejudiced connotations it has acquired over the years.

Toward a Definition

A highly potent force in much of human life, "religion" has no global consensual definition; it varies vastly according to the social experiences, moral consciousness, and vocations of the definers (Chance, 1988). Freud (1950), for example, defined religion as a need-driven quest for security and reassurance. He stated that the God of each of us is formed in the likeness of our human father. In contrast, Whitehead (1926) defined religion as that which people do with their solitude; and Fromm (1963) said that in order to have a religion, people must be independent and free—they must be an end unto themselves, and not the means for any other person's purpose. Also from Fromm's perspective, our ability to love productively and without greed, to engage neither in submission nor domination, and to love with the fullness of our personality is a reflection of God's love that expresses itself out of strength, not weakness. Tillich (1963) proposed that religion is a state of "being," with our ultimate concern for the meaning of life. Thus, to Tillich, God is the absolute religious receptacle for the content of life.

In the concepts of thanatology and existential philosophy, confrontation with our own mortality can lead us to more authentic life styles that quicken our spiritual sensitivities and precipitate an understanding of our humanity (Acklin et al., 1983). Traditional American religionists cite the belief in God, the teachings of the Bible, acceptance of the preexistence and immortality of the soul, and involvement within a church community as characteristics of a religious person. Scholars who study mainstream religious denominations define religion (1) *vertically* as faith in God, fear of God, devotion to God and observance of the laws of God, and (2) *horizontally* as a sense of our humanity and of loving our neighbors as ourselves. Inherent in both the horizontal and vertical relationships are overwhelming implications of "thou shalt not."

St. Thomas Aquinas (1947), greatly influenced by the thinking of Aristotle, described God as pure form. We infer His existence from the facts of creation—everything that moves must have a mover; there is movement in the universe, and the ultimate source of this movement is an Unmoved Mover, or God. In 1874, Mill (1885), the great utilitarian philosopher, appealed to the human heart when he stated that religion and poetry address themselves, at least in one of their aspects, to the same part of the human constitution: They both supply the same want, that of an ideal life grander and more beautiful than we see in the prose of human life.

As there is a disparity in what constitutes religion, so too is there a wide variety of beliefs in what constitutes "health." In 1864, Bentham (1879) defined health as the absence of disease and of pain, which is the symptom of disease. He proposed that we are healthy when we are not conscious of any uneasy sensations in the body. Mary Baker Eddy (1915), the founder of Christian Science, defined health as a condition of the mind, not matter. Thoreau (1920) said we should measure our health by our sympathy with the morning and the spring. Others have described health as a sound mind in a sound body, as equilibrium of the physical elements of the body, as the absence of pain and suffering, and as a sense of simultaneous calm and enlivenment. Whatever our definition of health, having been born we are immediately subject to accidents, disease, and death.

Health care practitioners should understand a patient's illness in terms of his or her religious beliefs. More than any other institution, religion attempts to lift humans above pain, illness, and death. Countless persons in extreme physical pain have refused a cure or medical help because it is not consonant with their religious beliefs. Some individuals, such as Christian Scientists, refuse blood transfusions. For some patients and health care professionals, it is very difficult to reconcile a loving God with suffering humanity. Scientists and artists have attended with great interest to the interrelatedness of religious values and health care, and to the question regarding the kind of health which should be given precedence: existence or quality of life. This chapter will examine the relationships of religious beliefs and health care, mental health and religion, and conflicts of religious beliefs and health protocols (See Table 5-1).

Religious Beliefs and Health

The genesis of Western religions is generally attributed to Egypt and Mesopotamia, where animism influenced a complex polytheism which,

Table 5-1. Death-related beliefs and practices of selected religious groups

Group	Afterlife	Rituals/Funerals	Autopsy	Organ Donation	Prolonging Life
American Indian	Beliefs vary	Practices vary; most want family present	Prohibited		
Black Muslim		Special procedures for washing and shrouding the dead; special funeral rites			
Buddhist in America	Reincarnation: after reaching state of enlightenment, may attain nirvana	Last rite; chanting at bedside	No restriction		Permit euthanasia in hopeless illness
Church of Christ Scientist	Yes	No last rites	Only in sudden death	No	
Church of Jesus Christ of Latter Day Saints (Mormon)	Yes	Baptism essential; preaching gospel to dead also practiced	No restriction	No restriction	
Eastern Orthodox (Greek and Russian Orthodox)	Yes	Last rites (administration of Holy Communion obligatory)	Discouraged		Encouraged
Episcopal (Anglican)	Yes	Last rites not mandatory	No restriction	No restriction	
Hindu	Reincarnation; after leading a perfect life, may join Brahma	Priest pours water into mouth of corpse and ties string around wrist or neck as sign of blessing; string must not be removed; family washes body	No restriction	No restriction	
Islam (Moslem, Muslim)	May join Allah by being a good Moslem and observing rituals daily	Dying person must confess sins and ask forgiveness in presence of family; family washes and prepares body (female body cannot be washed by male) and turns body toward Mecca	Prohibited unless required by law	Prohibited	Encouraged
Jehovah's Witness			Prohibited unless required by law. No body parts may be removed	Prohibited	
Judaism	Dead will be resurrected with coming of Messiah; man lives on through survival of memory	Body ritually washed by members of Ritual Burial Society; burial as soon as possible after death; dead not left unattended; five stages of mourning extending over a year; no embalming; no flowers at funeral because flowers are a symbol of life	Orthodox prohibit; some liberals permit; no body parts removed	Beliefs vary	
Lutheran	Yes	Last rites optional	No restriction	No restriction	
Roman Catholicism	Yes; resurrection with second coming of Christ	Rites for annointing the sick not mandatory; receiving Holy Communion mandatory	Permitted, but all body parts must be given appropriate burial	No restriction	Discouraged
Seventh Day Adventist	Dead are asleep until return of Christ, when final rewards and punishments will be given				
Unitarian	Beliefs vary		No restriction	Encouraged	Preferred

Source: H. M. Ross, Societal/cultural views regarding death and dying, *Nursing 77*, December 1977, 7:64-70.

in turn, gave way to the belief in one supreme God, Yahweh (Smith, 1971). From Yahweh, Moses eventually received the Ten Commandments —a contract or covenant under which Yahweh would protect the Hebrews. In return, the Hebrews were to serve Yahweh forever by living out the terms of the contract. Judaism's contribution to Western religions also includes its aggressive and theistic tone, as well as its body of literature. The documented religious history of Jews, as recorded in the Old Testament of the Bible, provides us with a picturesque look at ways in which religion has affected both personal and community behaviors.

There are many difficulties in trying to use the Bible as a point of reference. It is not a single book; it is a large collection of eclectic writings. Its name is derived from the Greek word *biblia,* which means "books." The Bible consists of at least sixty-six books written by many authors over a period of approximately one thousand years. Furthermore, there are several different Bibles, including the Hebrew, the Greek Orthodox, the Catholic, and various Protestant versions. Despite their differences, three broad principles and five basic beliefs characterize Christian religions. The *principles* are: (1) there is a spiritual ground of all reality, (2) there is a moral order in the world, and (3) the good life is an aspect of religion. The *beliefs* are: (1) God is Creator and Father, (2) Christ is Lord and Savior, (3) the Church is the body of Christ and the community of believers, (4) the Bible has unique religious value, and (5) Christianity is relevant to personal and social ethics.

The most obvious Christian contributions to healing practices evolve around the teachings of Christ. The essence of Christ's wisdom is contained in the Sermon on the Mount, the Lord's Prayer, and the parables. Jesus was concerned with the healing of souls, and he taught psychological principles, many of which are embodied in 20th century approaches to psychological health. "The Kingdom of Heaven," he said, "is within you, and whosoever shall know himself shall find it." The foremost Christian concept to human relations is the concept of *love.* The Greeks emphasized self-love, and the Old Testament portrayed Yahweh as a God of fear and justice. But Jesus said, "God is love." Faith in the power of love has deeply affected the Western world. Social conflicts have sent many supporters of Christian religious morality back to their theological foundations in an attempt to accommodate Judeo-Christian traditions. In this age of scientific exploration of outer space, psychological probing of inner space, and sociological delineation of personal space, religious leaders have become increasingly hard pressed to make relevant interpretations of standard religious doctrines that are applicable to such controversial subjects as abortion, racism, sexism, homophobia, drug abuse, poverty, and euthanasia.

In most Christian denominations, there is a tendency to downplay the solemn, suffering aspects of human existence and, instead, to concentrate on the joyful prospect of participating in eternal life. Pentecostals are prominent among those expressing such a cheerful attitude toward the human condition. Their perspective is not a denial of pain and suffering; rather, it is an affirmation that God is always at hand to solve all problems and to assume all human burdens (Fichtes, 1981, p. 17). This attitude is the essence of faith healing, which no longer resides exclusively among lower-class fundamentalists. Charismatics now abound in mainline Protestant churches as well as among Roman Catholics and Episcopalians. The central motif of this attitude of cheer is that God wants humans to be well and that He can truly heal anyone who is suffering. To "true believers," pain and suffering are redemptive—they precipitate the seeking of religious convictions, and are thus positive in value.

Freud (1950) observed that hardships, terror, and suffering cause some people to turn to religion. Hume (1969) speculated that all of us hang in personal suspense between life and death, health and sickness, affluence and poverty, which are distributed among the human species by secret and unknown forces whose behavior is often unexpected and always unaccounted. Hippocrates, the earliest renowned physician of record, is said to have delved deeply inside himself to discover the cause and meaning of sickness and suffering, and the nature of healing. He concluded, for example, that epilepsy was of divine origin. Frankl (1972) noted that in the quest for religious meanings, it is often physicians, not the clergy, of whom patients ask the ultimate questions of life. Psychiatrists are frequently asked questions concerning the meaning of illness and suffering by their patients. These philosophical questions can be more difficult to answer than inquiries concerning physical illness.

Health care is affected, both positively and negatively, by the religious beliefs of patients. Most hospital patients suffer from a diagnosable injury, infection, or disease and perceive a majority of their disabilities as personal, unexpected, and undeserved. Some of the problems associated with their responses to illness are the result of patriarchal religious traditions that have been superimposed on medicine. In searching for the meaning of pain and suffering, many people with religious beliefs and values conclude that God is punishing them. This, in turn, may lead to feelings of guilt. The responses and decisions of caregivers, which are often colored by their own religious health care values, can complicate the problem. Raymond (1982) hypothesized that medicine is a patriarchal religion, and throughout history both the art and science of medicine have been closely patterned after the idea of sacred religious practices. Medicine is sometimes construed to be a religion because it deals with questions of ultimate concern and meaning, as well as questions of bodily and spiritual integrity. Raymond further stated that the effects of medicine as a patriarchal religion have disproportionately affected women. Statistics seem to bear this out. For most types of medical care, women visit doctors twice as often as men. Over 70 percent of the population in mental institutions are female; over 70 percent of those undergoing electroshock treatment are women; and over 70 percent of behavior modification and control therapies are practiced on females.

Similar to religious practitioners, medical practitioners have their costumes, props, taboos, and rituals. One important medical rite is that of instilling in the patient a proper attitude toward disease, death, and dying. Patients are expected to trust the doctor; the parallel expectation of some religions is a complete willingness to trust God. In medicine, patients must follow the doctor's orders; in some religions, followers must accept and adhere to the will of God. In medicine, patients must endure the consequences of medical procedures; in some religions, followers must endure sin, suffering, and the uncertainty of fate. There is a tacit understanding that without compliance to medical procedures, they will be ineffective; in some religions, sinners cannot be healed if they challenge the supernatural order and purpose of the universe. In medicine, the physician does not want to fail; in religion, God does not fail. Medicine has successfully appropriated many of the sacraments of religion. For example, the Roman Catholic Church is centered in the dictum that outside the church, there is no salvation; the medical hierarchy projects the attitude that outside of orthodox, licensed medicine, there is no safe healing.

Christianity and Judaism share the traditional belief that there is only one God, and that this God is the creator, or maker, of the world. In early religious myths, the natural world was God-created and, thus, good. Health was embraced as a moral and physical good because of the intrinsic value placed on anything created by God. From these principles, it was inferred that the study of nature can yield morally binding rules or principles. The symbolism of God, creation, and nature have been very influential in the relationship between physician and patient—both to the benefit and the detriment of the relationship (Shelp, 1983). From the Christian perspective, health care relationships are privileged ways to encounter other persons—a way to encounter Christ (McCormick, 1983). Christians believe that physicians must envision Christ in all people, whether they are close associates or strangers. If health care professionals define their calling in this way, the result will be an expanded will to nourish, protect, and support, and every medical encounter will be viewed as a religious experience, not just a technological exercise. This attitude exemplifies a commitment to compassion, honesty, generosity, and self-denial. When health care becomes deeply penetrated by people of such faith and disposition, one must ask whether healing will be transformed to loving service. Health care providers can flourish in a religious way by applying, without proselytizing, the positive values inherent in various religions. This requires of health care providers a spirituality, which is both a personal and professional commitment to acquiring and enhancing the belief in a higher power as its basic foundation, particularly as this power is defined within a healing context. Jewish religion and medical traditions support this approach.

The Jewish Healing Tradition

In the first century, a pagan asked Rabbi Hillel, a contemporary of Jesus, to instruct him concerning the values of the entire Torah while standing on one foot. The rabbi replied: "That which is hateful to you, do not inflict on your fellow beings. All the rest is commentary." This particular example of the Jewish perspective is cited to note the similarity between the values in early Jewish thought and the Christian admonition "Do unto others as you would have others do unto you." Today, Christian and Jewish communities still possess common religious dimensions. The key concepts that govern the values of both Judaism and Christianity are "affirmation of human conscience," "freedom," and "responsibility." A foremost contribution of Judaism to healing and helping is its emphasis on judgment as a value, and on contracts that govern areas of personal and professional relationships.

In the medieval period, Jewish doctors worked as translators and transmitters of Greek medicine throughout Europe. They were proficient in Greek, Latin, Arabic, and Hebrew. The close religious and family ties that linked together a variety of Jewish communities helped spread medical knowledge. But the large number of Jewish physicians is mainly attributed to the fact that the profession of medicine was regarded as a spiritual vocation, equal in stature to the career of a rabbi. Also, the curriculum of Talmudic schools often included the sciences and philosophies of the day. Maimonides was one of the most important Jewish physicians. In 1170 he became the personal physician of Sultan Saladin of Egypt and his family. In addition to his philosophy and legal-religious works, Maimonides wrote ten medical books. The disparate moral emphases in his life all meshed to form a concept of medicine based on the premise that a healthy soul requires a healthy body. A healthy body, he believed, can facilitate the development of one's intellectual and moral capabilities toward greater knowledge of God and an ethical life (Feldman, 1986). Maimonides proposed that physicians should acquire the technical knowledge, sensitivity, and intuition needed to relate to each patient's personality and life style. For him, the Talmud was the unquestioned ethical authority but, in addition to using it as a reference, he encouraged independent quest for medical knowledge. Jewish physicians earned a wide reputation for unselfish devotion to their profession, especially in times of epidemics.

There are several ways in which Judaic laws set forth the physician-patient relationship (Franck, 1983). Some of the terms of the relationship are set independently—for example, physicians decide when and how they can treat patients, and they determine the fee; patients decide what kind of treatment they will accept or reject. But the patient-physician relationship is governed by strict obligations and terms that are not always based on mutual consent. A questionable, or dangerous, treatment for higher fees is not an option, even if both parties agree. In the Jewish tradition, society's major role is to ensure that both parties enter the relationship when they should and behave as they should. Social custom necessitates paying for treatment; and the physician can demand payment from the community for treating an indigent patient. In Jewish ethics, *responsibility* is the fundamental value that governs the patient-physician relationship. The physician has the ethical responsibility to provide the best medical treatment, and society is obliged to fund the treatment when patients cannot.

An authentic patient-physician relationship is formulated in Judaic religious law. It is set forth as a dyadic relationship that is transactional in character. As conceived within Jewish law, however, in any medical encounter there is a third party—the omnipresent God who attends all medical endeavors. This is a covenantal triadic relationship between the patient, the physician, and God or God's Torah. The central goal is to collaborate with God in the process of His continuing effort to mend the imperfections of the world. God is the supreme healer. Unlike other professionals, those engaged in the practice of medicine are commanded to practice their craft as a *moral imperative*. In the triadic collaboration between the patient, the physician, and God, the special role of the physician is that of God's emissary.

Hebrew Scriptures provide the humanizing aspect of healing and helping. Rabbi Hillel's famous maxim "Do not do to others what is hateful to yourself" is a practical version of "love your neighbor as yourself" (Lev. 19: 18). From this perspective, patients should not have to demand that physicians respect them as fellow human beings; if they must demand it, something is wrong in the relationship. The Torah gives physicians the duty to heal. If they refrain from this duty, they are "shedders of blood." In the matter of physician payment, it is permissible for physicians to charge patients, but, as noted earlier, there is an expectation in the religious literature that they will not charge the poor for medical treatment. As for healing members of other ethnic groups, the Biblical injunctions derived from the experiences of Jews enslaved in ancient Egypt caution: "The stranger that sojourneth with you shall be unto you as a native among you . . . ; for ye were strangers in the land of Egypt" (Lev. 19: 34); "And a stranger shalt thou not oppress. . . . " (Exod. 23:9). The lesson to be learned is that all physicians, and other health care professionals, must not discriminate against peoples of other cultures —we are all strangers or descendants of strangers.

The largest number of malpractice suits today reflect some of the ancient fears about the practice of medicine. Physician errors have been recorded from data going back as far as 2,000 B.C., but it has only been since the 1930s that medical malpractice litigation has begun to look like a patient revolt. Comprehensive studies of patient grievances reveal the following accusations: doctors are too rushed to listen to patients; technology has rendered doctors too specialized and too impersonal; patients resent the refusal of doctors to make house calls; doctors do not answer specific questions and rely too heavily on answering services; doctors profit excessively from human illness and become very wealthy from patient fees; and doctors send bill collectors. In summary, unlike their Jewish predecessors, a growing number of patients believe they are being abandoned by overburdened, overspecialized, overautomated, and overpaid physicians (Kahn, 1978).

The Christian Healing Tradition

American patients expect the doctor's services to be less impersonal than most other services. The question arises as to why patients expect doctors to be like fathers or mothers. Perhaps it is because ancient Christian beliefs held healing to be of divine origin, and physicians to be dispensing agents for God. Early Christian patients were penitents, convinced their sinfulness was the cause of their illness. The patient's relationship was that of a child reaching out to an omnipotent God through His intermediaries—the clergy of the church and physicians who healed by faith. Good health was a manifestation of God's love. And healing the sick became a manifestation of humankind's love.

Both medicine and religion are sacred duties that require self-sacrifice. In earlier times, monks in monasteries and hospitals risked death by contagion as they ministered to the sick and wounded. No one needing help was ever turned away and no fee was levied. This was an idealized concept that was probably superimposed on that of the benign and kindly stereotype known in the earlier days of our nation as "the family doctor." The earliest Christian healing was antiscientific. Fully committed to the powerful therapy of faith healing, the church sought to discredit secular practitioners by branding them charlatans who plied their trade for a fee.

The medical texts of Galen and Hippocrates were secretly preserved through two hundred years of suppression and, finally, found their way to monastic hospitals throughout Europe. Soon, monks began to change their emphasis from faith healing to the traditional teachings of ancient Greek medicine. Along with this change of perspective, the Christian ideal of free medical care diminished and fees for service again became standard procedure. As the services of physicians became broadly available for purchase, medical treatment became a private transaction between physicians and patients. By the 14th century, physicians had formed guilds to oppose illicit practitioners without licensure. This was to ensure that fee-charging would not be wiped out by a few old-fashioned Christian idealists. Gradually, people came to accept the fact that healing was a commodity that must be purchased with the coin of the realm.

As noted earlier, the most obvious contributions of Christianity to health care center on the teachings of Jesus. Although 2000 years of conflicting interpretations leave most investigators unsure of the role of Christianity in healing, it has influenced health care. For example, the belief that an individual's illness is "the will of God" has had profound implications on health care. Christians who follow this belief behave differently than those who do not. There is consensus among scholars about Jesus' concern for the sick. In the New Testament, the attention Jesus gave to the sick is closely tied to his ministry of forgiving sins. A residual effect of such thinking still exists in modern times; it is demonstrated when religious bodies sit in judgment and attach the label "sickness" to much that they assess as immoral. Some religious groups adopt a scientific posture that does not associate sickness with moral guilt, however. The scientific approach has no room for moral judgment or forgiveness— both of which are cornerstones of Christian beliefs.

It is helpful to understand the functions performed by Protestant ministers and Roman Catholic priests in health care settings, especially in hospitals. In addition to talking with patients, ministers may read from the Bible or pray with patients; Roman Catholic priests may hear confessions and distribute Communion. The Roman Catholic Church is not unlike Protestant churches. It too acts as a bulwark of conservatism placing obstacles in the path of medical progress and of emancipation from folk practices. The Catholic church teaches obedience to its doctrines, authority, and one's parents. Acceptance of adversity is taught as a virtue that, like patience, will be rewarded in Heaven: it is God's Will. A major difference between Catholic and Protestant religious treatment of illness is that the former tends to be more restrained. Compared with the Protestant minister:

> The work of a Roman Catholic priest is different in form, though it is essentially about the same things. . . . One difference which immediately catches the eye is that the work of the Roman Catholic priest is marked less by words than by actions. The minister is called a servant of the word of God (*verbi divini minister*), while the most characteristic task of the priest is the administration of the sacraments. Of course, the priest also talks with the sick—a great deal of emphasis is placed on this—and, of course, the minister is entitled not only to proclaim the word but to administer the sacraments of baptism and the last supper (the two sacraments, sacred acts, which Protestants and Roman Catholics have in common). But the emphasis is different, more on the word with one, on the sacrament with the other. (Faber, 1971, p. 79)

Protestant and Roman Catholic words and sacraments are basically the same in that they are meant to help patients. This is true whether we are talking about washing away sin through baptism, lighting a candle to make visible the burning up of life, or feeding with bread in the Eucharist as a means of strengthening life.

When dealing with dying patients, ministers and priests focus on three aspects of the experience. First, there is a visible reaction in the dying person. During this phase the religious emphasis is on the faith in God. Second, after experiencing an initial reaction to dying, the patient may feel a fear of dying, which may give way to the fear of judgment. During this phase, religious leaders try to help patients to get their lives in order. The third phase is the desire for death. The religious emphasis is on returning to God. In ancient Judaic terms, dying is being gathered to one's fathers. Both the minister and the priest try to help the patient to understand how he sees life, what faith means for him, what significance it brings to his life and how that significance may grow deeper. One could perhaps say that the priest as much as the minister tries to accompany the patient to the point where the sacrament can convey its saving power most fully and bring the sick in touch with Christ (Faber, 1971).

Too often, health care professionals do not fully appreciate the impact of religious sects on health care. The importance of evangelistic groups is clear to social scientists who have studied them. Kaplan's article (1965), "The Structure of Adaptive Sentiments in a Lower-Class Religious Group in Appalachia," vividly describes the rituals of the Free Will Baptist Church. Although his study was of the Free Will Baptist Church, Kaplan described behavior characterizing many other Christian denominations: we are poor people but we have a mansion in Heaven; thou shalt not be angry; give your love to Jesus; we belong to the fellowship of sufferers—can be construed as doctrines for being sick. Indeed, a deep pride in suffering can be instilled in the faithful. This is not to imply that there is a religious scheme to support illness. Instead, it implies that religious sentiments are functional for individuals seeking to cope with physical and mental illness.

Within the Christian denominations, there are conflicting beliefs about such subjects as the right to die, medical termination of pregnancy, blood transfusion, and homosexuality. Logical arguments can do little to alter positions based on faith. But we can attempt to understand other people's viewpoints. After all, no single religion is accepted by all people.

Whatever a health care professional's religion, if any, he or she should focus on the ultimate goal in medicine: helping and healing patients.

Third World Cultures

Sometimes a physician will report that an operation was a success but the patient died, that is, the technical procedures were correctly followed but something more was needed for the patient to recover. American health professionals seem poorly educated regarding such intangibles as faith in the medical personnel, the will to live, and the ability to heal. Western medicine carves the patient into territorial pieces, and few health professionals are taught to handle the intangible portions. Conversely, most non-Western cultures tend to adopt a holistic approach to health care, viewing the patient as a biological, psychosocial, and spiritual whole existing in a specific environment. From this perspective, epidemiology rests side by side with folk medicine.

Table 5-2. Selected characteristics of six American ethnic groups

Ethnic group	Approximate time of United States population influx	Estimated population (1979)	Traditional family structure	Expression of pain	Folk healers
Black Americans	1600s	25,000,000	Extended/ matriarchal and egalitarian	Open, public	Hoodoo men and ladies Root doctors Blood doctors
Mexican Americans	400 B.C.	7,000,000	Extended/ patriarchal	Open, public	Curanderos
Puerto Ricans	1900s	1,700,000	Extended/ patriarchal	Open, public	Espiritistas
American Indians	13000-18000 B.C.	900,000	Extended/ patriarchal and matriarchal	Closed, private	Medicine men
Chinese Americans	1700s	500,000	Extended/ patriarchal	Closed, private	Herbalists Herb pharmacists Acupuncturists
Japanese Americans	1800s	700,000	Extended/ patriarchal	Closed, private	Herbalists

Many Third World people (Africans, Asians, and South Americans) feel comfortable with modern curers who understand, for example, that hypertension and cirrhosis of the liver are more than physiological conditions; that they are also manifestations of stresses that accrue at a higher rate in people of low social status than in those of high social status. Different foci differentiate Western and Third World health care practices. Some of the differences are more significant than others. For example, Western societies are usually characterized by dyadic relationships such as those of the physician-patient and nurse-patient. Multiperson health care networks, in which parents, nonparents, relatives, and nonrelatives are the care providers, are characteristic in Third World societies. Fortunately, multiperson networks are no longer dismissed by Western practitioners as being irrelevant; Western health care systems are shifting toward the multiperson perspective.

Ethnic diets are another aspect of human ecology that health care providers are beginning to understand and utilize. Each ethnic group must consume enough food to meet its nutritional requirements for energy, fat, protein, vitamins, and minerals. Relatively little is known about the range of human biological variability, among and within human populations, with regard to such common parameters as nutritional requirements, physiolog cal responses to malnutrition, and digestive capabilities (Rittenbaugh, 1978). This lack of knowledge has resulted in the prescription by Western-oriented health care providers of prescribing nonacceptable diets for Third World patients. Geographically related biological adaptations of some Third World people have rendered them unable to digest certain Western foods.

Third World people are likely to explain their illness in terms of an imbalance between the individual and his or her physical, social, and spiritual worlds. In short, health and illness are believed to come from supernatural sources. Although all medical systems focus on preventive and curative medicine, "good health" among most Third World people centers on *personal* rather than scientific behavior. From this perspective, it makes sense to burn incense, or to avoid certain individuals or cold air, or evil eyes. Kay (1978) was correct in saying that one person's religion is another's magic, witchcraft, or superstition. It is difficult for some health professionals to see the study of religion, witchcraft, and magic, as directly relevant to their practice. It is equally difficult for them to realize that, for some people, religion is an equivalent of science.

All religious systems have elaborate rules that determine appropriate and inappropriate health care behavior, particularly in regard to giving and receiving care. Religious experiences may include blessings from spiritual leaders, apparitions of dead relatives, and miracle cures. Heal-

ing power may be found in animate as well as inanimate objects. The key
concept in religious systems is "faith." The distinction between the shaman,
whose powers derive from the supernatural, and the priest, who learns a
codified body of rituals from other priests, is not always clear. Both may
engage in similar behavior. However, in traditional Third World societies,
some of the most significant religious rituals are those that mediate
between events "here," in this world, and "out there," in the nether world
(Morley & Wallis, 1978). In mediating between these worlds, folk practitioners may effect cures and work protective and evil magic. Many
names are given to individuals who utter charms, spells, supplications,
and incantations.

Both Third World and Western medical systems are functional. It is
important for health care practitioners to be aware of the strengths
possessed by Third World medical systems. Third World medical systems are comprehensive. They include the individual and his or her
family and community environment. The curer or healer tries to maintain
a balance between humans, their society, and their physical environment.
Relatives and friends are part of the curing rites. Third World therapeutic techniques, when effective, relieve pain, and frequently provide emotional catharsis and a sharing of guilt; one does not suffer alone. By
eliminating the division between physical and mental symptoms, indigenous therapies often achieve remarkable results.

Spiritualism is an integral part of folk medicine, especially among
Hispanics, Indians, and African Americans. For the purpose of our
discussion, spiritualism is defined as *the belief that the visible world also
includes an invisible world inhabited by good and evil spirits who influence our
behavior.* Spirits make their presence known through "mediums." The
failure of health care professionals to acknowledge and understand the
importance of spiritualism to millions of Americans can be detrimental
to health plans. In addition to conferring protection and enabling mediums to function, spirits cause and prevent illness (Fisch, 1968). Our
spiritual protection acts as a shield—it turns away evil spirits and hexes
while at the same time bringing good luck. If we lose spiritual protection,
we can become ill. And illness may be manifested by such signs as pain,
lethargy, nervousness, and bad luck.

Mediums treat both emotionally-related and physical illnesses. Unlike
Western-based approaches to health, Third World cultures do not distinguish sharply between physical and mental illnesses. Consequently, mediums treat the whole person. For example, in Puerto Rican culture,

psychological symptoms are frequently expressed as somatic illness. While most modern medical professionals tend to ignore psychosomatic illnesses, mediums do not. Mediums take for granted the dual nature of illness. Folk healers, due to the fact that most share the ethnic background, language, social class, and community of followers, have a distinct advantage when compared with modern healers and their helpers. Also, mediums are not bogged down with bureaucratic red tape. Perhaps the essence of their success resides in the faith that their followers have in them.

The belief in supernatural forces is expressed in magic, witchcraft, and religion. Several years ago, anthropologists observed that there is virtually no incompatibility between religion and spiritualism. Most religion, like spiritualism, is based on a belief in spirits. Furthermore, like that of the medium, a religious leader's authority is of a spiritual nature. Both magic and religion offer relief from suffering through the use of ritual and belief in supernatural forces.

Mental Health and Religion

Most mental health professionals and religious counselors are dedicated to a similar therapeutic goal—the enhancement of the quality of life for their patients. Whereas behavior changes can be attained by different clinical strategies, a growing number of psychologists and psychiatrists are beginning to recognize the fact that religious beliefs affect therapeutic outcomes. Several researchers have found success in cooperative treatment programs that incorporate both psychology and religion (Fichtes, 1981).

O'Malley and associates (1984) conducted a study of mental health professionals and ministers who lived in two large Rocky Mountain cities. The respondents classified themselves into either the "theological" or "therapeutic" category. The ministers were ranked as "fundamentalists," "orthodox," or "main-line Protestants"; and the mental health practitioners were classified as "psychodynamic," "behavioral," or "humanistic." The researchers concluded that all three religious groups declared a greater appreciation for the counseling process than did the psychological groups. Behaviorists, humanists, and Protestant ministers were more optimistic concerning the prospect of cooperation between religion and mental health than were psychodynamic, orthodox, and fundamentalist counselors. The schism between psychology and religion was reflected most clearly in the responses of psychodynamic therapists and fundamentalist counselors. Overall, the results of the survey are encouraging for those who anticipate a cooperative and beneficial exchange between psychology and religion.

McDonald and Luckett (1983) examined the relationship between religious affiliation and psychiatric diagnoses. They concluded that specific emotional stresses are significantly more prevalent in particular religious affiliations. For example, Jehovah's Witnesses were diagnosed as schizophrenics three times more often than members of the general population, and they were four times more frequently diagnosed as paranoid schizophrenics. Adolescent drinking was less frequent among fundamental Protestants and more frequent among liberal Protestants and Catholics. This study provides support for the premise that there are important interrelationships between religious affiliation and psychological dysfunction.

Glik (1986) differentiated religious affiliation into seven major groups: "no religious preference," "non-mainline Protestants," "mainline Protestants," "Catholics," "other Protestants," "unknown," and "sects." Psychoses were most prevalent among "sects"; substance abuse was highest in the "no religious preference" and "unknown religious preference" respondents. Very strong emphasis on marital maladjustments was indicated only among "mainline Protestants"; "non-mainline Protestants" had the greatest number of behavior disorders, especially in reaction to childhood experiences. "Catholic" respondents were characterized by excessive concern with control and self-absorption. The "other Protestant" respondents had more severe psychiatric disorders, childhood behavior disorders, and negative reactions to the stressful demands of life. This latter group was also described as being more compliant. Spiritual healing respondents had consistently higher scores on measures of psychosocial wellness than did the patients with no religious affiliation. From these data, it can be hypothesized that regular participation in religious healing groups results in a significantly higher percentage of feelings of wellness than does participation in nonreligious healing groups. Religious healing activities appear to reinforce a belief system that enhances the patient's feeling of self-worth and positive expectations of healing.

In another study, Kroll and Sheehan (1989) examined the religious beliefs and practices among 52 psychiatric inpatients in Minnesota. The study revealed that religious beliefs and practices were extremely important in the lives of most of the patients. Considerable data were collected because the patients replied in great detail regarding their religious beliefs and how they affected their lives. Results of the study indicate that religious beliefs and practices of patients deserve far more consideration than most psychiatrists customarily accord them. Additional research concerning the influence of particular religious beliefs on suicidal behavior would be beneficial. Does the belief in sin or immoral behavior precipitate illness? What are the influences of religious beliefs on the willingness of individuals to seek out psychiatric consultation? It is interesting to note that some psychiatrists and psychologists find much relevance in Eastern religions and philosophies—such as Buddhism, Hinduism, and Confucianism—but do not place much importance in Judeo-Christian religions.

In summary, physicians treat disease, but patients suffer illnesses that alter their sense of identity and meaning. Human beings construct meaning through four basic relationships: between their ideal self and their real self; between their self and the social world, between their self and the natural world, and between their self and the cosmos (Barnard, 1984). Illness can elicit new meanings from any or all of these dimensions. An illness alters our self-image, disrupts our societal relationships, interferes with our ability to manipulate the physical environment, and, most importantly, raises questions about our ability to survive in the cosmos. Mental health professionals who exhibit patience and religious tolerance serve their patients well in times of psychospiritual conflict, facilitating a healing relationship, if not a curing one.

Conflicts of Religious Beliefs and Health Laws

There are numerous instances when religious attitudes have conflicted with both state interests and prescribed health care protocols. Examples of such religious practices include handling poisonous snakes, ingesting poison during religious worship, using prohibited drugs during worship, and refusing blood transfusions for critically ill persons (Flowers, 1976). Religious freedom is held in high esteem in the United States—only very grave abuses that jeopardize the general welfare are occasions for limiting the First Amendment right of religious freedom. A continuing controversy centers on the use, sale, and distribution of narcotics, including hallucinogens for religious rituals.

The Native American Church uses peyote to achieve a mystical experience that is a part of its religious ritual. However, the principal constituent of peyote is mescaline, which is classified as a hallucinogen that causes visual enhancement and a heightened sense of friendliness toward other human beings. Other churches, in addition to the Native American Church, have petitioned courts for exceptions to drug laws. Members of the Neo-American Church have sought legal permission to use marijuana and LSD in their religious services; members of the Church of the Awakening want to legally use peyote; and some segments of the Universal Life Church have petitioned the courts to allow them to use marijuana in their rituals. The courts have ruled in favor of the Native American Church because of its long history of peyote use; the religion was not invented to justify the use of peyote. In the Native American Church, peyote is an object of veneration with prayers directed to it. Thus, it is a sacramental symbol similar to that of bread and wine in certain Christian denominations (*People v. Woody*, 1964). The other churches have not received court approval for their drug use.

The handling of poisonous snakes and drinking of strychnine during worship in some Appalachian churches is a very different matter. This form of worship bases its legitimacy on a literal interpretation of Matthew, verses 17–18, which state: "They shall take up serpents and if they drink any deadly thing no harm shall come to them and they shall lay hands on the sick and they shall recover." Believers in this practice argue that the activities in question are not carried out to test their faith, but to substantiate the Word of God. Generally, the courts have ruled against these practices on the basis that they constitute a public nuisance, and that the state has the right to protect people from themselves (*State ex rel. Swann v. Pack*, 1976).

A major area of controversy between religion and health care is the matter of blood transfusions. Principal litigants in this matter have been Jehovah's Witnesses. They believe transfusions are forbidden by God in his commandments in Genesis 9:3–4, Leviticus 17:10–14, and Acts 15:19–20 that forbid the "eating" of blood. Originally, these admonitions applied to eating improperly bled animals, but the proscription has come to be applied to blood transfusions, gamma globulin, and other serums containing blood components (Lebacqz, 1986). When Witnesses appear for medical care, their refusal to accept transfusions can present a potentially lethal outcome. Even though Witnesses sign statements relieving doctors and hospitals from liability, many doctors will petition the courts to allow them to proceed with transfusions (*Prince v. Massachusetts*, 1944).

This is especially prevalent in the treatment of children, and the *Prince* decision is unequivocal: "The right to practice religion freely does not include the liberty to expose . . . a child . . . to ill health or death. Parents may be free to become martyrs themselves. But it does not follow that they are free . . . to make martyrs of their children before they have reached the age of full and legal discretion when they can make that choice for themselves."

While Jehovah's Witnesses are mainly concerned with blood transfusions, followers of some other religions have theological objections to all medical procedures. The most well known of these is Christian Scientists, who believe that illness is unreal—an illusion—and God, spirit, is All-in-All. Being law-abiding people, they obey health laws that compel vaccination for communicable disease, but they work diligently to be exempted from them and are sometimes successful.

Health care providers often encounter conflicts of value in trying to mediate between patients' religious values and the larger community's medical values. In an effort to provide patients with maximum freedom, self-determination, and quality of life in health care, health care providers must ask themselves the crucial question "When should the practitioner seek to override, by legal means if necessary, a patient's decision, made on religious faith, that contravenes currently accepted practices of good medical care?" Health care in a democratic society requires respect for each person's religious beliefs, but the inability of members of some religious groups to accept crucial medical interventions has created dilemmas that can sometimes tear apart families and communities.

Rapprochement

At their most profound levels, medicine and religion often have much in common. Yet our laws do not always deal with these similarities—or differences. Through seeking a personal understanding of folk medicine traditions, health care practitioners often are able to reduce conflicts. This does not minimize the fact that religious beliefs can both kill and heal. Countless case studies illustrate this point. In folk medicine, mind and body are literally embodied in the human person; our body is mindful, and the central nervous system is the mediating processing agent between our mind and body. There are remarkable examples of this theory. In Australia, among some aboriginal peoples, pointing a bone at someone can result in his death. In Latin America and Africa, the belief that one is "bewitched" can lead to sudden "voodoo death." In more "civilized" countries, there are instances of rapid death during psychological stress. Negative thoughts, emotions, and expectations precede a wide range of morbid conditions, causing people to give up or adopt an attitude of inability to cope with their illness.

It is of great importance that we learn which religious beliefs weaken and kill; which heal; and what mechanisms produce these causal effects. Experts differ about these issues, but it is reasonable to suggest that positive results appear to be faith- and hope-related, and negative results appear to be hate- and fear-related. Each of us has an internal therapeutic system. Our biopsychosocial makeup can produce systemic positive catharsis and anxiety reduction—or the reverse: fear and despair can result in disease, illness, and death. When people hit bottom, e.g., alcoholics become sick of being sick, religious beliefs may cause them to place themselves within the reach of God (Spahr, 1987). Sometimes this results in a positive change in their behavior. When this happens, another of God's creatures becomes "well" in a most profound sense.

We have described how modern medicine was derived from ancient religious beliefs that place the power to heal in God. As countries become industrial, this view shifts from a metaphysical emphasis to a focus on scientific methods. Thus, medicine has become a scientific endeavor, and its practitioners have moved from the ideal of sacrificial care, with no charge to the patient, to a system of care for fees. And the medical profession has begun to transfer some of the responsibility for wellness to the patient. Relatedly, physicians and other health care providers appear to be legally empowered and reinforced when they accept patients' religious beliefs that do not endanger them. Recognition of their role as agents for an omnipotent, loving healing power is growing among some health professionals. The very presence of such persons has a calming and enlivening effect on many patients in their care. In 1530, Paracelsus declared, "Medicine is not only a science, it is also an art. It does not consist of compounding pills and plasters; it deals with the very processes of life, which must be understood before they may be guided" (Mencken, 1962, p. 775). Health care can profit by applying the values inherent in the Christian phrase, "As I have loved you."

Medicine and religion are inextricably interwoven; the values and beliefs that guide each of them can augment or diminish the covenance of the other. In a world where overwhelming problems, both natural and contrived, affect us all, faith is often a potent medicine, particularly when it is laced with the loving kindness that gives credence to the verity that we are all part of each other. Religious values can rouse patients to follow a medical regimen and substantiate a purpose for their existence. Unlike religious leaders, medical practitioners work tirelessly to destroy the reason for their existence: ill health. Practitioners bestirred by religious values have made significant contributions to health care through the exigency to love and heal. Paraphrasing Einstein, medicine without religion is incomplete, and religion without science is narrow-minded.

REFERENCES

Acklin, M. W., Brown, E. C. & Mauger, P. A. (1983). The role of religious values in coping with cancer. *Journal of Religion and Health, 4:* 322–333.

Aquinas, T. (1947). *Compendium of theology.* Trans. by C. Vollert. St. Louis: B. Herder.

Bahm, A. J. (1964). *16 world's living religions.* New York: Dell.

Barnard, D. (1984). Illness as a crisis of meaning: Psychospiritual agendas in health care. *Pastoral Psychology, 2:* 74–82.

Bentham, J. (1879). *An introduction to the principles of morals and legislation.* Oxford, England: Clarendon Press.

Chance, S. (1988). Gods, patients and psychiatrists. *Psychiatric Annals, 18:* 432–435.

Eddy, M. B. (1915). *Christian healing, and the people's idea of God.* Boston: A. V. Stewart.

Faber, H. (1971). *Pastoral care in the modern hospital.* Philadelphia: Westminister Press.

Feldman, D. M. (1986). *Health and medicine in the Jewish tradition.* New York: Crossroad.

Fichtes, J. H. (1981). *Religion and pain: The spiritual dimensions of health care.* New York: Crossroad.

Fisch, S. (1968). Botanicas and spiritualism in a metropolis. *Milbank Memorial Fund, 41:* 370–378.

Flowers, R. B. (1976). Freedom of religion versus civil authority in matters of health. *Annals of the American Academy of Political and Social Science, 446:* 149–161.

Franck, I. (1983). Jewish religious law as a model of the patient-physician relationship, pp. 141–148. In E. E. Shelp. (Ed.), *The clinical encounter.* Boston: D. Reidel.

Frankl, V. (1972). *Man's search for meaning.* New York: Simon & Schuster.

Freud, S. (1950). *Totem and taboo.* New York: W. W. Norton.

Fromm, E. (1963). *The dogma of Christ, and other essays on religion.* New York: Holt, Rinehart & Winston.

Glik, D. C. (1986). Psychosocial wellness among spiritual healing participants. *Social Science and Medicine, 22:* 579–586.

Hume, D. (1969). Origin of religion, pp. 19–22. In N. Birnbaum & G. Lenzer (Eds.), *Sociology and religion.* Englewood Cliffs, NJ: Prentice-Hall.

Hunsberger, B. (1985). Religion, age, life satisfaction and perceived sources of religiousness: A study of older persons. *Journal of Gerontology, 40:* 615–620.

Kahn, D. (1978). Religious roots of a medical crisis. *Harvard Magazine, 1:* 42–46.

Kaplan, B. H. (1965). The structure of adoptive sentiments in a lower-class religious group in Appalachia. *Journal of Social Issues, 21:* 126–141.

Kay, M. (1978). Clinical anthropology, pp. 2–10. In E. E. Baywens (Ed.), *The anthropology of health.* St. Louis: C. V. Mosby.

Kroll, J. & Sheehan, W. (1989). Religious beliefs and practices among 52 psychiatric inpatients in Minnesota. *American Journal of Psychiatry, 146:* 67–72.

Lebacqz, K. (1986). Faith dimensions in medical practice. *Primary Care, 13:* 263–269.

McCormick, R. A. (1983). *Health and medicine in the Catholic tradition.* New York: Crossroad.

McDonald, C. B. & Luckett, J. B. (1983). Religious affiliation and psychiatric diagnoses. *Journal for the Scientific Study of Religion, 22:* 15–37.

Mencken, H. C. (1962). *Dictionary of quotations.* New York: Alfred A. Knopf.

Mill, J. S. (1885). *Three essays on religion.* London: Green.

Morley, P. & Wallis, R. (Eds.). (1978). *Culture and curing.* Pittsburgh: University of Pittsburgh Press.

O'Malley, M. N., Gearhart, R. & Becker, L. A. (1984). On cooperation between psychology and religion: An attitudinal survey of therapists and clergy. *Counseling and Values, 28:* 117–121.

People v. Woody, 394 P. 2d 813 at 816–817 (1964).

Prince v. Massachusetts, 321 U.S. 158 (1944).

Raymond, J. G. (1982). Medicine as patriarchal religion. *Journal of Medicine and Philosophy, 7:* 197–216.

Rittenbaugh, C. (1978). Human foodways: A window on evolution, pp. 110–113. In E. E. Bauwens (Ed.), *The anthropology of health.* St. Louis: C. V. Mosby.

Shelp, E. E. (Ed.) (1983). *The clinical encounter.* Boston: D. Reidel.

Smith, J. (1971). *The book of Mormon.* Salt Lake City: Desert Book.

Spahr, J. H. (1987). The role of the conversion experience in alcoholism recovery. *Studies in Formative Spirituality, 8:* 220–223.

State ex rel. Swann v. Pack, 527 S.W. 2d 99, cert. denied U.S. 954 (1976).

Whitehead, A. N. (1926). *Religion in the making.* New York: Macmillan.

Tillich, P. (1963). *Christianity and the encounter of the world religions.* New York: Columbia University Press.

Thoreau, H. D. (1920). *Walden; or life in the woods.* New York: Macmillan.

SUGGESTED READINGS

Batson, C. D. & Ventis, W. L. (1982). *The religious experience.* New York: Oxford University Press.

Braverman, E. C. (1987). The religious medical model: Holy medicine and the Spiritual Behavior Inventory. *Religious Medical Model, 80:* 415–420, 425.

Conwill, W. I. (1986). Chronic pain conceptualization and religious interpretation. *Journal of Religion and Health, 25:* 46–50.

Cousins, N. (1982). *Healing and belief.* Cincinnati: Mosaic Press.

Desai, P. N. (1988). Medical ethics in India. *Journal of Medicine and Philosophy, 13:* 231–255.

Dominian, J. (1983). Doctor as prophet: Medicine and religion. *British Medical Journal, 287:* 24–31.

Griffith, E. E. H., English, T. & Mayfield, V. (1980). Possession, prayer, and testimony: Therapeutic aspects of the Wednesday night meeting in a black church. *Psychiatry, 43:* 120–128.

Gupta, A. (1983). Mental health and religion. *Asian Journal of Psychology Education, 11:* 8–13.

Guy, J. R. (1982). The Episcopal licensing of physicians, surgeons and midwives. *Bulletin of History and Medicine, 56:* 528–542.

Hall, C. M. (1986). Crisis as opportunity for spiritual growth. *Journal of Religion and Health, 25:* 46–53.

Idler, E. L. (1987). Religious involvement and the health of the elderly: Some hypothesis and an initial test. *Social Forces, 66:* 226–237.

Kerewsky-Halper, B. (1985). Trust, talk and touch in Balkan folk healing. *Social Science and Medicine, 21:* 319–325.

Koenig, H. G., George, L. K. & Siegler, I. C. (1988). The use of religion and other emotion-regulating coping strategies among older adults. *The Gerontologist, 28:* 303–310.

McCormick, R. A. (1989). Theology and bioethics. *Hastings Center Report, 19:* 5–10.

Meadow, M. J. & Kahoe, R. D. (1984). *Psychology and religion.* New York: Harper & Row.

Nanji, A. (1988). Medical ethics and the Islamic tradition. *Journal of Medicine and Philosophy, 13:* 257–275.

O'Doherty, E. F. (1978). *Religion and psychology.* New York: Alba House.

Osmond, H. (1982). God and the doctor. *New England Journal of Medicine, 302:* 555–558.

Ratanakus, P. (1988). Bioethics in Thailand: The struggle for Buddhist solutions. *Journal of Medicine and Philosophy, 13:* 301–312.

Rosner, F. (1984). *Medicine in the Mishneh Torah of Maimonides.* New York: KTAV.

Shriver, D. W. (Ed.). (1980). *Medicine and religion: Strategies of care.* Pittsburgh: University of Pittsburgh Press.

Qiu, R. (1988). Medicine—the art of humaneness: On ethics of traditional Chinese medicine. *Journal of Medicine and Philosophy, 13:* 277–300.

Weinberger, M., Tierney, W. M., Greene, J. Y. & Studdard, P. A. (1982). The development of physician norms in the United States: The treatment of Jehovah's Witness patients. *Social Science and Medicine, 16:* 1719–1723.

Chapter 6

PAIN AND SUFFERING

"Suffering passes, but to have suffered never passes."

Leon Bloy

"After crosses and losses, men grow humbler and wiser."

Benjamin Franklin

Values are the driving force in human life. To a large extent, a person's values determine his or her perception of the world, what decisions are made, and which path is taken. By exploring values, we can gain an understanding of pain and suffering.

Each person measures things and experiences by his or her own scale of values. Each person creates a personal hierarchy of values, which reflects one's personal preferences and goals, but is also influenced by circumstances. Each person's hierarchy of values is shaped by the influence of society and culture. Pain and suffering, therefore, have different meanings in different cultures.

Human suffering is a negative emotional experience that takes place when what we value most is lost or threatened or prevented from growing (Kozielecki, 1978). Pain, on the other hand, is primarily a cognitive process. Pain is important to us because it is a signal of impending danger. In this way, pain serves as a protective mechanism of the body. The main function of pain is to cause withdrawal from the source of danger or damage.

Although pain and suffering are not identical, the line that separates them is thin and often indistinguishable. An understanding of the nature, functions, and causes of pain and suffering, both in relation to each other and separately, is important for health professionals who need to comprehend the attitudes and behavior of patients in pain and know how to relate to them. The purpose of this chapter is to provide insights into the processes of pain and suffering so that we, as health care professionals, can do more than understand and treat the symptoms of these phenomena.

153

Indeed, we can be more effective listeners, and provide information when appropriate.

Pain and Suffering: Definitions

Pain, such as that caused by a cut on a finger, can be present in one's body without suffering. Conversely, one can suffer from anxiety or fear in the absence of physical pain. It is difficult to define either term. Descriptions of pain and suffering are highly personal and lack any reliable method for verification or measurement, which does not make personal definitions generalizable. Operational definitions of pain and suffering can be offered for purposes of discussion. Pain is the stimulation of some part of the body which the mind perceives as an injury or threat of injury to that portion of the body or the self as a whole (Boeyink, 1974). Suffering is an anguish that is experienced, not only as a pressure to change, but as a threat to one's composure, integrity, and the fulfillment of one's intentions (Williams, 1969).

Prevalence of Pain and Suffering

Pain can be an intensely private and unique experience, yet, at the same time, can provide a common, shared frame of reference, and may have a profound effect on the development and shaping of our lives. Pain is also a social problem, being the most common presenting symptom in doctors' offices, a major cause of absenteeism from work, and a cause of loss of national productivity and income. Bonica (1974) states that pain is an epidemic, costing from $40 to $50 billion yearly for drugs, health care, disability compensation, and lost wages.

A national study states that at least 40 million Americans suffer from chronic headaches, on which $4 billion are spent for medication alone, which result in a loss of 65 million workdays each year (U.S. Department of Health, Education, and Welfare, 1979). Lower back pain affects 15 million adults, with $5 billion spent in direct medical costs and 93 million workdays lost every year. Arthritis affects 20 million Americans resulting in over $4 billion in health care costs as well as lost income and productivity. Hundreds of thousands suffer from pain associated with cancer, phantom limb pain, chronic joint disease, neuralgia, and other types of pain. In spite of the evidence, much of this epidemic remains hidden from public awareness. Those who experience pain appear to be reluctant to make it known to others as the response to a person with chronic pain is often one of avoidance and social isolation. Golden and Steiner (1981) state that some of the factors that contribute to the social reluctance to accept pain in others are: (1) there is no way to prove that pain actually exists; (2) many of the causes of pain are not clear; and (3) it is often impossible to cure pain. Thus, it is difficult to distinguish real pain sufferers from those who might be using their pain for psychological and social gain.

Suffering is a concern that daily pervades the thoughts and conversations of every person. Grief is an example of suffering that is experienced many times by all of us throughout our lifetime. Suffering can also be experienced on the societal level. Mankind's most common and persistent problem is suffering as reflected in death, war, famine, violence, oppression, poverty, and sickness (Doughterty, 1982).

Meanings of Pain and Suffering

While pain is a universal human experience, it is not a single entity. Pain refers to a series of events and depends upon the interests and belief systems of the observer (Fordyce, 1986). Pain is a subjective personal experience. If pain is persistent, it becomes an experience actively created and fashioned by the self. Acute pain is usually a symptom of a bodily injury or illness. Chronic pain is often a sign that the sufferer wishes to occupy the sick role in the absence of illness (Szasz, 1975).

There is some tendency to conceptualize pain from a mind/body dualism approach (Sternbach, 1986). Mind/body dichotomies tend to focus on causes of pain that originate within the patient and ignore the crucial role played by the environment of the patient in the development and persistence of pain. What happens to the patient at home or at work may have a greater influence on the course of his/her disorder than does either mind or body.

The meaning and experience of pain is inseparable from the phenomenon of illness behavior. When one considers that pain is regarded as the most important initial warning sign of illness, illness behavior provides the bridge in attempts to delineate the individual and social factors which influence and shape the experience of pain. It is important to identify the sociocultural factors that influence patients' style and language when they communicate their pain experience as well as the more personal factors which determine the tendency to use pain and illness behavior as a way to cope with stress. The experience of pain covers a broad spectrum ranging from complaining of pain when no pain is experienced, e.g., children who cry before they are hurt, to living a life dominated by pain.

Although suffering often occurs in the absence of acute pain or other bodily symptoms, suffering extends beyond the physical. Generally, suffering is a state of severe distress associated with events that threaten the intactness of a person (Cassell, 1982). Everything unpleasant is not pain; thus, suffering is not always painful. Suffering is shaped by how a person responds to his or her experiences (Buytendijk, 1962). Goldberg (1986) points out that suffering is an interpersonal and learned process. We learn how to suffer at both individual and societal levels. Goldberg notes that the quality of the early bonding relationship between parent and child mirrors and models how the child will, in subsequent years, relate to others. Suffering comes from the lack of self-integration, lack of self-sufficiency, and lack of feeling that we are living up to our capacities.

The individual sufferer, through complaining, makes others witness his or her misfortune and induces others to show sympathy. Some sufferers surrender to circumstances, abandon hope, and live in a state of chronic depression. For others, voicing their feelings of suffering can mobilize sufficient social support and assistance from others to relieve their suffering.

Suffering often results in seeking someone or something to hold responsible. Some may blame others, bad luck, or God's punishment. A person's attitudes about the cause of suffering influence his/her willingness to do something to alleviate that suffering. People who feel that they have no control over a situation and are helpless to change it may become immobilized by their suffering. Lifton (1967), in his studies of survivors of Hiroshima, discovered that to protect themselves from the awful threat to their sanity, the survivors became psychically numb. At the other extreme, suffering can open new perspectives on life. Bovet (1973) proposes that suffering can lead to creative activity and new relationships with others. The intolerance of suffering can mobilize individuals to divert attention from their own needs and the trivia of daily life and assume responsibility for the survival and quality of life of others, e.g., environmental activists, fund-raising activities for farmers, food for Africa. Suffering can be personal and universal. It can range in form and scope from a concern about one's health to concern about the persecution of an entire nation. An individual gains purpose by grappling with his or her finiteness and mortality. Pain and suffering, in this sense, enables us to create a better world and a more developed self. It enables us to transcend pain and suffering to use our talents constructively. According to Goldstein (1959), we can achieve a higher degree of self-realization if we can endure suffering. He points out that health is related to a mental attitude by which an individual has to value what is essential for his or her life. Health is a value. It's value consists of the individual's capacity to actualize his or her nature to the degree it is essential. "Being sick," in pain, or suffering diminishes the value of health, of self-realization, and of existence. It is important to enable the sick person to make a choice which, in his/her view, makes life worth living. He or she may still suffer, but may no longer be immobilized by anxiety and feelings of helplessness (Seligman, 1975).

Cultural, Social, and Psychological Aspects of Pain

Cultural values are known to play an important role in the way a person perceives and responds to pain. One of the most striking examples of the impact of cultural values on pain is the hook-hanging ritual still practiced in parts of India (Kosambi, 1967). The ceremony derives from an ancient practice in which a member of a social group is chosen to present the power of the gods. The role of the chosen man is to bless the children and crops in a series of neighboring villages during a particular period of the year. What is remarkable about the ritual is that steel hooks, which are attached by strong ropes to the top of a special cart, are shoved under his skin and muscles on both sides of his back. The cart is then moved from village to village. Usually the man hangs on to the ropes as the cart is moved about. But at the climax of the ceremony in each village, he swings free, hanging only from the hooks embedded in his back, to bless the children and crops. There is no evidence that the man is in pain during the ritual, rather, he appears to be in a state of exaltation.

Except for trigeminal neuralgia, the incidence of other pain syndromes in China is lower than in Western countries (phantom pain, migraine and sciatica). Except for trigeminal all other pain syndromes are influenced by social and cultural factors. People in modern societies have a significant incidence of functional diseases with pain symptoms.

Modernization alienates people from nature because the conveniences brought about by modernization provide fewer opportunities for them to struggle physically for their needs. Sensory adaptability decreases and susceptibility to noxious stimuli increases. The pain threshold and pain tolerance decrease. In China, people are less alienated from nature and have fewer pain syndromes (Yu-huan & Neng-yu, 1989). Emotion can influence the pain threshold and pain tolerance. The Chinese are taught to be composed, hence affective psychoses, anxiety, and depression are rare. In addition, China has a different view of medical ethics. There is no consent obtained from patients for medical treatment. Doctors do not tell patients the truth in the case of terminal illness.

Zborowski (1969) studied the qualitative responses to pain among patients at a Veterans Hospital in Bronx, New York. The majority of the patients were amputees, had cancer, herniated discs, headaches, and various other disabilities. Zborowski was interested in how patients from different ethnic groups expressed their pain and their expectations about pain relief. He found that patients of Jewish or Italian origin tended to be more emotional while experiencing and expressing pain than did Anglo-Saxons. Emotional descriptions of pain experience occurred more frequently in interviews with Jewish and Italian patients than with Anglo-Saxon and Irish patients. This emotionality was expressed in the tendency of the Italian and Jewish patients to play up pain, whereas the Anglo-Saxon and Irish patients tended to play down pain. While the Irish and Anglo-Saxon patients said that they prefer to hide their pain, the Jewish and Italian patients admitted freely that they show pain by crying, complaining, and being more demanding. The expressive behavior was also manifest in motor responses to pain. Anxiety and worry were frequently expressed by Jewish patients. Jewish patients also expressed more concern about the symptomatic significance of pain. Italian patients tended to speak primarily of pain only and were less concerned with the future effects of pain.

Zola (1966) found differences in how Irish and Italian patients presented their complaints and expressed pain even when they had similar diagnoses. Koopman et al. (1984) compared patients over age 60 and found that Italian-Americans more frequently report pain than Anglo-Americans, but this difference was not found among the younger patients.

The complex sequences of behaviors appropriate to either the expression or suppression of pain, and the impact of the social environment, are seen in the religious rituals of some cultures. Penitents, flagellators, and others participating in religious acts involving self-inflicted pain require cultural training (Elton et al., 1983). For instance, in some cultures, when a child is born, the father takes to bed as if bearing the child and submits himself to fasting, purification, or taboos. This is called couvade (Kosambi, 1967). In Africa, during religious ceremonies, members of certain cults walk on burning coals, insert spikes into their flesh, and so on.

Contemporary Mediterranean peoples approve of free expression of pain and exhibit greater pain behavior than people of other cultures. The Anglo-Saxon cultures are somewhere between the two extremes of the free expression of pain and the repression of pain. Southern Negroes have been found to have a lower pain threshold than Americans of North European ancestry. Eskimos have been found to have higher pain thresholds than Alaskan Indians and whites. Woodrow et al. (1972) analyzed the pain tolerance scores of 41,119 subjects who took the Automated Multiphasic Screening exam at either the San Francisco or Oakland Kaiser Foundation Health Plan laboratories. They found that pain tolerance decreases with age, men tolerate more pain than women, and whites tolerate more pain than Orientals, while blacks occupy an intermediate position. In a study comparing the pain response of Afro-Asians and Whites, no differences were found. Flannery et al. (1981), found no difference in pain response to episiotomy among five ethnic groups— Black, Italian, Jewish, Irish, and Anglo-Saxon patients. Streltzer and Wade (1981) studied underuse of medication in the treatment of postoperative pain among Caucasians, Chinese, Japanese, Filipinos, and Hawaiians. They found that differences in pain responses among the groups were small. Lipton and Marbach (1984) studied patients' pain experiences in a facial pain clinic. The responses to pain reported by five ethnic groups (black, Italian, Jewish, Irish, and Puerto Rican) were similar, yet each group was quite different with regard to factors which influenced these responses.

It is often asserted that variations in pain experience from person to person are due to different "pain thresholds." However, there are several thresholds. Typically, thresholds are measured by applying a stimulus like an electric shock or radiant heat to a small area of the skin and gradually increasing the intensity. There is new evidence that all people, regardless of cultural background, have a uniform *sensation threshold*. Cultural background, however, has a powerful effect on the *pain perception threshold*. Levels of radiant heat that are reported as painful by people of Mediterranean origin are described as warm by Northern Europeans. The most striking effect of cultural background, however, is on *pain tolerance levels.* Sternbach and Tursky (1965) report that the levels at which subjects refuse to tolerate electric shock (even when encouraged by experimenters) depend, in part, on their ethnic origin.

Wolff and Langley (1975), in a review of the literature on the effects of ethnocultural factors on the response to pain, revealed a paucity of information. The few existing experimental studies yield equivocal results as to the significance of such factors and suffer from anthropological naiveté. Consequently, the question as to whether or not there are basic differences between ethnocultural groups in the response to pain remains unanswered. However, there is some experimental evidence that attitudinal factors do influence the response to pain within cultural groups. There is need for cultural anthropologists to combine efforts with medical investigators to add to our knowledge about cultural differences in pain responses.

Bates (1987) has noted that there is well documented cultural variability in the ways in which patients express pain symptoms, in their anxiety levels accompanying pain, and in their responses to different strategies in relieving pain. Yet, clinicians do not incorporate ethnic nor cultural differences as part of their diagnosis and treatment. She suggests that the gate-control theory of pain strongly suggests that psychological and cognitive variables have an impact on the physiological processes in human pain perception and response. Bates proposes that clinicians use a biocultural model in their practices.

There is considerable evidence to show that people also attach variable meaning to pain-producing situations and that the meaning greatly influences the degree and quality of the pain they feel. Beecher (1959) observed that most American soldiers who were wounded at Anzio in World War II either denied the existence of pain or expressed so little pain that they did not want any analgesics. When brought to combat hospitals, soldiers in only one out of three cases asked for morphine for their pain. When Beecher returned to clinical practice as an anesthesiologist, he asked civilians who, in major surgery, had incisions similar to the wounds received by the soldiers, whether they wanted morphine to alleviate their pain. In contrast to the wounded soldiers, four out of five claimed that they were in severe pain and needed morphine.

If a person's attention focuses on a potentially painful experience, he tends to perceive pain more intensely than he would normally. Distraction of attention can diminish pain. The influence of suggestion on the intensity of perceived pain is demonstrated by studies of the effectiveness of placebos (Melzach & Wall, 1982).

The evidence that pain is influenced by cultural factors leads to an examination of early experiences related to pain. It is commonly accepted that children are deeply influenced by attitudes of their parents toward pain. The influence of early experience on the perception of pain has been demonstrated experimentally by Melzach and Scott (1957). They found that Scottish terriers reared in sensory isolation booths did not seem to suffer pain after being released. The dogs did not avoid painful stimuli, such as a lighted match, even if burnt by it previously. This could be attributed to the effect of sensory deprivation per se. An alternative explanation might be that these dogs did not learn the fear of pain, or anxiety over pain, and were thus devoid of both.

Childrearing practices may determine future processing of pain experience. Melzack (1973) stated that children of families who disregard their pain behavior grow up more stoical in their approach to pain than children who are given undue attention by their parents for every minor childhood hurt. These children may grow up using pain as an attention-getting device and, therefore, may actually feel pain more.

Social modeling with families points out individual differences in pain experience (Craig, 1978). Parents teach their children ways of avoiding pain and injury. They also provide positive or negative reinforcement systems for the display of pain behaviors and the coping strategies in response to pain. Craig (1983) argued that in order to protect a child from harm, modeling of pain experience is essential. It substitutes vicarious experience for direct suffering, and teaches avoidance of potentially painful situations. At the same time, it trains the individual in a specific pattern of illness behaviors (Mechanic, 1962; Pilowski, 1980).

Sternbach (1968) noted that first born children and only children appear to have a lower tolerance to experimental pain, measured by electric shock stimulation. A possible explanation is that these children get more attention from their parents. On the other hand, children from large families seem to complain more about pain. This may be attributed to their need to attract parental attention.

Craig (1978) argued that there was a close correlation between the type of presenting complaint and a family history of the complaint; for example, children of families whose members suffered from recurrent abdominal pain also showed a tendency towards abdominal pain. Minuchin et al. (1975) proposed a conceptual model of psychosomatic illness in children. They argued that the onset of a situation, coupled with the personality of the individual, was critical in the development and maintenance of psychosomatic symptoms. They also suggested that disorganizing events within the family, such as death, negative parental attitudes, or parental struggles, may contribute to a child's psychosomatic illness. Certain types of family organizations are closely related to psychosomatic complaints in children. Psychosomatic symptoms may play a major role in maintaining family homeostasis (Bruhn, 1977).

Most studies concerned with the measurement of pain threshold and tolerance in different age groups indicate that there is a progressive increase in reports of pain as individuals grow older (Elton et al., 1983). Weisenberg (1977) pointed out that, clinically, age can be an important factor in assessing pain reaction and treatment approach. It seems that there is a significant correlation between age and responses to pain. Mersky (1965) found that in a psychiatric population, the complaints of persistent pain were most frequent in the older age groups, and conversely, the denial of pain was associated with younger patients.

The data on sex differences in the experience of pain is controversial. Some authors have found there is no difference in pain threshold between the sexes. Other authors have claimed that females have a lower pain tolerance than males (Elton et al., 1983). The data are equally puzzling as there seem to be sex differences in the propensity for certain types of complaints; for example, women seem to suffer more from migraine and facial pain, whereas men seem to suffer more from lower back pain. There have also been some interesting reports of differences in the attitude of hospital staff towards the administration of analgesics to men and women. Females were more likely to be offered analgesics on the staff's own initiative; males generally had to complain about their pain before they were given analgesics (Pilowsky & Bond, 1969).

Hypochondriasis and psychogenic pain are often associated with lower socioeconomic status (Mersky, 1965; Pilowsky, 1968). Several researchers have observed that patients from the lower socioeconomic group had a tendency to see the presenting problem as physical rather than emotional. Mersky (1978) described a personality profile of hypochondriacal patients based upon socioeconomic distinctions. Generally, they were married, yet unsuccessful in their marriages, came from large families, were skilled or semi-skilled workers, and placed an emphasis on bodily complaints. Lower back pain traditionally has been associated with men who are skilled and unskilled workers who come from large families.

These men are viewed as routine-minded, obsessional types. Many suffer from poor sexual adjustment or impotence.

Social factors can also play a role in maintaining chronic pain. Pain can become an object of attention, concern, and care and, therefore, provide a reinforcer for the maintenance of pain and disability. Excessive economic pressures may predispose an individual to maintain pain. The family plays a part in the maintenance of symptoms. Pain may become the central point of interactions and may bring about a redistribution of roles among family members. The attitude of the spouse is crucial in the maintenance of pain. A spouse who is anxious or depressed may produce greater anxiety or depression in the patient or, on the other hand, may withdraw support and seek it for him/herself. This may exacerbate the patient's pain symptoms. Sometimes the spouse will report suffering from pain and may present symptoms similar to those of the patient. A sense of guilt in family members may result in overconcern and produce increased symptomatology. Other factors, such as the need for control, escape from conflicts, hidden animosities between family members, all help to maintain pain (Elton et al., 1983). Mirowsky and Ross (1986) point out that alienation, authoritarianism, and inequity produce distress and that distress is reduced by control, commitment, support, meaning, flexibility, trust, and equity. Pain changes people. Sternbach (1974) noted that the effect of pain is to cause emotional disturbance and this changes a person's perception of the world, his/her relationship with others, and his/her preoccupations and activities. People in pain have unique needs.

Individuality in Pain and Suffering

A friend told me that he didn't know what pain and suffering really meant until his daughter was diagnosed with manic-depressive illness. Over the past ten years, she has been maintained on lithium, but about once each year, she has to be hospitalized when she fails to take her lithium. Recently, my friend and his wife were going on a much needed vacation and asked their daughter whether she would like someone to stay with her while they were gone. The daughter wished to stay alone. Upon returning from vacation, my friend and his wife found that the daughter had done about $125,000 damage to the house "cleaning out old things," including my friend's prize stamp collection, which he had

STRONG, SILENT AND SUFFERING
Stephen R. Morris

My neighbor Max had his heart attack in silence. The rescue squad arrived shortly after dawn on Saturday morning. Max's wife, Lillian, was back home that afternoon. "He's getting the best care he can get," she told me. "After that, it's in God's hands."

Lillian was stunned, but talkative. And in her detailed chronology of the day's events she kept returning to Max's reticence. "I don't understand why he didn't say anything earlier," she lamented. The rescue workers were shocked when they found him, sweating profusely, his face ashen, hardly able to breathe. Why hadn't she called earlier, they demanded, with the reflexive exasperation the young in this community feel for the old. She had, of course, called within seconds of waking to the sound of Max's breathless coughing, pausing only to administer her own bedside oxygen mask to him, and to dry his sopping face.

Max had said nothing. Throughout much of the night he sweated and struggled with the oppressive weight on his chest, somehow convincing himself that it would pass, or that it was not serious enough for him to wake his companion of over 35 years. This she could not understand. "You'd think an intelligent man, college educated,

a professional—you'd think he'd know better," she said later. "Or maybe his mind was too cloudy. Or he just cared too much."

I didn't mention to her a fourth possibility. I didn't mention how natural Max's conduct seemed to me, how I was seeing stoic resistance where she saw at best a foolish solicitude. And I didn't mention how Max's silence seemed to me a simple manifestation of a prevalent male habit: the impulse to suffer alone.

I imagined Max's agonized denials, so resonant with similar inner dialogues I have recited to myself. "Perhaps I had better wake her. But don't be ridiculous—it's 3 in the morning! It would just upset her—and then me. And it's not so bad. I can deal with it; it'll pass . . ."

Max's silence, so disturbing and inexplicable to his wife, struck a deep chord. Pain is best left unspoken—an ideal with roots at least as deep as Plato, who writes that "it is finest to keep as quiet as possible in misfortune." Our culture has encoded many values that are heir to Plato's sentiment: the "stiff upper lip" we admire as a hallmark of English breeding; the athlete who "plays with pain" and without excuses; even the (male) child who suppresses his tears. These values are learned, and go on to become traits of character.

Of course we hesitate to see anything heroic about Max's silent endurance of his heart attack, even as we rain plaudits on the football player who continues to play after a mild concussion. But both acts stem from the same ethos: the first is simply the second in a mundane, relational dimension. Both Max and the player must play the role of the strong, silent type. The player, of course, plays on a stage, before an audience, sometimes for stakes that are the stuff of a schoolboy's dreams. Max, by contrast, plays out of habit. Far from relishing, as the player does, the heady intoxication of the state, he engages in elaborate rationalizations to convince himself he is acting rightly by telling no one how he feels.

Rational thing: Surely Lillian is right: Max should have told her sooner. He should have thought to share with her the profound disturbance he was experiencing. But I shudder at drawing from this conclusion a call to men to "communicate their feelings" better. For one thing, traits of character are stubborn things, no matter how much exposed to the cool light of reason. Max was silent because he is habitually silent about such things—that's the way he is.

For another, it should give us pause to advocate eradicating an ethi-cal standard that has thrived since, and for long before, Plato. This is not to say that a standard is merely a function of age and lineage. It is to urge that we not forget the reasoning that first implanted the standard in the Western psyche, so deeply that both Max and I, and millions of other men and women alike still find our lives swayed by it. Plato argued that to keep quiet in pain was the only deliberate, rational thing to do, the fastest way, as he put it, of "Banishing threnody by therapy."

No doubt some middle ground can be reached, as the issue is thrashed out in those silent dialogues Max and I conduct with ourselves, and in particular as some of those dialogues are given reluctant voice in marriages that can no longer bear the weight of silence. Max is gradually gaining a new lease on his life. When his recovery has proceeded enough, Lillian will take up with him more earnestly what remains for her the incident's central perplexity. Max, perhaps, will learn something new. He will not change much—if anything, surviving a heart attack will make him even more of a stoic. But perhaps his wife will impress a new impulse on his soul—to turn to her the next time his life hangs in the balance.

I wonder if the male ethic of lone suffering is tied to an equally pervasive but more insidious male ethic; to exclude women from life-

and-death decision making. (Here the cultural antecedents are even more venerable, beginning with Abraham's decision not to consult Sarah when God told him to sacrifice his son, Isaac, on a mountaintop). If so, it is a deep-rooted linkage, one not subject to alteration in physical struggle with a heart attack. And one just as hard to disentangle from the dialectic of dependency and autonomy that makes a marriage such a complex and difficult thing.

Reprinted from *Newsweek*, April 3, 1989, with permission of the author.

assembled since age eight, antique furniture, original scores of music, and other family treasures. The fact that my friend was a psychiatrist and understood the psychodynamics of manic depressive illness did not lessen his pain and suffering.

What pain and suffering mean to us individually, how we experience and cope with them, are personal and, therefore, unique. Le Shan (1964) regards pain as a form of communication, although our vocabulary for the description of pain is poor and usually contains metaphors of violence (e.g., stabbing pain, shooting pain, burning pain, etc., Mersky, 1968). Melzach and Tongerson (1971) have provided a comprehensive vocabulary for patients to choose words descriptive of pain across a variety of disorders.

Pain is a way of stating a psychological situation and feeling. How pain is expressed gives others a message. It can be a way to ask for social support, empathy, or to call attention to a predicament creating the need for financial or other help. It can be a way to express one's limits of tolerance with a life situation or stress. Pain can also be a way of communicating one's inner needs and feelings, such as guilt, frustration, ambivalence, hurt pride, or fear. The hardest task for a health professional is to help the patient make sense of his/her pain and suffering.

It is clear that we must recognize the psychological contribution to pain, but we must maintain a balanced view of it. Psychological factors contribute to pain, and pain may be influenced by psychology. This does not deny the existence of people who need their pain and whose lives derive meaning from it. Perhaps the most convincing evidence that chronic pain is usually the cause rather than the result of neurotic symptoms derives from studies of patients who are eventually relieved of their pain. Typically, these patients, while they are suffering from chronic pain, show evidence of psychological disturbance on the Minnesota Multiphasic Personality Inventory (MMPI). In particular, they have elevated scores on hysteria, depression, and hypochondriasis. Some investigators have argued that these personality characteristics lead to pain or to susceptibility to chronic pain after minor injuries that would have little effect on people who do not have these characteristics. A chronic emotional problem is assumed to become manifest as chronic pain. However, the evidence points in the other direction: pain produces the elevations in these emotional characteristics. In one study, it was found that patients who had pain of more than six months duration—due to special injuries, postherpetic neuralgia, and other problems—showed significant decreases in several indices of psychological disturbance when their pain was abolished by successful surgery (Sternbach and Timmermans, 1975). Similarly, patients suffering several forms of chronic pain, including headache and abdominal pain, were found to have lower self-esteem than pain-free control groups. However, after these patients underwent several therapeutic procedures that significantly reduced their pain, they showed a striking improvement in their self-esteem ratings (Elton et al., 1978). It is unreasonable to ascribe chronic pain to neurotic symptoms. Patients with thick charts are often considered neurotic and that their neuroses are the cause of their pain. Indeed, patients whose pain complaint can be understood in physical terms have been found to be undistinguishable from patients whose pain complaint is psychological in presentation. All too often the diagnosis of neurosis as the cause of pain hides our ignorance of the many aspects of pain because we do not want to take time to talk with the patient about his/her pain. This lack of a "healing partnership" is why patients may seek out nontraditional types of healers, e.g., religious healers, chiropractors, to relieve their pain, in addition to or in lieu of, traditional medical treatment.

How an individual experiences pain and suffering now is closely related to how he/she has experienced them in the past (Murray, 1975). Anticipation and attitude help shape new pain experiences. Hall and Stride (1954) showed that subjects' attitudes influenced the amount of pain response. When the researchers used the word "pain" in their instructions to the subjects of their experiment, the subject's anticipations were translated into greater sensitivity, or lower thresholds for pain than those of similar subjects who received the same stimulus, but with a neutral instructional set. The term "pain experience" has been suggested as a substitute for "pain" because it includes an individual's reaction to the threat of pain.

Pain is a barometer which helps us monitor our health. We expect pain to follow certain behavior, for example, aching legs after a long hike. If pain is not present when we expect it, we become alarmed that something is wrong. Dr. Paul W. Brand, the noted leprosy expert who was chief of the rehabilitation branch of the leprosarium in Carville, Louisiana, had a frightening experience one night when he thought he had contracted leprosy. Dr. Brand arrived in London one night after an exhausting transatlantic ocean trip and long train ride from the English coast. He was getting ready for bed, had taken off his shoes, and as he pulled off a sock, discovered there was no feeling in his heel. To most anyone else this discovery would have meant very little, a momentary numbness. But Dr. Brand was world famous for his restorative surgery on lepers in India. He had convinced himself and his staff at the leprosarium that there was no danger of infection from leprosy after it reached a certain stage. The numbness in his heel terrified him.

In her biography of Dr. Brand, *Ten Fingers for God* (1965), Dorothy Clarke Wilson says, "He rose mechanically, found a pin, sat down again, and pricked the small area below his ankle. He felt no pain. He thrust the pin deeper, until a speck of blood showed. Still he felt nothing. Like other workers with leprosy, he had always half expected it. In the beginning probably not a day had gone by without the automatic searching of his body for the tell tale patch, the numbed area of skin.

All that night the great orthopedic surgeon tried to imagine his new life as a leper, as outcast, his medical staff's confidence in their immunity shattered by this disaster. And the forced separation from his family. As night receded, he yielded to hope and in the morning, with clinical objectivity, 'with steady fingers he bared the skin below his ankle, jabbed in the point—and yelled.'

Blessed was the sensation of pain! He realized that during the long train ride, sitting immobile, he had numbed a nerve. From then on, whenever Dr. Brand cut his finger, turned an ankle, even when he suffered from "agonizing nausea as his whole body reacted in violent self-protection from mushroom poisoning, he was to respond with gratitude, 'Thank God for pain!' " (pp. 142–145).

Pain and Suffering as Adaptation

Kotarba (1983) points out that in the course of coping with pain and suffering, people develop a meaning for the pain and suffering they are

MOST OF ALL, JOHN HENRY WAS JUST A FRIEND
John Whitmire

The Houston Post Staff

The thought of never seeing another sunrise—or hearing the voice of his wife and the laughter of his children—made John Henry Faulk break down and cry one day last month.

John Henry Faulk knew he was dying that day. A cancer was eating away at his insides, and the pain had been fierce and unforgiving weeks before he died Monday.

He was with a friend—Austin satirist Cactus Pryor—and they were cruising around Austin, talking about life and how fine it could be sometimes.

"When you loved life as much as John Henry did, he had good reason not to want to say goodbye to it," Pryor said in a telephone interview from his Austin home on Tuesday.

John Henry Faulk was 76 when he succumbed to throat cancer. Funeral services for the humorist and folklorist have been set for Saturday at University Methodist Church in his hometown of Austin.

Despite his yearning to live, the pain had grown so intense during the last few weeks of his life that he briefly considered suicide.

Another close friend, Houston businessman Randy Parten, remembers the day five or six weeks ago that Faulk talked openly about ending it all.

"He told me he was really suffering," Parten said. "And then some of his loved ones told him that as long as his heart was still beating—no matter what his quality of life was—he owed it to them to go on living.

"I remember he called himself a chicken. I told John Henry that—over his lifetime—a lot of folks had called him a lot of things, but chicken was not one of them."

That was the last time Parten saw his friend.

And these are the last words Faulk spoke to him: "I really am a very lucky man. I chose the hard road for myself. I had some rough and tumble times along the way. But in the end, I think it was a pretty good life."

Wednesday, April 11, 1990, *Houston Post*

experiencing and define or redefine themselves in terms of the pain and suffering. This is, perhaps, most profound in the case of a life-threatening illness which evokes questions of ultimacy. Modes of adapting are as varied as those experiencing it. People may become depressed, others react with anxiety and fear, others react with denial, others with anger and hostility, others with a determination to fight, and some give up (Slaby and Glicksman, 1985). Many who survive a life-threatening illness experience a change in values. We are all familiar with persons who have changed their priorities for daily life following a near death experience, such as a heart attack, or who survived an illness that was supposed to be terminal (Cousins, 1979, 1983). Chronic illness, pain, and suffering can make individuals and families stronger, or they can create further strife. Individuals who are not happy or whose marriages are filled with tension or unsatisfying love affairs, may be so consumed with conflict that there is little energy left to fight their disease. Depressed people become more so when struck with life-threatening illness, and are more vulnerable to the disease and complications of treatment. Crises created by husbands who walk out on their wives after mastectomies, by men or women who walk out on their lovers following a colostomy, and by the sudden withdrawal of family members or friends from patients wasting away from cardiac or pulmonary disease or AIDS; work against whatever biological successes may be hoped for with medical treatment. Specific stresses confront individuals with life-threatening illnesses. These include loss of autonomy, beauty, potency, friends and family, fear of death, mutilation, loss of job and income, treatment, limited functioning, pain, greater dependence on others, change in body image, uncertain prognosis, mood changes, cognitive deterioration, and medical complications of the illness (Slaby and Glicksman, 1985).

Life can become dominated by pain or pain can be dominated by life (Kleinman, 1988). We all know persons who live life from one pain to the next. Living has become so painful for them that they choose to live everyday as a struggle. On the other hand, we also know persons who experience continual pain (physical and/or social-psychological) and who seem to transcend it by living life in spite of their illness or limitations of life style. Pain and suffering, at both extremes, are real to those involved. However, the former persons derive meaning for their life through pain and suffering, while the latter persons do not permit pain and suffering to take meaning from their lives.

Everyone experiences loss, depression, pain, and suffering at points throughout their lives. Seligman (1975) notes that persons who are most resistant to developing helplessness are those who feel they have control of their lives and can manipulate sources that provide reinforcement to deal with traumas as they arise. Similarly, Wood (1986) claims that we have been led to believe that common unhappiness is an illness called neurosis, which people have used as an excuse for their inadequate approach to problems and unrealistic expectations of what life should bring them. He states that life is tough and frequently unpleasant, but that we should not become slaves to our predicament and seek to change ourselves for the better. As Sontag (1978) has said, "Everyone who is born holds dual citizenship in the kingdom of the well and in the kingdom of the sick. Although we all prefer to use only the good passport, sooner or later, each of us is obliged, at least for a spell, to identify ourselves as citizens of that other place" (p. 3).

Acute and Chronic Pain

The terms "acute" and "chronic" sometimes are used to mean "reversible" and "irreversible" respectively, but they can also mean short-term and long-term pain. Some reports, which make a distinction between acute and chronic pain, refer to a variable time of four to six months or longer when using the word "chronic" and a shorter period of time when "acute" is used. Time is closely associated with different psychological reactions to pain. Figures 6-1 and 6-2 contrast the different emotions that emerge depending upon the length of time pain has persisted. Woodforde and Mersky (1972) concluded that the effect of chronic pain is to cause emotional disturbance. Studies tend to support the notion that when normal persons experience organic pain, they develop patterns of emotional responses which, over time, look increasingly similar to those whose pain is psychogenic. The degree of similarity seems partly determined by the severity and duration of the pain and partly by the patient's preexisting neuroticism, which, in turn, determines the severity of the pain experienced (Sternbach, 1977). Different diagnoses are made in the acute and chronic stages of pain. In general, acute pain patients show test patterns and mental status responses that are normal or that show a tendency to an anxiety reaction or a hysterical defense against anxiety. On the other hand, as pain persists over time, anxiety appears to give way to depression.

Chronic pain is rarely life-threatening. Unlike acute pain, or pain associated with terminal illnesses, chronic pain is benign. Chronic pain becomes an unpleasant, if not emotionally growing, context for an individual's everyday life. Medicine's common prescription for chronic

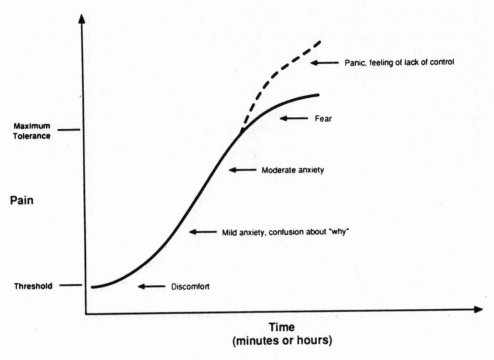

Figure 6-1. Sequence of reactions to acute pain.

pain is to "learn to live with it." An individual's strategy for coping with chronic pain is shaped largely by the degree to which that person accepts the inevitability of suffering (Kotarba, 1983).

The pattern of illnesses that occur with age are, for the most part, chronic, and many are associated with discomfort, pain, and suffering. A recent report concerned with new-pain visits in over 70 million patient visits indicated that first-time pain complaints occur mainly in patients 15 to 44 years of age. First-time pain visits to office-based physicians are at their lowest in the elderly, in whom the pain complaint has been a recurrent or chronic problem. Little is known concerning the impact of recurrent or chronic pain on the older individual. The old are very underrepresented at major chronic pain centers. This is surprising considering that as many as 80 percent of the old are estimated to have at least one chronic ailment that is likely to be a source of pain and suffering. In another regard, this may not be surprising. Chronic pain is a major stress. The frail, older person with a reduced capacity to cope with stress may not survive the time period used to define chronic pain. More likely, individuals are not referred to specialty care and pain

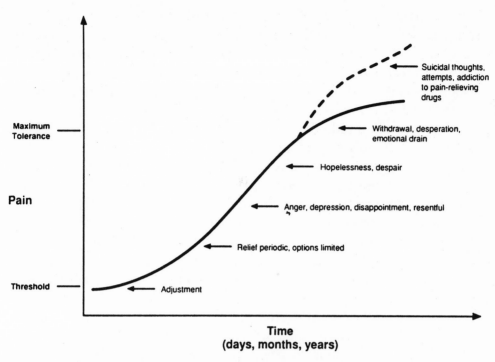

Figure 6-2. Sequence of reactions to chronic pain.

clinics. And, indeed, the older person and the health care practitioner may accept the presence of pain as a "normal" consequence of aging (Harkins, 1988).

The Ethics of Pain Management

The goal of pain management will often be to make pain less evocative of suffering, even when the pain itself may remain. Ethical issues in pain management can be analyzed using the contrast between medical and nonmedical models of care, and the patient-therapist model of pain management versus the client-service provider model of pain management (Engelhardt, 1980). These dyads signal differences in the amount of active participation in pain management ranging from the patient who accepts the management provided by the therapist to the patient who decides upon the form and circumstances of the management to be provided. Depending upon this spectrum, there are different ethical issues. There can be profound value conflicts with respect to pain management because of the different ways in which one can view the place of patient/client participation in pain management. There are also religious values regarding pain and suffering and their expression. Kotarba (1983) points out that Christianity is most notable for attributing a positive meaning to physical pain. Whereas the Old Testament repeatedly speaks of pain as a form of punishment, the New Testament ascribes a religious significance to suffering within the framework of God's plan of salvation for mankind. For the Christian believer, pain and physical suffering are God's way of testing, strengthening, and purifying his children. The good Christian is expected to endure pain patiently.

The ethical questions raised by pain management can be put into two categories. One concerns free and informed consent. It involves the ways in which free individuals may agree on joint projects. The second involves hierarchies of values in which the good of pain control is balanced against such risks as permanent physical damage and addiction. The ethical dilemmas of pain management reflect the general problems of moral conduct, that is, how to allow free agents to create their own ways of living and dying (Engelhardt, 1980).

The usual response to pain, suffering, and death in our society is to subject these phenomena to technical management and control. The medicalization of pain, suffering, and dying eliminates the need for individuals to assume responsibility and frees the family from the responsibility of caring and sharing. There are many ways in which people transcend pain and suffering—alcohol, drugs, tranquilizers, and television. Moller (1986–1987) states that the denial of suffering diminishes human loving, decreases the meaningfulness of human experience in suffering, and anesthetizes a person to the suffering of others and the suffering they cause others.

Once a patient is in pain, there are broad humanistic ethics which apply to the domain of medical care, which give patients a strong *prima facie* right to freedom from unnecessary pain, and which place upon health professionals, two moral obligations to patients. First, is the duty not to inflict pain and suffering beyond that which is absolutely necessary for effective diagnosis, treatment, and research. Next, is the duty to do all that can be done within the limits of current medical knowledge and available resources to relieve all the pain and suffering that can be alleviated. Attempts to fulfill these obligations must be subject to the informed consent of the patient and must be compatible with the goal of an ultimate restoration of health where there is hope of a cure, with the patient's own plans and desires for living and dying where there is no such hope, or with conditions that override patients' preferences. Edwards (1984) discusses seven conditions which set aside or override the principle of informed consent and the right to refuse treatment: where the patient is unconscious, confused, or overwhelmed by pain so that he/she is not rational; when the patient's condition presents a clear danger to others because of assault or serious communicable disease; where other persons depend so heavily on the patient that the state has a compelling interest in preserving the patient's life; when the patient is a minor; where the patient is mentally incompetent; where sufficient efforts have not been made to ensure that the patient is adequately informed or where it appears that the patient is acting under duress; and where a review committee considers the patient's prospects for suffering and for a meaningful future existence.

The Duty to Relieve Suffering

Suffering, like happiness, fear, and hope, has always formed a part of human fate and, therefore, is an ineradicable part of human life. (Kozielecki, 1978). Suffering is a culturally and personally distinctive form of affliction of the human spirit. James (1982) discusses the arguments proposed regarding our duty to relieve suffering including the proposal that we have a duty to relieve suffering because it is evil, that people must relieve suffering whenever they are in a position to do so, and that people must, at least, give up their resources to the point where they would sacrifice something of moral importance if they were to give more. James discusses our responsibility for harm. She notes that if each of us were to assume responsibility for all the suffering we could relieve, we would acquire an enormous burden of responsibility and guilt. A role for health professionals, which is equally as important as relieving suffering, is the prevention of suffering. Health professionals have a moral responsibility to advise and even warn patients about the consequences of certain behaviors and life styles on their future health, just as much as they have a professional responsibility to minimize the pain and suffering of patients who are sick, disabled, and dying.

The issue of the responsibility of individuals, and collectively of a country, to prevent suffering is evident in the current export and promotion of American cigarettes to other countries, while it is well established that smoking cigarettes is hazardous to one's health. The responsibility for prevention clashes with the economic value of free enterprise and the career interests of politicians from tobacco growing states. The United States, by permitting the marketing of tobacco in other countries while there are continuous attempts to limit its use at home because it is a health hazard, is permitting the unnecessary suffering of millions of individuals throughout the world. Some people would argue that individuals should have free choice of what habits and behavior they wish to engage in as long as their behavior does not harm others. This argument could be extended to say that harm and suffering extends beyond an individual to his/her family.

The theory of responsibility we use to assess blame deals with the actions of private individuals and aims to specify the types of circumstances in which people are morally responsible for harm they have caused and those in which they are excused. But private individuals are not the only agents of harm and the theory loses clarity at this level. A striking example is the policy adopted by the Occupational Safety and Health Administration (OSHA) toward the use of organophosphate pesticides. These chemicals are known to be extremely dangerous to humans, but ever since the banning of DDT in 1972, they have been widely used by farmers growing fruits and vegetables, despite the considerable risk to which this exposes their employees. In 1970 the Environmental Protection Agency recorded 5,729 cases of severe poisoning among pesticide formulators, airplane loaders and spreaders, and field workers, who suffered from dizziness; sweating; headaches; cramps; loss of appetite; sores; bloody urine; muscle spasms in the esophagus; bleeding from the eyes, nose, and mouth; and respiratory arrest (Zwerding, 1975). An official from the U.S. Department of Agriculture estimated that there are 80,000 poisonings and 800 deaths from pesticides each year. Some attempts have been made to ban the use of organophosphate sprays. Faced with stricter rules, a number of growers pressed for a policy known to cause harm, the OSHA approved it and some workers fell ill or died as a result. It might be argued that the farmers had no choice but to lobby for the legalization of these pesticides. OSHA repealed its own regulations and thus exposed workers to harm and failed in their duty to protect them. Harm resulted from both omissions and commissions.

Acquired immune deficiency syndrome (AIDS) vividly illustrates the range of suffering from the individual to the societal level. Like tuberculosis, cancer, and leprosy, AIDS is an affliction of a person and of society. The way in which a person, a family, or a community responds to AIDS reveals a great deal about core cultural values. AIDS can be viewed as suffering from several standpoints (Farmer & Kleinman, 1989). AIDS is suffering because it is compounded by the inappropriate use of resources. For patients with chronic illness, routine biomedical treatment should be complemented by humane care that affirms the illness experience and its meaning. Certain practical clinical strategies can, when given with the attitude of compassion for illness as a burden of the human spirit, improve health care for those who cannot be cured. AIDS is suffering because it is magnified by discrimination. Discrimination has been evident in employment, housing, granting of visas, and health care. The "victims" of such discrimination are not only people with AIDS and positive HIV infection, but those thought to be in "risk groups." AIDS is suffering because it is augmented by fear. Despite facts about how AIDS is transmitted, people's behavior toward individuals with AIDS has been one of social withdrawal and avoidance. Fear has created suspicion and doubt between possible sexual partners. No one can be sure who knowingly or unknowingly carries the HIV virus. AIDS is suffering amplified by social death. The diagnosis of AIDS is also a death sentence. Shame, stigma, guilt, humiliation, and outright rejection can encourage suicide or giving up. Indeed, many persons with AIDS die socially before they die physically. AIDS is also suffering generated by inequities. AIDS emerges from and contributes to social cycles of human misery, such as drug addiction, sexual promiscuity, alienation, and neglect of personal health. Many of the causes and consequences of AIDS lie outside of traditional medical intervention. The public's response to AIDS has been divided and ambivalent and has constrained the natural response of the human spirit to alleviate suffering (Farmer & Kleinman, 1989).

The Right to Die

Bakan (1968) has said, "there are two major points in life which are beyond the scope of individual will. One is conception; the other is death. Between these, but not including them, the will of the individual has its proper sphere" (p. 128).

It is the promise of medicine that doctors should be healers and caregivers; that they must work for the patient's well-being; that if they cannot cure, they should at least do no harm. For many physicians and other health professionals, the actions they take often depend more on circumstance than on moral certainty. How far is the patient from death? How great is the pain? How clear is the patient's will to live? The American College of Neurology argues that the doctor's duty is to continue treating unconscious patients as long as there is some chance of improvement. When hope is gone, then duty ends (Gibbs, 1990).

Nancy Cruzan, at age 32, had done nothing for seven years. Since her car crashed on an icy night, she had lain so still for so long that her hands curled into claws; nurses wedged napkins under her fingers to prevent the nails from piercing her wrists. "She would hate being like this," said her mother. "It took a long time to accept that she wasn't getting better." If they chose, the Cruzans could have slipped into Nancy's room, disconnected her feeding tube, and faced the consequences. Instead, they asked the U.S. Supreme Court for permission to end their daughter's life.

Nancy was not dying, she could have lived for years. Since she was awake, most doctors agreed that she was not suffering. But her parents were suffering. They were so convinced Nancy would not want to go on this way that they asked the court for authorization to "let her go." A lower court judge gave that permission, but the Missouri Supreme Court, affirming the "sanctity of life," reversed the ruling. The U.S. Supreme Court avoided ruling on whether the federal Constitution's liberty guarantees a right to die for mercy's sake until July, 1990, when the court reached a narrow decision. By one vote, the Justices said Missouri could use the lack of "clear and convincing evidence" of Nancy Cruzan's wishes to block removal of a feeding tube that had kept her alive in a vegetative state for seven years. But in handing legislative leeway to states, the Court recognized for the first time a "constitutionally protected liberty interest in refusing unwanted medical treatment," a finding that could lead toward euthanasia for millions with ailments from Alzheimer's disease to dementia. In its broad outline, the Cruzan ruling reflects growing public sentiment for the right to die. In December, 1990, the Missouri Supreme Court agreed that the feeding tube could be removed from Nancy Cruzan. Twelve days later she died.

The Association of American Physicians and Surgeons argue that the obligation of the physician to the comatose, vegetative, or developmentally disabled patient does not depend upon the prospect for recovery. The physician must always act on behalf of the patient's well-being. This principle can mean ignoring or overriding the patient's express wishes.

MAN SUES HOSPITAL FOR SAVING HIS LIFE

By David Margolick

New York Times

CINCINNATI—In some ways, Edward H. Winter is a prototypical miracle of modern medicine.

He would probably have died of a heart attack in May, 1988, when he was 82, if a nurse at St. Francis-St. George Hospital had not revived him through electric shock.

He has just marked his 84th birthday, and his daughters and grandchildren brought him a cake.

It is not the fate he wanted.

A few months before his heart attack, he watched the slow death of his wife of 55 years, who had suffered brain damage after shock resuscitation from a heart attack of her own, and he resolved that nothing like that would happen to him.

When his time came, he told his children, they should let him die. He told his doctor the same thing.

Things have turned out even more nightmarish than Winter could have imagined, and he has filed a lawsuit accusing the hospital of wrongfully saving his life.

Two days after he was revived, he suffered a debilitating stroke.

He is now partly paralyzed and largely confined to his nursing home bed. Although he can still speak, he can utter only a few words before he begins to cry, in despair.

The lawsuit, brought in November in the Hamilton County Court of Common Pleas, charges the hospital with negligence for failing to follow Winter's instructions and with battery for giving him a jolt of electricity without his authorization.

But for the hospital's intervention, he has charged, he could have died, and in dignity.

His medical bills now total about $100,000 and are rising. His life savings are just about depleted.

His doctors see scant chance for physical improvement. They say he could live for years.

"There are in fact some things worse than death, and what has happened to Mr. Winter is one of them," said his lawyer, William C. Knapp of Cincinnati.

The hospital's motion for dismissal of the lawsuit is pending.

Its lawyers said Winter's version of the facts was incorrect, but they declined to be specific.

The facts do not really matter, they add since saving a life can never be considered, in legal terms, an injury that can be compensated.

"There is no case directly on point, but the case law suggests that if you save someone's life you cannot be held liable," said Deborah R. Lydon, who teaches health care law at the University of Cincinnati College of Law.

Winter was visiting friends at a

Cincinnati center for the elderly May 1988 when he felt chest pains and collapsed.

In the hospital's coronary care unit, he told his doctor, George E. Russo, he did not want to be resuscitated if his condition worsened.

Winter gave the same instructions to his daughters, Lynn Kroger and Joan Muenchen, both of Cincinnati, and Ann Wessel of Syracuse, N.Y.

Russo entered those instructions on Winter's chart. But, Knapp said the instructions were not recorded on the monitor by Winter's bed.

Thus, three days later, when he began experiencing ventricular fibrillations that signal sudden death, a nurse applied electrodes to his chest and revived him.

Kroger said even before his stroke her father was angry over what had happened.

"He said he could have died in peace if they had left him alone and that now he was completely dependent," she recalled. "He was upset being the way he was. My father is a pretty staunch Catholic, and would never have taken his own life, but he didn't believe in dragging people back to life."

She said her father asked to see a lawyer.

In his conversations with Winter, Knapp said, the octogenarian knew he had told the hospital not to revive him, he knew it had done so, "and he knew what shape he ended up in."

The hospital argues any damages Winter has suffered resulted from "an act of God" over which the hospital had no control.

Winter spends most of his time in his room at Hillebrand Nursing Home in Cheviot, Ohio, where he does little but lament his fate.

Recently he showed a visitor his limp right arm and described how it was useless even though "it looked all right."

He appeared unable to cope with questions about his lawsuit. He seemed unable to recognize his lawyer.

Sunday, March 18, 1990, *Houston Chronicle*

When Dax Cowart was critically burned in a propane gas explosion, he begged a passing farmer for a gun with which to kill himself. On his way to the hospital, he pleaded with the medic to let him die. For weeks his life hung by a thread. For more than a year, against his will, he endured excruciating treatment: his right eye and several fingers were removed, his left eye was sewn shut. His pain and protests were unrelenting. One night he crawled out of bed to try to throw himself out of a window, but was discovered and prevented from doing so.

That was 17 years ago. Cowart is now a law school graduate, married, and managing his investments. Yet he argues that doctors violated his right to choose not to be treated. "It doesn't take a genius to know when you're in that amount of pain, you can either bear it or you can't," he says. "And I couldn't." He still resents the powerless of patients who are forced to live when they beg to die. "The physicians say that when a patient is in that much pain, he is not competent to make judgments about himself. It's the pain talking. And when narcotics are given to subdue the pain, they say it's the narcotics talking. It's a no-win situation." (Gibbs, 1990; Kliever, 1989).

Overtreatment of the terminally ill strikes physicians as both wasteful and inhumane. Patients living within sight of death often find themselves more concerned with the quality of life than with its quantity. Once reconciled to the inevitable, they want to die with dignity, not submerged in a battery of machines in an intensive care unit.

When her cancer was diagnosed three years ago, Diana Nolan, did not need much imagination to know what lay ahead. The disease had killed both of her parents. Surgeons removed part of her lung, but the cancer spread. Her physician next suggested that she try a potent chemotherapy but warned of the potential side effects—hair loss, nausea, and vomiting. She asked for a week to think and pray. In the end she told her doctor she wanted only pain-killers. Her two grown sons supported her decision, but some friends urged that she battle on. "They said, go for it at all costs, but I had seen my father, my mother, and several friends go through this." She preferred to stay at home to die and summoned her priest to administer unction. Nolan hopes she will leave a message for those considering decisions like hers. "I wish people wouldn't be frightened about knowing what they're up against. To have a part in my treatment has been so important. I'm part of the team, too."

But when doctors cannot consult the patient directly, the issue becomes much harder. Karen Ann Quinlan's was the most celebrated right-to-die case before Nancy Cruzan's. In 1975, after she had been comatose for seven months, Quinlan's father went to the New Jersey Supreme Court to have her respirator turned off. The court agreed, and the U.S. Supreme Court declined to consider the case further. After the ruling, Quinlan lived nine more years, breathing on her own. Nancy Cruzan was not on a life-support system. Her parents were asking doctors to remove a feeding tube.

When it is not high technology but basic care that is being withheld, doctors find themselves on shakier ground. Right-to-life proponents argue that food and water, even supplied artificially, are not medical treatment.

If doctors and other health professionals are uncomfortable about withholding food and water, they are more uneasy about actively assisting in a suicide. Some physicians and ethicists warn that active euthanasia could undermine the whole ethos of healing. Even hospice workers, who are more concerned with controlling pain than delaying death, are opposed to loading a syringe with an overdose of morphine. (Gibbs, 1990).

For active help with suicide, patients will have to look outside the realm of health care. The spread of AIDS has prompted some right-to-die activists to offer support and counseling about pills and lethal injections to people with the virus. As the costs of health care rise annually, and as new technologies promise higher bills, the questions grow about how to ration health care. In 1987, the Oregon legislature voted to deny organ transplants under its Medicaid program and to use that money for prenatal care. As the historic taboo regarding mercy killing gradually erodes, the courts and legislatures work to ensure that the vulnerable are protected, e.g., the severely disabled, so that the right to die does not become a duty to die. In the Baby Doe case in 1982, the Indiana Courts allowed a couple to refuse surgery for their baby, born with Down's Syndrome and an incomplete esophagus; after six days, the baby starved to death.

Religious groups differ in their views of suffering, death, and compassion. Furthermore, there are clash's between the religious view of the right to privacy and the court's view of the sanctity of life. The notion that life is sacred and worthy of the state's protection is embedded in the American legal tradition, right alongside the protection of individual liberty. Although the wishes of patients and families are often frustrated in court, lawmakers are not insensitive to their plight. William Webster, who has led the legal fight against the Cruzans, has endorsed new legislation in the Missouri legislature proposing that families of patients who have been continuously unconscious for three or more years could petition for withdrawing treatment, including food and water. If the family was unanimous that this is what the patient would want, and three independent physicians certified that the coma was irreversible, the patient would be allowed to die. That would put the decision in the hands of the family.

POLL: 80% OF AMERICANS FAVOR
GIVING SOME PATIENTS RIGHT TO DIE

Almost half believe suicide morally OK for the incurably ill.

Eight of 10 Americans believe patients should be allowed to die in some circumstances and about half say some incurably ill people have a moral right to commit suicide, according to a poll released Tuesday.

The poll, by the Times Mirror Center for The People and The Press, was conducted a month before Dr. Jack Kevorkian, a retired pathologist in Pontiac, Michigan, assisted in the June 4 suicide of Janet Adkins, who had been diagnosed as being in the early stages of Alzheimer's disease.

Diane Colasanto, a researcher for the Times Mirror Center who is based in Princeton, N.J., said the survey did not include any questions about physician-assisted suicide, but added, "I think what we found is relevant to the Kevorkian case."

The survey found that 80 percent of those polled believed there are some circumstances in which a patient should be allowed to die. Only 15 percent thought doctors and nurses should always do everything possible to save a patient's life.

Forty-nine percent said a person with an incurable disease has the moral right to commit suicide, compared with the 40 percent who expressed such a view in a 1975 Gallup poll.

Fifty-five percent said there is a moral right to commit suicide if a person is suffering great pain with no hope of improvement. Forty-one percent held such a view in the 1975 survey.

Susan M. Wolf, a lawyer with the Hastings Center, a research institute in Briarcliff Manor, N.Y., that studies medical ethics, said there is a clear distinction between a doctor withholding life support and a doctor assisting in a suicide.

"Both medical ethics and law treat those things as exact opposites of one another," she said. "In both ethics and law, it is very widely agreed now that the doctor is really mandated to stop life-sustaining treatment at the patient's request. On the other hand, when you get to the question of physician-assisted suicide, both medical ethics and the criminal law roundly condemn that as it stands."

Of 690 callers in a recent Houston Post poll on the subject 369, or 53.5 percent, favored the right to die, while 321, or 46.5 percent, were opposed.

Many states have right-to-die laws, but the question has remained a controversial one. The Supreme Court is expected to rule soon on the efforts of a Missouri couple to remove life support from their 31-year-old daughter, Nancy Cruzan, who was severely brain-damaged in a car crash. The Justice Department has sided with the state of Missouri in attempting to block removal of the life-support equipment.

In 1985, the Lou Harris polling organization asked whether a patient who was terminally ill, with no hope in sight, had the right to ask a doctor to be put out of misery. Sixty-one percent said yes; 31 percent said it would be wrong.

Colasanto said the percentage of affirmative responses was an increase over previous polls on the same question.

A poll last year by Opinion Research Associates said that 66 percent of people surveyed believed a physician should be allowed by law to end the life of an incurably ill patient, she said.

Wednesday, June 13, 1990, *The Houston Post*

Hope: An Antidote for Pain and Suffering

Selye (1976) has said, "It's not what happens that matters, but how you take it." The list of awful things that happen to good people is imposing, yet, the majority of individuals, families, communities, or nations that have suffered a tragedy survive and continue to live productive lives. Veninga (1985) has noted several characteristics of such survivors: (1) a sense of hope and social support; (2) a reason to live; (3) overcoming regrets; and (4) understanding and accepting loss.

Although hope does have therapeutic value, it also has limits. Creech (1975) has suggested that when caregivers are aware of their own feelings about death and evaluate them realistically, they will feel more comfortable in dealing truthfully with the issues of giving or withholding hope. The matter is not so simple as that. The clinical progress of some conditions varies greatly, as may a patient's hopefulness. Too often, caregivers rely on drugs or the latest therapy to express hopefulness to a patient. By doing this, the caregiver avoids having to discuss the limitations of his healing power or of his hope.

Giving hope does not end with a patient's hospital discharge. It is important to realize that even cured patients need active psychologic support long after therapy has been terminated. All patients will be aware of the homily, "Where there is life, there is hope." Perhaps a safer approach would be to assume also that where there is hope, there is life, and that the proper role of the health professional is to nurture both (Motto, 1975).

Social Support and Hope

It has been said that "to keep life we must strengthen all our links with life and living" (Hutschnecker, 1951). To remain hopeful, patients need to retain communication with their relatives, friends, jobs, and other activities in which they have invested themselves. Social support is the gratification of a person's social needs for approval, esteem, and succor through environmental sources (Kaplan et al., 1977). Social support is an expression of hope. The linking of sources of social support has come to be known as networking. There is evidence that supportive interactions among people protect against the consequences of life stress on health. Social support also seems to reduce the amount of medication required, accelerate recovery, and facilitate compliance with prescribed medical regimens (Cobb, 1976). The social support of the caregiver is important, especially if other sources of support for the patient are weak or absent.

In the case of hospitalized patients, the environment can convey a sense of hope and support or the opposite. Caregivers may become so accustomed to the environment they work in that they become insensitive to the cues that patients sense in the physical environment and in the interaction among staff and between staff and patients (Kastenbaum and Kastenbaum, 1971). For example, patients may deduce much about their condition by observing how they are cared for in contrast to other patients with a similar condition in a coronary care or intensive care unit. Unspoken hopelessness may be communicated by the patient's refusal to eat, or by restlessness, frightening dreams, and crying spells.

Religion and Hope

Vanderpool (1977) has observed that religion gives valued emotional or psychologic support to those who are religiously oriented; their faith or trust gives them a sense of well-being and hope. Sevensky (1981) pointed out that religion serves at least three functions in the life of sick or dying patients. It provides an understanding of illness and mortality; it provides patients with various resources in coping with sickness, suffering, and mortality, especially through confidence and faith; and it gives them hope for an ultimate victory, despite sickness and inevitable death.

Some would propose that people become sick when they lose their hope or faith. Whatever the nature of illness, sick people do need to have their hope restored or replenished. For this reason, it is difficult for the sick and for their family to accept the statement, "There is no more hope, there is nothing more that can be done." Some sick persons turn, in desperate hope, to methods of healing or to healers who work from the standpoint that there is always hope (Jourard, 1974). The shrine at Lourdes, France, attracts millions in search of medical miracles. Psychic surgery, practitioners using experimental drugs, and evangelical clergymen who carry out healing ceremonies using prayer and the laying on of hands draw millions of sick in search of hope (Jourard, 1974; Nolen, 1974). Changing one's life style through the help of a healer's charisma is a common denominator in nonmedical approaches to healing. Guidance on how to become and how to remain healthy, and the agent's expression of hope that the patient can do this, seem to be essential elements that instill hope. Perhaps the inherent function of hope is simply the promotion of health and happiness (Obayuwana, 1980).

Hope and the degree of effectiveness of treatment are not determined by the characteristics of the patient or caregiver alone, but by their interaction in the context of a caring environment. Although we know little about the dynamics of hope and how it is given or lost, there is evidence that "hope, like faith and a purpose in life, is medicinal" (Wolff, 1957, Bruhn, 1984).

Caregivers Who Care

Hope is an expectation, usually that something positive will happen. It is difficult, but not impossible, to give hope to another person. A person comes to believe in or trust another through experience. Hope is more than optimism; it is an expression of values that are reinforced or altered by the way other people behave toward us. Patients expect that caregivers will express a caring or hopeful attitude. Caregivers also expect that patients will show a caring or hopeful attitude and, in addition, will become partners in the healing process. An uncaring or hopeless attitude on the part of the patient presents a barrier for the caregiver. The patient's attitude may be more injurious to recovery than the illness itself. Hope is intricately tied to the caregiver's image. Sometimes, this image is the only evidence of hope a patient has. Patients who grasp for evidence of hope from sources external to themselves are likely to experience only fleeting periods of hope. Caregivers cannot be expected to carry the burden of hopelessness expressed by some patients or to feel guilty because some patients have given up hope. On the other hand, caregivers need to be sensitive to how their behavior can convey the hope or hopelessness their patient comes to live.

In Retrospect

Health professionals must come to terms with pain for several reasons. First, they must explain pain. They must gather what the patient tells them about pain and fit it into a nosologic category. They must do something to relieve pain. Finally, if the pain is recurring, the health professional needs to develop a plan to follow the patient. Pain is one of the most common experiences leading to help-seeking. Pain, like anxiety, serves a protective function. It is a subjective experience that cannot be shared. The management of pain requires a comprehensive approach involving biological, psychological, and social factors.

We feel sure that health professionals are aware of their mission to deal with human suffering, even if, at times, little can be done to bring about relief. The health professional has a special obligation toward the incurable and toward patients facing death. Because of the ever-changing nature of life, pain, suffering, and grief happen, interrupting otherwise good health and relative stability in life. Whether it is through an illness, an injury, a divorce, or a death, we all experience loss. Many of our current symptoms are related to unresolved losses of the past. Compassion and understanding on the part of the health professional is essential if the patient is to let go of sorrow, anger, and self-pity. The management of pain and suffering requires the health professional to mobilize the support of the family and/or other community support systems.

REFERENCES

Bakan, D. (1968). *Disease, pain, and sacrifice. Toward a psychology of suffering.* Chicago: University of Chicago Press.

Bates, M.S. (1987). Ethnicity and pain: A biocultural model. *Social Science & Medicine, 24*, 47–50.

Beecher, H.K. (1959). *Measurement of subjective responses.* New York: Oxford University Press.

Boeyink, D.E. (1974). Pain and suffering. *Journal of Religious Ethics, 2*, 85–98.

Bonica, J.J. (1974). Therapeutic acupuncture and implications for American medicine. *Journal of the American Medical Association, 228,* 18–27.

Bovet, T. (1973). Human attitudes toward suffering. *Humanitas, 9,* 5–20.

Bruhn, J.G. (1977). Effects of chronic illness on the family. *Journal of Family Practice, 4,* 1057–1060.

Bruhn, J.G. (1984). The therapeutic value of hope. *Southern Medical Journal, 77,* 215–219.

Buytendijk, F.J.J. (1962). *Pain: Its modes and functions.* Chicago: University of Chicago Press.

Cassell, E.J. (1982). The nature of suffering and the goals of medicine. *New England Journal of Medicine, 306,* 639–645.

Cobb, S. (1976). Social support as a moderator of life stress. *Psychosomatic Medicine, 38,* 300–314.

Cousins, N. (1979). *Anatomy of an illness as perceived by the patient.* New York: Norton.

Cousins, N. (1983). *The healing heart.* New York: Norton.

Craig, K.D. (1983). Modelling and social learning factors in chronic pain. In J.J. Bonica, V. Lindblom & A. Iggo (Eds.) *Advances in pain research and therapy* (pp. 813–827). Vol. 5. New York: Raven Press.

Craig, K.D. (1978). Social modeling influences on pain. In R.A. Sternbach (Ed.) *The psychology of pain* (pp. 73–109). New York: Raven Press.

Creech, R.H. (1975). The psychologic support of the cancer patient: A medical oncologist's viewpoint. *Seminars in Oncology, 2,* 285–292.

Doughterty, F. (Ed.). (1982). *The meaning of human suffering.* New York: Human Sciences Press.

Edwards, R.B. (1984). Pain and the ethics of pain management. *Social Science & Medicine, 18,* 515–523.

Elton, D., Stanley, G. & Burrows, G. (1983). *Psychological control of pain.* New York: Grune & Stratton.

Elton, D., Stuart, G.V. & Burrows, G.D. (1978). Self-esteem and chronic pain. *Journal of Psychosomatic Research, 22,* 25–30.

Engelhardt, H.T., Jr. (1980). Ethical issues in pain management. In H.W. Kosterlitz and L.Y. Terenius (Eds.) *Pain and society* (pp. 461–480). Weinheim: Verlag Chemie.

Farmer, P. & Kleinman, A. (1989). AIDS as human suffering. *Daedalus, 118,* 135–160.

Flannery, R.B., Jr., Sos, J. & McGovern, P. (1981). Ethnicity as a factor in the expression of pain. *Psychosomatics, 22,* 39–50.

Fordyce, W.E. (1986). Learning processes in pain. In R.A. Sternbach (Ed.) *The psychology of pain* (pp. 45–65). New York: Raven Press.

Gibbs, N. (1990). Love and let die. *Time, 135,* (March *19*), 62–71.

Goldberg, C. (1986). Concerning human suffering. *The Psychiatric Journal of the University of Ottawa, 11,* 97–104.

Golden, J.M. & Steiner, J.R. (1981). Unique needs of people with chronic pain. *Health and Social Work, 6,* 47–53.

Goldstein, K. (1959). Health as a value. In A.H. Maslow (Ed.) *New knowledge in human values* (pp. 178–188). New York: Harper and Brothers.

Hall, K.R.L. & Stride, E. (1954). The varying response to pain in psychiatric disorders: A study in abnormal psychology. *British Journal of Medical Psychology, 27,* 48–60.

Harkins, S.W. (1988). Issues in the study of pain and suffering in relation to age. *International Journal of Technology and Aging, 1,* 146–155.

Hutschnecker, A.A. (1951). *The will to live.* Englewood Cliffs, NJ: Prentice Hall.

James, S. (1982). The duty to relieve suffering. *Ethics, 93* (October), 4–21.

Jourard, S.M. (1974). *Healthy personality: An approach from the viewpoint of humanistic psychology.* New York: Macmillan.

Kaplan, B.H., Cassel, J.C., Gore, S. (1977). Social support and health. *Medical Care, 15,* 47–58, 1977.

Kastenbaum, R., & Kastenbaum, B.A. (1971). Hope, survival, and the caring environment. In E.E. Palmore, F.C. Jeffers (eds). *Prediction of life span* (pp. 249–270). Lexington, KY: Heath Lexington Books.

Kleinman, A. (1988). *The illness narratives: Suffering, healing & the human condition.* New York: Basic Books.

Kliever, L.D. (Ed.) (1989). *Dax's case: Essays in medical ethics and human meaning.* Dallas: Southern Methodist University Press.

Kozielecki, J. (1978). Suffering and human values. *Dialectics & Humanism, 5,* 115–127.

Koopman, C., Eisenthal, S. & Stoeckle, J.D. (1984). Ethnicity in the reported pain, emotional distress and requests of medical outpatients. *Social Science & Medicine, 18,* 487–490.

Kosambi, D.D. (1967). Living prehistory in India. *Scientific American, 216,* 105–114.

Kotarba, J.A. (1983). *Chronic pain: Its social dimensions.* Beverly Hills, CA: Sage.

Kotarba, J.A. (1983). Perceptions of death, belief systems and the process of coping with chronic pain. *Social Science & Medicine, 17,* 681–689.

LeShan, L. (1964). The world of the patient in severe pain of long duration. *Journal of Chronic Disease, 17,* 119–126.

Lifton, R.J. (1967). *Death in life: Survivors of Hiroshima.* New York: Random House.

Lipton, J.A. & Marbach, J.J. (1984). Ethnicity and the pain experience. *Social Science & Medicine, 19,* 1279–1298.

Mechanic, D. (1962). The concept of illness behavior. *Journal of Chronic Diseases, 15,* 189–194.

Melzack, R. (1973). *The puzzle of pain.* New York: Basic Books.

Melzack, R. & Scott, T.H. (1957). The effects of early experience on the response to pain. *Journal of Comparative and Physiological Psychology, 50,* 155–161.

Melzack, R. & Torgerson, W.S. (1971). On the language of pain. *Anesthesiology, 34,* 50–59.

Melzack, R. & Wall, P.D. (1982). *The challenge of pain.* New York: Basic Books.

Mersky, H. (1978). Pain and personality. In R.A. Sternbach (Ed.) *The psychology of pain* (pp. 111–127). New York: Raven Press.

Mersky, H. (1968). Psychological aspects of pain. *Postgraduate Medical Journal, 44,* 297–306.

Mersky, H. (1965). The characteristics of persistent pain in psychosomatic illness. *Journal of Psychosomatic Research, 9,* 291–298.

Minuchin, S., Baker, L., Rosman, B.L., Liebman, R., Milman, L., & Todd, T.C. (1975). Conceptual model of psychosomatic illness in children. *Archives of General Psychiatry, 32,* 1031–1038.

Mirowsky, J. & Ross, C.E. (1986). Social patterns of distress. *Annual Review of Sociology, 12,* 23–45.

Moller, D. W. (1986–1987). On the value of suffering in the shadow of death. *Loss, Grief & Care 1,* 126–137.

Motto, J.A. (1975). Hope, suicide and medical practice. *Journal of the American Medical Association, 234,* 1168–1169.

Murray, J.B. (1975). Psychology of pain experience. In M. Weisenberg (Ed.) *Pain: Clinical and experimental perspectives* (pp. 36–44). St. Louis: Mosby.

Nolen, W.A. (1974). *Healing: A doctor in search of a miracle.* New York, Random House.

Obayuwana, A.O. (1980). Hope: a panacea unrecognized. *Journal of the National Medical Association, 72,* 67–69.

Pilowsky, J. (1980). Abnormal illness behavior and sociocultural aspects of pain. In H.W. Kosterlitz & L.Y. Terenius (Eds.). *Pain and society* (pp. 445–460). Weinheim: Verlag Chemie.

Pilowsky, J. (1968). The response to treatment in hypochondriacal disorders. *Australian and New Zealand Journal of Psychiatry, 2,* 88–94.

Pilowsky, J. & Bond, M.R. (1969). Pain and its management in malignant disease. Elucidation of staff-patient transactions. *Psychosomatic Medicine, 31,* 400–404.

Seligman, M.E.P. (1975). *Helplessness: On depression, development, and death.* San Francisco: W.H. Freeman.

Selye, H. (1976). *The stress of life.* New York: McGraw-Hill.

Sevensky, R.L. (1981). Religion and illness: An outline of their relationship. *Southern Medical Journal, 74,* 745–750.

Slaby, A.E. & Glicksman, A.S. (1985). *Adapting to life-threatening illness.* New York: Praeger.

Sontag, S. (1978). *Illness as a metaphor.* New York: Farrar, Straus, and Giroux.

Sternbach, R.A. (1968). *Pain: A psychophysiological analysis.* New York: Academic Press.

Sternbach, R.A. (1974). *Pain patients: Traits and treatment.* New York: Academic Press.

Sternbach, R.A. (1977). Psychophysiology of pain. In Z.J. Lipowski, D.R. Lipsitt & P.C. Whybrow (Eds.) *Psychosomatic medicine: Current trends and chemical applications* (pp. 355–365). New York: Oxford University Press, 1977.

Sternbach, R.A. (Ed.). (1986). *The psychology of pain.* 2nd edition. New York: Raven Press.

Sternbach, R.A. & Timmermans, G. (1975). Personality changes associated with reduction of pain. *Pain, 1,* 177–181.

Sternbach, R.A. & Tursky, B. (1965). Ethnic differences among housewives in psychophysical and skin potential responses to electric shock. *Psychophysiology, 1,* 241–246.

Streltzer, J. & Wade, T.C. (1981). The influence of cultural group on the undertreatment of postoperative pain. *Psychosomatic Medicine, 43* (October), 397–403.

Szasz, T.S. (1975). *Pain and pleasure: A study of bodily feelings.* New York: Basic Books.

U.S. Department of Health, Education, and Welfare, Public Health Service and National Institutes of Health (1979), *Report of the panel on pain to the national advisory neurological and communicative disorders and stroke council.* Washington, D.C.: U.S. Government Printing Office.

Vanderpool, H.Y. (1977). Is religion therapeutically significant? *Journal of Religion and Health, 16,* 255–259.

Veninga, K. (1985). *A gift of hope: How we survive our tragedies.* Boston: Little, Brown.

Weisenberg, M. (1977). Pain and pain control. *Psychological Bulletin, 84,* 1008–1044.

Williams, D.D. (1969). Suffering and being in empirical theology. In B.E. Meland (Ed.) *The future of empirical theology.* (pp. 175–194). Chicago: University of Chicago Press.

Wilson, D.C. (1965). *Ten fingers for God.* New York: McGraw-Hill.

Wolff, B.B. & Langley, S. (1968). Cultural factors and the response to pain: A review. *American Anthropologist, 70,* 494–501.

Wolff, B.B. & Langley, S. (1975). Cultural factors and the response to pain: A review. In M. Weisenberg (Ed.) *Pain: Clinical and experimental perspectives* (pp. 144–151). St. Louis: Mosby.

Wolff, H.G. (1957). What hope does for man. *Saturday Review,* January 5.

Wood, G. (1986). *The myth of neurosis: Overcoming the illness excuse.* New York: Harper and Row.

Woodforde, J.M. & Mersky, H. (1972). Personality traits of patients with chronic pain. *Journal of Psychosomatic Research, 16,* 167–172.

Woodrow, K.M., Friedman, G.D., Sielgelaub, A.B., & Collen, M.F. (1972). Pain tolerance: Differences according to age, sex, and race. *Psychosomatic Medicine, 34,* 548–556.

Yu-huan, H. & Neng-yu, F. (1989). Report from China. Social and ethical influence on pain: The causes of lower incidences of some pain syndromes in Chinese people. *Bioethics, 1,* 236–244.

Zborowski, M. (1969). *People in pain.* San Francisco, CA: Jossey-Bass.

Zola, J.K. (1966). Culture and symptoms—an analysis of patients' presenting complaints. *American Sociological Review, 31,* 615–630.

Zwerding, D. (1975). The new pesticide threat. In C. Lerza and M. Jacobson (Eds.) *Food for people, not for profit* (pp. 93–98). New York: Random House.

SUGGESTED READINGS

Kushner, H.S. (1981). *When bad things happen to good people.* New York: Avon.

Bradley, L.A., Prokop, C.K., Gentry, W.D., Van der Heide, L.H., and Prieto, E.J. (1981). Assessment of chronic pain. In C.K. Prokop and L.A. Bradley (Eds.) *Medical Psychology: Contributions to behavioral medicine* (pp. 91–117). New York: Academic Press.

Lynch, N.T. and Vasudevan, S.V. (1988). *Persistent pain: Psychosocial assessment and intervention.* Boston: Kluwer Academic.

Philips, H.C. (1988). *The psychological management of chronic pain: A treatment manual.* New York: Springer.

Sternbach, R.A. (1987). *Mastering pain: A twelve-step program for coping with chronic pain.* New York: Putnam & Sons.

Stein, J.J. (1978). *Making medical choices: Who is responsible?* Boston: Houghton Mifflin.

Petrie, A. (1967). *Individuality in pain and suffering.* Chicago: University of Chicago Press.

Chapter 7

CHOICE AS A VALUE

Death is not the worst; rather in vain to wish for death, and not to compass it.

Sophocles, *Electra*, c.495–405 B.C.

One of the fundamental rights on which the United States government is based is that of free choice within the limits of reason. The First Amendment in the Bill of Rights is about choice—the freedom to choose a religion or none at all; the freedom to voice opinions; the freedom to print any nonslanderous and nonlibelous ideas; the freedom to assemble peaceably to discuss what we choose to be concerned about; and the freedom to petition U.S. courts for a redress of the grievances which we believe have curtailed our right to choose. Within this framework, freedom means little apart from the ability of individuals to live their lives as they choose, making personal decisions without fear of coercion.

The choosing of values is a central concern and a goal toward which all persons must move if they are to become integrated as human beings (May, 1953). Whether we are involved in a helping relationship as professionals or friends, it is inevitable that, at some point in the relationship, choices must be made. Human beings not only *can* make such choices of values and goals, but we are the only animal who *must* do so. For the value—the goal we move toward—serves us as a psychological center, a kind of emotional energy which draws together our powers as a core of a magnet draws the magnet's lines of force together. Knowing what we want is the hallmark of mature persons. The realm of medicine is one which tends to make most people doubt their capacity to make wise decisions. Modern medicine, with its awesome technology and almost superhuman demands on practitioners, tends to bewilder individuals who are faced with making choices about something as serious as a threat to their health, perhaps even to their lives. Thus, patients ask physicians and other health care providers to make for them the choices that will determine the treatment and outcome of their illness. Through-

193

out the history of medicine, healers have been the dominant decision makers, and patients have largely been submissive followers.

Within recent years, issues such as quality of life, informed consent, and the right to die have led to a major reevaluation of the rights of patients in health care. The resolution of each issue has given patients substantially greater autonomy in choosing their treatment. In the last two decades, the patient's right to choose has been revolutionized, and health care providers' ethical and legal responsibilities have been delineated in greater detail than ever before. This change has been accelerated by state and federal court decisions that ensure patients' freedom of choice in their health care.

Quality of Life

Because our values as well as those of our healers can precipitate actions that are harmful to our well-being, we should carefully examine them. Actually, this is a process of reexamination—of listening with less certainty and critically analyzing health care values with the end goal of gaining a clearer sense of rightness. But it is not easy to comprehend what, in the final analysis, may be more knowledge about our inner selves than about our illness. "You would not find out the boundaries of the soul, even by traveling along every path; so deep a measure does it have," Heraclitus wrote. When critically ill, we tend to "lose" ourselves while walking philosophically along the footpaths of our souls. Common belief has it that modern Western medicine can rescue us from disasters, disease, and death.

> Surely everyone should have recognized by now that medicine is (to use a metaphor from game theory) engaged in a "no-win game." At its very best it can offer only palliative treatment. Its subject will surely die, and it will sooner or later lose its never-ending struggle to ameliorate if not indeed overcome the afflictions of mortality. Medicine can repair, and nowadays, sometimes even replace, damaged parts; it can make detours around otherwise dead-end obstructions; but it cannot really remedy. It can care, and sometimes (as survivors of heart attack will testify) it can rehabilitate, but it cannot cure. (Smith, 1987, p. 705)

It is generally agreed that health care has two basic objectives: (1) to increase patients' life expectancy and (2) to improve the quality of their lives during the remaining years. Neither disease cures nor mortality rates are the major criterion of good health. Improved patient care frequently has little influence on the death rate, and some debilitating illnesses such as arthritis do not significantly decrease a patient's life span. There is a stark realization that there is more to life than not dying (Taylor, 1989). The phrase "a sound mind in a sound body" reflects an ideal that has remained constant from ancient to modern times, and medical research has brought us closer to this goal. Enormous improvements have been made in diagnostic procedures, surgical techniques, and both prophylactic and therapeutic medicine. Unfortunately, the delivery of health services has not kept pace with medical research. This is true despite unusually large expenditures for health care delivery services.

In an age of dwindling public and private health care resources, the allocation of those resources must be based on something more than subjective personal decisions. Lately, quality of life data have been employed more frequently by individuals who make assessments of the cost effectiveness and cost utility of particular health programs. One of the most crucial questions now being asked by health care resource allocators is: Which competing programs and treatments will most improve the quality of patient's lives within a cost containment system? At the same time that we seek answers to the question, it is important to remember that health care decisions must be made with two beneficiaries in mind—the individual patient and the community. When managing greatly limited resources, health care allocators often apply the economist's concept of *opportunity cost* —the cost of using resources in a health care program is the value of the benefits that would have been generated in their best alternative use.

The following medical advances illustrate the potential values and costs of new technologies: (1) Erythropoitin, a hormone that stimulates the production of red blood cells, is an effective treatment for severe anemia associated with chronic renal failure. Approximately 80,000 patients who are currently undergoing chronic dialysis are suitable for treatment, and the cost is $10,000 per patient year. (2) AZT can delay the onset of AIDS in people who test positive for human immunodeficiency virus. The estimated annual cost is $5 billion. (3) The automatic implantable cardiac defilibrillator, a device that is activated when the heart develops life-threatening arrhythmia, could help approximately 20,000 persons annually at a cost of about $46,000 per patient.

The real cost of high technology diagnostic aids, however, is not solely the money spent on equipment and staff; it can also be calculated by the cost of programs that were *not* given funds (Drummond 1987). Nor is the decision to allocate health care resources easier when made in terms of optimum extended life or *quality adjusted life years.* For example, the cost per quality adjusted life year gained in 1986 U.S. dollars for coronary artery bypass surgery for left main coronary artery disease was $4,796, compared with $36,316 for neonatal intensive care for an infant weighing 500–900 grams (Patrick & Deyo, 1989). Which is the best investment?

It is in geriatrics that quality of life data may prove most useful. During the last twenty years, there has been a large increase in the proportion of elderly persons in the American population. Because of new discoveries in medication and medical technology, a large number of Americans can look forward to a longer life. This means that health care professionals will be seeing a greater number of patients with chronic diseases over a longer period of years. And the major treatment objectives for these patients will be (1) to improve their functioning through the reduction of their medical symptoms, (2) to reduce the severity of their illness, and (3) to limit the advancement of diseases. Currently, the prevention and control of chronic diseases among the elderly receives the largest allocation of health care resources. In fact, more than 80 percent of U.S. health care resources are targeted for clinical management and biomedical research involving chronic diseases in the elderly (Revicki, 1989).

Frequently, in the management of chronic illnesses, health care practitioners face the problem of patient noncompliance. In order to improve compliance, practitioners must be cognizant of the effect of therapy on each patient's physical, psychological, and social functioning. This is being knowledgeable about how each therapy may affect a patient's quality of life. Prescribing treatment is not enough. Noncompliance will render the best medical decisions useless. Revicki (1989) gave a cogent illustration of the interrelationship between quality of life and compliance: an antihypertensive drug can reduce blood pressure but if it creates difficulties for patients in terms of sleep and general sense of well-being, it probably will not be taken, thereby increasing the risk of cardiovascular disease. Generally, compliance is directly associated with a treatment's effect on a patient's quality of life. Although the side-effects of therapy and quality of life are not synonymous, the former may affect the latter in crucial ways.

What is quality of life if it is not side-effects? One of the major difficulties in discussing quality of life is that its definition is elusive.

Table 7-1. Dimensions of quality of life

Dimension	Examples
Physical functioning	Mobility, self-care ability to perform activities of daily living
Psychological functioning	Depression, anger, anxiety, helplessness
Social functioning	Participation in social activities, family relations, recreational activities
Cognitive functioning	Memory, alertness, judgment

Most clinicians make a distinction between "depth" of life versus "length" of life (Eiseman, 1981). Qualitatively, they define life as the combination of social, biomedical, and behavioral outcomes—the total psychosocial and physical well-being of a person. The term has also been defined as an individual's ability to function normally within society; and it has more narrowly been defined as the patient's functional capacity, perceptions, and symptoms (Hume, 1989) (see Table 7-1). In addition to these definitions, we could include the concept of "reintegration to normal living." From this perspective, quality of life is the readjustment of our physical, psychological, and social characteristics into a coherent whole so that we can have the best possible life after an incapacitating illness or trauma (Wood-Dauphinee & Williams, 1987). In summary, we could define health-related quality of life as *the ability of a patient to do as he or she wishes within individually tailored physical and psychological limitations.* Whichever definition we select, we can be sure of this: We must treat the patient, not just the tumor (Tannock, 1987).

Measuring Quality of Life

Those who question the emphasis on quality of life as a factor in health care and treatment usually cite a lack of "hard" data. When advocates of various medical treatments and programs compete for health dollars, the interventions which improve patients' quality of life usually will receive funds only if their proponents can show that promising results have been demonstrated in research studies. There are two basic types of instruments for measuring quality of life effects. One type, the *generic measure,* comprises a broad group of health concepts that are applicable to many different impairments, illnesses, patients, and populations. The major characteristics of such an instrument are that it allows a comparison of different patient populations and programs; it is applicable across various types and severities of diseases, different medical interventions, and demographic and cultural subgroups (Patrick & Deyo, 1989).

The second type of instrument, the *disease-specific measure,* concentrates on problems connected with individual diseases, particular patient groups, and specific areas of function. The major characteristics of such an instrument is that it can identify important concerns of patients with particular conditions and can measure small, clinically important changes from specific treatments. Disease-specific measures have been developed for several conditions such as cardiovascular disease, chronic lung disease, arthritis, and cancer. The major disadvantages of a disease-specific measure is that it is not comprehensive and investigators cannot use it for comparing different conditions or making interprogram treatment comparisons. The choice of using generic or disease-specific measures is made on the basis of the research objectives.

Several measures assess various quality of life characteristics. For example, the Sickness Impact Profile assesses illness-related dysfunction in physical functions (i.e., social interaction, alertness behavior, emotional behavior, and communication). It also assesses independent categories such as work, eating, sleep and rest, home management, and recreation or pastime. In a study of the effects of antihypertensive therapy on the quality of life, Croog et al. (1986) used an assessment based on five measures: (1) sense of well-being and satisfaction with life, (2) physical state, (3) emotional state, (4) intellectual functioning, and (5) the ability to perform social roles, including the degree of satisfaction derived from those roles.

The most important measure in quality of life assessments is the *perspective of the patients* —their values, feelings, desires, and personal assessment of physical capabilities. There is no advantage in the imposition of someone else's values on a patient if they do not coincide to a large extent with the patient's. A major guide for surgeons' clinical decisions, for example, is the patient's subjective feelings and physical capabilities (Troidl et al., 1987). Using this approach, decisions regarding surgery, the goal being to improve the patient's quality of life, are based on face-to-face interviews with patients, not solely on physical evaluation (Fowler et al., 1988). For this reason, a psychologist should be a member of the health care team when quality of life decisions are made (Hollandsworth, 1988). The special training of psychologists prepares them to elicit patients' true values and feelings.

Because most attempts at quantifying the effects of therapeutic intervention on health-related quality of life have been relatively recent, research data have had little impact on clinical practice (Taylor 1987). Nor have quality of life measures played a major role in court decisions. In one particularly important case concerning withdrawal of life support, the *Conroy* case, the court held that while several aspects of the patient's quality of life had a bearing on the case, pain was the only matter it considered. Everything else, it held, was too subjective. The dissenting opinion stated that other aspects of quality of life should have been considered, but it does not suggest what else should be measured. To date, *measures* of quality of life, have little significance for judges in cases regarding life support for terminally ill patients or for neonates with malformations that would necessitate extensive surgery to maintain life (Mosteller, 1987).

Some of the most ethically relevant uses of quality of life judgments are those concerning elderly patients who are critically ill. What decisions should be made by the patient, his or her family, and the physician when the end of life seems near? A study by Yinnon et al. (1989), conducted in a community hospital with a predominantly geriatric patient population, indicates that when patients enter the intensive care unit (ICU) with a low quality of life, care in the ICU will not give them more than a few weeks or months of life, and the majority of such patients will not leave the hospital alive. The same study found that most patients who had a good quality of life before they entered the ICU episode which necessitated their critical care, were long-term survivors with a quality of life after release that was comparable to what it had been before admission.

There seems to be very little correlation between elderly patients' assessments of their quality of life and their wish to undergo cardiopulmonary resuscitation (Starr et al., 1986). Only when patients are asked to consider circumstances of extreme disability (i.e., stroke with immobility, dysarthria, and inability to care for themselves) is there a significant correlation between the quality of life they had attained prior to treatment and their desire for resuscitation. A study of 160 patients over 55 years of age, who were representative of individuals who entered intensive care during the same year, found that elderly patients with previous ICU hospitalizations were willing to undergo intensive care again regardless of their age, functional status, perceived quality of life, hypothetical life expectancy, or the nature of their previous ICU experience (Danis et al., 1988). Family members who acted as proxies for incompetents, or patients who later died, agreed to have their relatives undergo intensive care. Seventy percent of patients and their family members were willing to undergo intensive care again or to approve it for relatives. Only 8 percent of the respondents were willing to undergo intensive care to achieve prolongation of life at a greatly diminished quality.

Quality of life judgments by someone other than patients themselves or members of their families must be made with extreme care. Research data suggest that even individuals who consider themselves skilled at assessing quality of life cannot always assume that their concept of quality of life is a good predictor of a patient's desire for it. Furthermore, there sometimes can be a conflict between the principle of patient autonomy and the principle of maximum societal welfare. We have yet to be able to accurately predict which patients will receive optimum benefit from intensive care. Even so, the concept of quality of life is one which health care professionals must keep in mind if they are to maintain medicine's high ethical standards. In choosing from among alternative therapies, it is important to make an evaluation of how each therapy might affect the quality of life of a patient. And the patient must give informed consent.

Informed Consent

In daily practice, the theoretical model of informed consent assumes that health care professionals will convey information to a competent patient who comprehends it and who voluntarily makes a decision to accept or reject a recommended procedure or treatment (Sprung & Winick, 1989). This process is followed in order to ensure joint decision-making by both the care provider and the patient. The goal is to help patients make rational decisions that reflect their personal values. Ideally, a patient will weigh the benefits of a suggested procedure or treatment against the risks, while comparing them to the benefits and risks of alternative procedures or treatment, with the option to reject all procedures. After all, the patient owns the illness. The doctrine of informed consent does not eliminate the moral problems inherent in matters of life and death. Upon close examination, each medical case has significant moral dimensions. Generally, there is no single right answer. And the legal requirement to disclose information to patients and obtain their voluntary, informed consent often results in conflicting values—respecting patients' autonomy and acting in their best interest. For the health care professional, this conflict usually culminates in respecting the patient's autonomy—even if this does not bring about the best possible medical outcome.

Much of the research concerning informed consent indicates that physicians often do not give patients much information about their treatment, and that patients do not understand much of the information they are given. As noted in other chapters, it appears that much of the information patients get from their doctors is given to them in such a way that they cannot understand it (Lidz et al., 1985). Taylor and Kelner (1987) reported that of 68 American physicians in the areas of medical oncology, surgery, and radiotherapy who were surveyed, only 13 percent said that they had been taught the technique of explaining informed consent to patients. Yet, the President's Commission for the Study of Ethical Problems in Medicine and Biomedical and Behavioral Research (1982) recommended informed consent and shared decision making as the legally and ethically acceptable processes by which decisions about health care should be reached.

Until about 1957, most physicians believed that their primary responsibility was to provide medical benefits for their patients, respect for patient autonomy was a secondary matter. The case of *Salgo v. Leland Stanford Jr. University Board of Trustees* (1957) changed the relationship between physicians and patients in a major way. Using the now famous phrase, "informed consent," the court decided that in order to make a valid choice of medical treatment, each patient must receive from the physician the following information about his or her treatment: its nature, consequences, harm and benefits, risks, and treatment alternatives. The court also ruled that patient choice, or consent, was "informed" only when it was made with such information in mind.

The problem of medical consent found its way to the courts more than fifty years before *Salgo*. In *Mohr v. Williams* (1905), a Minnesota court held that an operation performed without a patient's consent was a battery—intentional, nonconsensual touching of a person. Furthermore, the court said that the plaintiff was not required to show that the defendant meant to do harm, only that there was an intent to touch. Dramatically stated, a patient's consent is the characteristic differentiating surgery from assault with a knife (Kaufmann, 1983). This point was driven home forcefully in *Schloendorff v. Society of New York Hospital* (1914) when Judge Benjamin Cardozo upheld the patient's right to autonomy in medical decision-making: "Every human being of adult years and sound mind has a right to determine what shall be done with his own body and a surgeon who performs an operation without his patient's consent commits an assault for which he is liable in damage."

Three years after *Salgo*, a Kansas decision in the case of *Nathanson v. Kline* (1960) clarified the legal meaning of informed consent. The court said that the doctor providing treatment had a duty to inform the patient of the nature of the treatment and its possible risks. It further held that the physician's failure to relay information about risks meant that the patient did not give informed consent to the treatment. The court broke new ground by deciding that a failure to receive knowledgeable patient consent to treatment constituted negligence, no matter how ably the treatment was administered. The court ruled against the defendant, not because he had failed to obtain the consent of the patient to the treatment, but because the consent obtained was of "low quality" and did not meet the "standards of conduct of prudent, reasonable physicians." The decision said that the patient, at a minimum, had to be informed as to what he was consenting to and the risks associated with the proposed treatment. The absence of consent constitutes an action of assault and battery, and failure to inform the patient adequately constitutes negligence.

By 1972, two standards were emerging to spell out the physician's responsibility to disclose information to the patient: the "professional community" standard and the "reasonable person" or "lay" standard. Under the professional community standard, the scope of the physician's duty to disclose information is predicated on the custom of physicians in the same or in a similar community. Under this standard, a doctor cannot be held liable unless the omission of information varies from the professional practice common in the community. Also, under the professional standard, the patient must prove what the routine practice of disclosure is and that the disclosure given by the doctor did not conform to the customary practice. Professional medical testimony is necessary to reveal the professional standard common in the community. The second standard of disclosure, the lay standard, necessitates that the doctor give the patient all the information a reasonable person in the patient's place would consider material to the process of medical decision-making.

Business as Usual

Legal relief for physicians in the matter of informed consent came in *Cobbs v. Grant* (1972), which reached the California Supreme Court. The court held that during an emergency or when the patient is a minor or incompetent, the physician has "therapeutic privilege," a term that had been employed in 1962 by an Alabama court (*Roberts v. Wood*) and which means that a doctor may be exempted from the requirements of informed consent. However, in *Cobbs* the court did require, as a minimum under normal circumstances, physician disclosure of risks of death and serious bodily harm from a procedure in accordance with the reasonable person standard. The court also incorporated the professional standard in mandating disclosure of additional information.

In the same year as *Cobbs*, the Washington, D.C. Circuit Court ruled in *Canterbury v. Spence* (1972) that the medical profession alone does not establish the scope of the standard of disclosure. Also, the court ruled that the doctor cannot restrict the information given to patients, even if he or she believes that divulgence may cause patients to reject treatment which the doctor believes is necessary. The court further held that only if the doctor feels that a patient would become so ill or emotionally agitated on disclosure as to prevent a rational decision, can information be withheld. The *Canterbury* decision meant that the conduct of doctors in giving information can be appraised in terms of standards established by the courts, rather than solely upon the ordinary practice standards in the community. The traditional legal protection given the medical profession was restricted, and as one authority said, the decision "implied that physicians were subject to judicial review and sanction not only in regard to the techniques and outcomes of treatment, but in the quality of interactions with patients" (Kaufmann, 1983, p. 1661).

Although it seemed, in the early 1970s, that many courts were following the *Canterbury* decision in rejecting the professional standard measure in favor of the lay or reasonable person standard, a few years later, a number of states established laws based on the professional standard. And a majority of the states now adhere to it. Even so, in Massachusetts, a "physician's failure to enable a patient to give or withhold consent constitutes professional misconduct" (*Harnish v. Children's Hospital Medical Center* (1982). The Texas law is the most stringent regarding informed consent. It mandates disclosure on a procedure by procedure basis, and it requires a yearly update of the list of medical and surgical treatments or procedures and the measure of disclosure demanded. Yet, by 1980, all states had made modifications of their statutory laws to permit signed and written consent forms to represent evidence of adequate information disclosure in the event of legal action.

In spite of its complex legal history, informed consent is a gray area of professional ethics. Many physicians are still unwilling to adhere to the doctrine's guidelines. Perhaps these doctors view informed consent as an empty charade because they feel secure in their skill of manipulating patient consent (Brody, 1989). The observation has been made that while physicians tend to keep information from patients, the tendency to do so varies directly with the status distance between them and those under their care. It is probable that upper- and middle-class patients will get more answers to their questions than patients of lower socioeconomic status (Kaufmann, 1983). Language is another barrier between health professionals and less affluent patients. Medical practitioners usually couch their information in terms that are all but unintelligible to the less educated. It is very difficult for a functionally illiterate person to understand information concerning alternative choices, or even the choice that the health care provider recommends. Compliance with the practitioner's wishes regarding medication also varies appreciably with patients' abilities to comprehend what they have been told.

Some physicians argue that there exist no clear guidelines or comprehensive rules to which they can adhere in deciding what is acceptable disclosure in an emergency, or when they are legally protected in invoking therapeutic privilege. Although the courts have ruled on many occasions about the legal doctrine of informed consent, they seldom convey to physicians exactly what the law demands of them (Sprung & Winick, 1989). The following guidelines seem reasonable:

1. A patient must agree to an intervention based on an understanding of relevant information.
2. Consent must not be controlled by influences that would engineer the outcome.
3. The consent must involve the intentional giving of permission for an intervention (Silverman, 1989).

It is evident that progress has been made in the matter of informed consent. In the 1960s, nearly all doctors believed as a general rule, that they should not tell patients their diagnoses. In the 1980s, almost all doctors surveyed believed that they should reveal diagnoses to patients (Sprung & Winick, 1989). The more effective health professionals communicate with their patients and accept their judgment after proper information has been conveyed to them. The willingness to be as honest as conditions allow is a major characteristic of an ethical health care provider. Such a practitioner has little to fear, either from the courts or from peers.

Clinical Trials

There is another important application of informed consent in medical practice. Health caregivers and researchers must get patients' written consent prior to entering them in randomized clinical trials. These trials are valuable because they provide a way of generating scientific data when there is no single recognized best treatment for a disease. In such a case, the clinical trial may be used to compare the present treatment with a new, possibly better, but unproven treatment alternative. Clinical trials can elicit information from particular patients, which may then be extrapolated to large populations of patients suffering from similar diseases. The consent form is a legal document which states that patients have been informed of their disease, the risks of treatment, and the possible side effects, and that they agree to random assignment to one of the trial's treatment options.

Notwithstanding the legal and moral necessity of patient consent forms for clinical trials, this often presents physicians with serious ethical problems. Some clinical trials have used a disproportionate number of ethnic minority groups, mainly children, as subjects, both in the United States and abroad. The representatives of these groups are usually from the lower classes. One of the reasons for this is that researchers are often situated in teaching hospitals that are utilized by poor patients. The National Commission for the Protection of Human Subjects of Biomedical and Behavioral Research (1977) recommended that children who take part in research projects should be chosen so that the burdens of participation are shared among all parts of society in a just manner. However, the report says nothing about how this recommendation will be implemented. Silverman (1989) hypothesized that the selection process for clinical trials automatically excludes affluent adults of society and their children—they are the ones who are most likely to understand what is requested in the consent form and to opt out. It is mainly those persons who do not understand who "consent."

Currently, American pharmaceutical companies are conducting clinical trials in the United States and several Third World countries. How much protection for these subjects is there? How much do they really comprehend about the risks involved? Do many of the subjects feel coerced by local civil and medical authorities? This is a major moral issue which should awaken the conscience of all health professionals, many of whom reap the benefits of such research.

To Die or Not to Die

Concern about the needs of terminally ill patients has increased during the past twenty years. Nelson and Bernat (1989) list four related factors that influence the ethical issues centering on the withholding or terminating of a patient's treatment: (1) most people die after an extended period of gradually deteriorating health; (2) there is almost always an additional therapy available to prolong a patient's life; (3) most hospital deaths follow decision making at the end of life, so someone must decide how long life will be prolonged and at what quality; and (4) usually there is time for patients, family members, and physicians to discuss the appropriate date to terminate or withhold treatment to hasten a person's death.

Beauchamp and Childress (1983) delineated three ethical principles relevant to the issue of withholding or terminating treatment: (1) *autonomy* —the right of patients to make decisions for themselves, which other persons must respect; (2) *nonmaleficence* —the concept of "do not harm"; (3) *beneficence* —the duty to promote good. These principles respectively have the following corresponding moral rules: "do not deprive people of freedom," "do not kill," "do not cause pain or disability," and "do no evil." Attempts to apply these ethical principles and moral rules are complicated by the fact that clinicians and researchers do not agree on definitions for "well-being," "quality of life," "health status," and "functional status."

The most stressful part of medicine for health caregivers is making life-death decisions. It is common for people who have been trained to save lives to become angry and frustrated when a patient's condition worsens to the point that there is no hope, either from medicine or a skilled practitioner. They wonder why medicine, with all its marvelous advances, cannot keep a human being from extinction after they have given the sick patient the benefit of all their years of training and dedication. The worst situation in which caregivers can find themselves is that in which they have to decide whether to continue treating the patient who has no possibility of recovery and yet is not legally dead. What could be more emotionally devastating for a spouse, child, relative, or friend than to have to make a choice between keeping a comatose loved one alive artificially or letting him or her die as painlessly and quickly as possible.

During the last decade, one of the most crucial questions confronting physicians has been whether to withdraw life-support systems from patients whose only future condition can be that of vegetation. The general public has given its opinion by a substantial margin. An Associated Press/Media General poll conducted in 1985 showed that 68 percent of the respondents stated that "people dying of an incurable painful disease should be allowed to end their lives before the disease runs its course." That this opinion is gaining in support, can be seen in the 1987 decision by the California Department of Health Services to become the first state agency to develop clear guidelines for the removal of life support, including tube feeding, in the state's 1500 nursing homes and convalescent hospitals (Wanzer et al., 1989).

The widespread use of end of life directives suggests that attitudes regarding the termination of life have changed. The "living will," a legally nonbinding instrument in its generic form, is a legally binding instrument when properly executed under a state's "terminal care document" or "natural death act" statutes. These directives protect the right of incompetent patients to reject life-sustaining measures when they are terminally ill and have no reasonable expectation of recovery. Although a living will instrument is better than no indication of the wishes of an incompetent patient, it has a very limited application because its language is not specific, and its purpose is applicable only to terminal situations. A more effective directive is the "durable power of attorney for health care" (DPAHC). This instrument allows any adult to name a person authorized to make surrogate medical decisions if he or she becomes incompetent. The value of the DPAHC is its flexibility to adapt the individual's value system to any particular medical situation.

DECLARATION

Declaration made this _____ day of _____ (month, year).

I, _____ , being of sound mind, willfully and voluntarily make known my desire that my dying shall not be artificially prolonged under the circumstances set forth below, do hereby declare:

If at any time I should have an incurable injury, disease, or illness certified to be a terminal condition by two physicians who have personally examined me, one of whom shall be my attending physician, and the physicians have determined that my death will occur whether or not life-sustaining procedures are utilized and where the application of life-sustaining procedures would serve only to artificially prolong the dying process, I direct that such procedures be withheld or withdrawn, and that I be permitted to die naturally with only the administration of medication or the performance of any medical procedure deemed necessary to provide me with comfort care.

In the absence of my ability to give directions regarding the use of such life-sustaining procedures, it is my intention that this declaration shall be honored by my family and physician(s) as the final expression of my legal right to refuse medical or surgical treatment and accept the consequences from such refusal.

I understand the full import of this declaration and I am emotionally and mentally competent to make this declaration.

Signed _____

City, County and State of Residence _____

The declarant has been personally known to me and I believe him or her to be of sound mind.

Witness _____

Witness _____

Figure 7-1. A sample "living will" developed by the Society for the Right to Die.

Several states now have DPAHC laws that give legal authority for designating a surrogate (Nelson & Bernat, 1989, p. 761).

In 1989, thirty-eight states and the District of Columbia had laws pertaining to living wills and 15 states specifically approved a patient's health care proxy authorization for withholding or withdrawing life support (Wanzer et al., 1989). Some courts accept informal written documents that specifically convey the patient's wishes about life support, while other courts accept as evidence verbal statements that convey a clear wish regarding life support. Prior to 1988, all courts that ruled on the matter held that court involvement was not mandatory in a decision to withdraw life support from a comatose patient (Davenport, 1989). The states whose courts have dealt with the question of the withdrawal of nutrition and hydration from incompetent patients have treated it in the same way as the withdrawal of advanced life support (Ruark et al., 1988).

The legal history of the right to die in the United States is lengthy and complex. In *Canterbury v. Spence* (1972), the District of Columbia Circuit Court held that a competent adult has the right "to forgo treatment or even cure, if it entails what for him are intolerable consequences or risks, however unwise his sense of values may be in the eyes of the medical profession." In *Barber v. Superior Court* (1983), two physicians were charged with murder when they withdrew intravenous nourishment and hydration from an irreversibly comatose man with the informed consent of the patient's family. A California intermediate appellate court dismissed the charges and used the concept of *proportionality* as the criterion to be used in deciding whether to withdraw life support. The *Barber* court stated: "Proportionate treatment is that which, in the view of the patient, has at least a reasonable chance of providing benefits to the patient which outweigh the burdens attendant to the treatment." The court went on to say that, in such cases, doctors must identify a surrogate to make a substituted judgment on behalf of the patient. The court also held that, without legislation to the contrary, it is legal to bypass formal conservatorship proceedings. Relatedly, an Ohio appellate court held in the case of *Estate of Leach v. Shapiro* (1984) that a physician may be sued for placing and maintaining a patient on life-support systems without the informed consent of the patient or his guardian (see Areen, 1987).

In a landmark decision, *Bartling v. Superior Court* (1984), the California Court of Appeals ruled in favor of William Bartling, who was competent, and neither comatose nor terminal, and whose death was not necessarily imminent. He refused to accept the quality of life that necessitated an endotracheal tube and respirator from which he could not be weaned. Citing the Constitutional right to privacy, the court said: "If the right of the patient to self-determination as to his own medical treatment is to have any meaning, it must be paramount to the interests of the patient's hospital and doctors." The court concluded that the life-support systems should have been removed as the patient requested (see Abrams, 1987, p. 78).

In the case of *In re Jobes* (1986), the New Jersey Supreme Court was petitioned by a guardian to allow the removal of a gastrostomy tube. The young woman in the case, who was in a nursing home, had been in a permanent vegetative state for six years, and her physicians agreed there was absolutely no hope for a better condition. The court held that artificial feeding by means of a nasogastric tube or intravenous infusion was equivalent to artificial breathing by means of a respirator because both extend "life through mechanical means when the body is no longer able to perform a vital bodily function of its own." The court went on to say that the guardian ad litem did not have to argue for continuation of the incompetent ward's life in each and every case.

One of the most significant cases in the matter of the right to die is that of Elizabeth Bouvia, a young and fully competent quadriplegic secondary to cerebral palsy (*Bouvia v. Superior Court,* 1986). Ms. Bouvia petitioned the court to allow removal of an involuntarily placed nasogastric tube, but her request was rejected on grounds that the state's interest and the physician's duty to preserve life overrode her right of privacy. In April 1986, the appeals court overruled the lower court and stated that the right to refuse treatment is not confined to terminal patients because it is a personal, not a legal or medical, decision. The Superior Court in Riverside, California, went on to say that it was immaterial if the decision hastened death. In a concurring opinion, Judge Compton wrote: "The right to die is an integral part of our right to control our own destinies so long as the rights of others are not affected. That right should, in my opinion, include the ability to enlist assistance from others, including the medical profession, in making death as painless and as quick as possible."

In 1983, William Drabick, then thirty-nine years old, suffered a severe head injury that resulted in a subdural hematoma. Although the hematoma was evacuated, Drabick remained in a coma, sustained by nasogastric feeding. His electroencephalogram showed some brain activity; thus, he was not brain dead. All of his physicians believed that he had no chance of regaining consciousness. Drabick's brother was appointed conservator, and in 1985 he petitioned a California superior court to order nasogastric feeding stopped. The court refused to so order, and the conservator petitioned the appellate court to review the case. The appellate court ordered the feeding stopped and said that doctors may stop life-supporting treatment when surrogates agree with them that continued treatment is not likely to materially improve the patient's prognosis for recovery. The court further asserted that without legislative guidance, no prior court sanction was necessary before a decision to withdraw treatment was made. The court ended by stating that "courts are not the primary decision makers in the area of medical treatment" (see Davenport, 1989).

However, two court decisions in 1988 added to the confusion in the issue of the right to die. In the case of *In re O'Connor*, the New York Court of Appeals said that Mary O'Connor, a comatose patient, could not have treatment in the form of a feeding tube withheld from her unless there was unequivocal evidence that she would have chosen to refuse it. The ruling held that previous statements by a patient might not indicate "reflection and resolve" or address the current situation directly, and the patient may have changed her mind. Lo et al. (1990) said that "this decision set a standard of proof so strict that few patients are likely to satisfy it" (p. 1228). In August, 1989, Mary O'Connor died at the age of 78 with the feeding tube in place.

A Landmark Case

In Chapter Six, we discussed the case of Nancy Cruzan, who remained in a type of coma known as a "persistent vegetative state" for seven years. The legal and social impact of her case merits a closer review. In July 1988, Jasper (Missouri) County Probate Judge, Charles Teel, ruled the feedings could end. But, in November 1988, the Missouri Supreme Court ruled that families cannot order life support stopped without "the most rigid formalities" such as a living will or clear and convincing evidence that the patient would have rejected artificial feedings. On June 25, 1990, the United States Supreme Court ruled in the case of *Cruzan v. Harmon* (1988), which was the Court's first right-to-die decision, that the state of Missouri could sustain Ms. Cruzan's life because her parents had not shown by "clear and convincing evidence" that she would have wished the feeding treatment withdrawn.

Eight of the justices, with Justice Scalia dissenting, concurred that a Constitutional right exists, as part of the "liberty" guaranteed by the 14th Amendment, to refuse unwanted medical treatment. But when a permanently unconscious individual has not left clear instructions, the state is free to assert its interest in "the protection and preservation of human life" by rejecting a family's request to end treatment. The four justices who favored the right of the Cruzan family to have feeding withdrawn stated that the majority opinion did not take into consideration the patient's quality of life or that of her family. However, it was the issue of Ms. Cruzan's wish that ultimately determined the outcome. The case was returned to Judge Teel to determine if Ms. Cruzan would have wanted to die. On December 14, 1990, Judge Teel ruled that there was clear and convincing evidence that Ms. Cruzan would want to end her life. And he ruled that her parents may have the feeding tube removed. The director of the Missouri Rehabilitation Center in Mount Vernon, where Ms. Cruzan was being cared for, carried out the order. On December 26, 1990, Nancy Cruzan died.

After Nancy Cruzan

The Cruzan case has had a far-reaching effect. Earlier in 1990, U.S. Senator John Danforth, of Missouri, sponsored a federal law requiring health care institutions that accept Medicare and Medicaid funds to give adult patients written information explaining their right-to-die options under their state laws. Also, hospital personnel and other health caregivers must note on medical records whether patients have received legal directives on treatment. The goal is to ensure compliance with patients' wishes to accept or refuses medical care in the event they become incapacitated. Implicit in the law is the right to live and die with dignity. This was a bittersweet victory for Ms. Cruzan's parents, who lobbied Congress for passage of the law.

It is particularly important for physicians to discuss end-of-life treatment with patients while they are competent. At the same time that they encourage their patients to make directives concerning terminal care, they can counsel them about possible medical situations they could face at the end of life. Hospitals and nursing homes should also inquire of all patients whether they have signed living wills or other such directives. Physicians who work in nursing homes should check regularly to see if end-of-life instruments have been filled out and if they are up to date. In this instance, we can see why physicians should get to know their patients' values.

Physicians and other health professionals should bear in mind that patients near the end of life need reassurance that they will not be abandoned. Whether dying patients are in a hospital, nursing home, or their own home, physicians must devise a careplan for each individual. Always, the caregiver should ask patients if the benefits of a particular treatment are worth the discomforts it produces. Allowing dying patients to suffer needlessly is unethical, and most practitioners strongly recommend that narcotic doses which produce a reliable pain-free state, be administered. Because adequate narcotic management is a difficult area for many doctors, it has been suggested that educational materials from a noncommercial source be given to them (Wanzer et al., 1989). Chemical addiction in dying patients usually does not present an ethical problem for physicians; alleviation of intense suffering associated with terminal illness is the main concern. Ruark et al. (1988) recommends a six-step plan for physicians to carry out before the decision to withdraw life-support measures is made:

1. Exercise reasonable clinical judgment about the likelihood of medical benefit from further treatment.
2. Assess the patient's competence.
3. Seek unanimity among members of the health care team. Consult regularly with attending nurses, since they usually spend hours by the bedside of the patient and often have information about patients and families physicians may not have.
4. Vigorously solicit the patient's judgment regarding withdrawal of treatment.
5. Do not rush decision-making with families.
6. Establish time-limited goals, based on clinical judgment and information such as the Acute Physiologic Assessment and Chronic Health Evaluation (Apache II). (p. 29)

An excellent way for a physician to inform patients and families that he or she believes life support should be withdrawn is to say, "It is my best judgment, and that of the other doctors and nurses, that your relative has essentially no chance to regain a reasonable quality of life. We believe that life support should be withdrawn, which means that your relative will probably die." This statement has two advantages. First, it is realistically qualified in a manner which suggests that the decision must be shared. Second, it makes explicit the fact that death will be the probable result of the suggested course. If this knowledge is not conveyed, there is no true informed consent.

The preceding guidelines do not stop physicians from being reluctant to do what the courts allow regarding withdrawal of life-sustaining treatment. Perhaps one of the reasons for this reluctance is that physicians often do not know how to deal with patients and families at the end of life. Some doctors believe that under certain conditions it may be appropriate to withhold treatment, but that it should not be withdrawn once it has been begun. The distinction is not ethically valid. As a general practice, a treatment is started based upon its potential benefit and the agreement of the patient. If the benefits are less than projected or if the risks are greater than foreseen and the competent patient reasonably rejects the treatment, it should be abandoned. However, if health care professionals have deep ethical objections to taking part in such treatment plans, they have a right to refuse to assist in carrying them out. A health care professional is not obligated to accede to the patient in a way that violates the provider's own moral beliefs.

Euthanasia

Euthanasia, which means "good death" or "happy death," refers to either the commission of some act that shortens a person's life or the omission of an act that would prolong it. This is not a recent phenomenon. Aristotle believed that there should be a law prohibiting deformed children to be reared. In the 5th century B.C., Euripedes encouraged people enduring long illnesses to "quit this life" and make room for healthy youth. Thomas More, a Utopian writer, wanted priests and magistrates to urge persons who suffer painful incurable illnesses to end their misery or let someone else release them from it. Seneca summed up these views: "If one death is accompanied by torture, and the other is simple and easy, why not snatch the latter?"

Modern efforts to legalize euthanasia began in 1938, when the Euthanasia Society of America was organized. The three major recommendations of the Society were: (1) compulsory euthanasia for the aged, incurably diseased, and the insane, (2) compulsory euthanasia for genetically defective persons in the early stages of their lives, and (3) voluntary euthanasia for dying persons. Questions which frame the issues of euthanasia include the following: If death is legally and morally preferred to intense suffering, is it also preferred to drugged stupor? What is an individual dying of a terminal disease obliged to do? What is a physician treating a terminal patient obliged to do? Are our obligations toward a terminal patient being kept alive artificially different from those toward patients not being kept alive artificially?

Euthanasia is a very different issue from that of withholding or withdrawing life-sustaining measures. In 1988, a Roper Poll of 1,982 Americans, taken for the National Hemlock Society, asked the question: "Should a physician be lawfully able to end the life of a terminally ill patient at the patient's request?" Of those polled, 58 percent said yes, 27 percent said no, and 15 percent were undecided (Wanzer et al., 1989). Nevertheless, since patients seek health, they have a right to believe that a physician will provide medical treatment to make them well, or as well as they can become. Treatment to cause death does not heal and it is thus basically contradictory to the physician's role in the patient-physician relationship (Orentlicher, 1989). Whenever physicians or other caregivers agree to kill, there is usually a strong negative impact on society's perception of them, and this in itself leads to disapproval of euthanasia.

What To Choose?

Within recent years, a new concept has been introduced into the healer-patient relationship—quality of life. It has brought health care professionals to the realization that they must be cognizant of their patients' values. What possible effects, they must ask themselves, will their choice of treatment have on the future life of a patient? What kind of life does a particular patient choose to live after treatment? A patient's choice will be conditioned by the values he or she holds. Thus, the health care practitioner's treatment decision should be based largely on the particular quality of life that a patient desires. If treatment condemns the patient to an existence that he considers a living hell, even though it has brought about a "cure," does it really "heal" him? What worth does longevity of existence have if that existence is devoid of all meaning and pleasure for a particular individual? If quality of life has a different meaning for each individual, ethical practitioners will make treatment decisions for a particular patient only after they have learned of that patient's choice concerning life after treatment.

In order for patients to make such a choice, they must have proper information about the risks and benefits of a proposed method of treatment, as well as the risks and benefits of alternate therapies. It is here that one of the health care providers' major ethical responsibilities lies. They must make certain that each patient receives all the information necessary for making informed choices. Courts of law in the United States, for the last eighty-five years, have tried to spell out what "informed consent" means for patients and physicians. That the courts' attempts have sometimes led to confusion does not obscure the fact that physicians and other health care professionals are ethically and legally bound to make patients aware of what a proposed course of treatment entails, insofar as they are able to do so. The legal necessity of informed consent, although often neglected by many practitioners, has a beneficial effect on the patient-practitioner relationship. It has empowered patients to assume the major responsibility for their treatment and their future.

And what if the future holds for a patient only the certainty of a long, cruelly painful effort to sustain his or her life when there is no hope for recovery? Should the patient and his or her family be forced to undergo the traumatic experience such an effort entails? Many health care professionals would argue that life-sustaining measures in such an instance should be withheld or, if already begun, withdrawn. The question is simple, yet complex: What choice should be made?

REFERENCES

Abrams, F. R. (1987). Withholding treatment when death is not imminent. *Geriatrics,* 42: 77–84.

Areen, J. (1987). The legal status of consent obtained from families of adult patients to withhold or withdraw treatment. *JAMA, 258:* 229–235.

Associated Press/Media General. (1985). *Poll No. 4:* Richmond, VA: Associated Press.

Barber v. Superior Court, 147 Cal. App. 3d 1006 (1983).

Bartling v. Superior Court, 209 Cal. Rptr. 220 CA of App. 2d Div. 5 (1984).

Beauchamp, T. L. & Childress, J. F. (1983). *Principles of biomedical ethics.* 2d ed. New York: Oxford University Press.

Bouvia v. Superior Court, 179 Cal. App. 3d 1127 (1986).

Brody, H. (1989). Transparency: Informed consent in primary care. *Hastings Center Report 19:* 5–9.

Canterbury v. Spence, 464 F. 2d 772, 787 (D.C. Cir.), *cert. denied,* 409 U.S. 1064 (1972).

Cobbs v. Grant, 8 Cal. 3d 229, P.2d 1 (1972).

Croog, S. et al. (1986). The effects of antihypertensive therapy on quality of life. *New England Journal of Medicine, 314:* 1657–1664.

Cruzan v. Harmon, 760 S.W. 2d 408 (1988).

Danis, M. et al. (1988). Patients' and families' preferences for medical intensive care. *JAMA, 260:* 797–802.

Davenport, J. (1989). Common questions about withdrawal of life support. *American Family Physician, 39:* 201–205.

Drummond, M. F. (1987). Resource allocation decisions in health care: A role for quality of life assessments? *Journal of Chronic Diseases, 40:* 605–616.

Eiseman, B. (1981). The second dimension. *Archives of Surgery, 116:* 11–13.

Estate of Leach v. Shapiro, 13 Ohio App. 3d 393, 469 N.E. 2d 1047 (1984).

Flight, M. R. (1986). Informed consent: The physician's dilemma. *The Professional Medical Assistant, 19:* 11–13.

Fowler, F. J. et al. (1988). Symptom status and quality of life following prostatectomy. *JAMA, 259:* 3018–3022.

Greenhouse, L. (1990). Justices find a right to die, but the majority sees need for clear proof of intent. *New York Times,* June 26: A-1 ff.

Harnish v. Children's Hospital Medical Center, 387 Mass. 152, 439 N.E. 2d 240 (1982).

Hollandsworth, J. G. (1988). Evaluating the impact of medical treatment on the quality of life: A 5-year update. *Social Science and Medicine, 26:* 425–434.

Hume, A. L. (1989). Applying quality of life data in practice: Considerations for antihypertensive therapy. *Journal of Family Practice, 28:* 403–406.

In re Jobes, No. C4971-85 E. N.J. Sup. Ct. Ch. Div. Morris Cty (1986).

In re O'Connor, 72 N.Y. 2d 517, 531 N.E. (1988). 2d 607, 531 N.Y. S. 2d 886.

In the Matter of Claire Conroy, 3457A, 2d 1232, N.J. Sup. C Ch. Div. (1983).

Kaufmann, C. L. (1983). Informed consent and patient decision making: Two decades of research. *Social Science and Medicine, 17:* 1657–1664.

Lidz, C. W., Meisel, A. & Munetz, M. (1985). Chronic disease: The sick role and informed consent. *Culture, Medicine, and Psychiatry, 9:* 241–255.

Lo, B. Rouse, F. & Dornbrand, L. (1990). Family decision making on trial: Who decides for incompetent patients? *New England Journal of Medicine, 322:* 1228–1232.

May, R. (1953). *Man's search for himself.* New York: W. W. Norton.

Mohr v. Williams, 95 Minn. 261, 104 N.W. 12 (1905).

Mosteller, F. (1987). Implications of measures of quality of life for policy development. *Journal of Chronic Diseases, 40:* 645–650.

Nathanson v. Kline, 186 Kan. 393, 350 P.2d 1093, 1104 (1960).

National Commission for the Protection of Human Subjects and Behavioral Research. (1977). *Research involving children.* Washington, D.C.: U. S. Government Printing Office.

Nelson, W. A. & Bernat, J. L. (1989). Decisions to withhold or terminate treatment. *Neurologic Clinics: Ethical Issues in Neurologic Practice, 7:* 759–774.

Orentlicher, D. (1989). Physician participation in assisted suicide. *JAMA, 262:* 1844–1845.

Patrick, D. L. & Deyo, R. A. (1989). Generic and disease-specific measures in assessing health status and quality of life. *Medical Care, 27:* 5217–5232.

President's Commission for the Study of Ethical Problems in Medicine and Biomedical and Behavioral Research. (1982). *Making health care decisions: The ethical and legal implications of informed consent in the patient-practitioner relationship.* Vol. 1. Washington, D.C.: U.S. Government Printing Office.

Revicki, D. A. (1989). Health-related quality of life in the evaluation of medical therapy for chronic illness. *Journal of Family Practice, 29:* 377–380.

Ruark, J. E. et al. (1988). Initiating and withdrawing life support: Principles and practice in adult medicine. *New England Journal of Medicine, 318:* 25–30.

Salgo v. Leland Stafford Jr. University Board of Trustees, 154 Cap. App. 2d 560, 317 P. 2d 170 (1957).

Schloendorft v. Society of New York Hospital, 211 N.Y. 125, 105 N.E. 92 (1914).

Silverman, W. A. (1989). The myth of informed consent: In daily practice and clinical trials. *Journal of Medical Ethics, 15:* 6–11.

Smith, H. L. (1987). Medical ethics in the primary care setting. *Social Science and Medicine, 25:* 705–709.

Sprung, C. L. & Winick, B. J. (1989). Informed consent in theory and practice: Legal and medical perspectives on the informed consent doctrine and a proposed reconceptualization. *Critical Care Medicine, 17:* 1346–1354.

Starr, T. J., Pearlman, R. A. & Uhlmann, R. F. (1986). Quality of life and resuscitation decisions in elderly patients. *Journal of General Internal Medicine, 1:* 373–379.

Tannock, I. F. (1987). Treating the patient, not just the cancer. *New England Journal of Medicine, 317:* 1534–1535.

Taylor, K. & Kelner, M. (1987). Informed consent: The physicians' perspective. *Social Science and Medicine, 24:* 135–143.

Taylor, T. R. (1989). Commentary. *Journal of Family Practice, 28:* 407–411.

Troidl, H. et al. (1987). Quality of life: An important endpoint both in surgical practice and research. *Journal of Chronic Diseases, 40:* 523–528.

Wanzer, S. et al. (1989). The physician's responsibility toward hopelessly ill patients: A second look. *New England Journal of Medicine, 320:* 844–849.

Wood-Dauphinee, S. & Williams, J. I. (1987). Reintegration to normal living as a proxy to quality of life. *Journal of Chronic Diseases, 40:* 491–499.

Yinnon, A., Zimran, A. & Hershko, C. (1989). Quality of life and survival following intensive medical care. *Quarterly Journal of Medicine, 71:* 347–357.

SUGGESTED READINGS

Appelbaum, P. S. & Grisso, T. (1988). Assessing patients' capacities to consent to treatment. *New England Journal of Medicine, 319:* 1635–1638.

Battin, M. P. (1985). Non-patient decision-making in medicine: The eclipse of altruism. *Journal of Medicine and Philosophy, 10:* 19–44.

Bedell, S. E. et al. (1986). Do-not-resuscitate orders for critically ill patients in the hospital: How are they used and what is their impact? *JAMA, 256:* 233–237.

Brennan, T. A. (1988). Ethics committees and decisions to limit care: The experience at the Massachusetts General Hospital. *JAMA, 260:* 803–807.

Bulkin, W. & Lukashok, H. (1988). Rx for dying: The case for hospice. *New England Journal of Medicine, 318:* 376–378.

Degner, F. & Beaton, J. (1987). *Life and death decisions in health care.* Washington, D.C.: Hemisphere.

Faden, R. & Beauchamp, T. L. (1986). *A history and theory of informed consent.* New York: Oxford University Press.

Ferrell, B. R. et al. (1989). Quality of life as an outcome variable in the management of cancer pain. *Cancer, 63:* 2321–2327.

Fletcher, A. E. et al. (1987). Evaluation of quality of life in clinical trials of cardiovascular disease. *Journal of Chronic Diseases, 40:* 557–566.

Gillett, G. R. (1989). Informed consent and moral integrity. *Journal of Medical Ethics, 15:* 117–123.

Guyatt, G. H. et al. (1989). Measuring quality of life in clinical trials: A taxonomy and review. *Canadian Medical Association Journal, 140:* 1441–1448.

Hull, R. T. (1985). Informed consent: Patient's right or patient's duty? *Journal of Medicine and Philosophy, 10:* 183–197.

Kaplan, R. M. et al. (1988). The quality of well-being scale. *Medical Care, 27:* 27–43.

Kapp, M. B. (1989). Enforcing patient preferences: Linking payment for medical care to informed consent. *JAMA, 261:* 1935–1938.

Katz, S. (1987). The science of quality of life. *Journal of Chronic Diseases, 40:* 459–463.

Lane, D. (1987). Utility, decision, and quality of life. *Journal of Chronic Diseases, 40:* 585–591.

Lo, B. et al. (1986). Patient attitudes to discussing life-sustaining treatment. *Archives of Internal Medicine, 146:* 1613 ff.

Lynn, J. (1986). *By no ordinary means,* Bloomington, IN: University of Indiana Press.

Mulley, A. G. (1989). Assessing patients' utilities: Can the ends justify the means? *Medical Care, 27:* 69–81.

O'Young, J. & McPeek, B. (1987). Quality of life variables in surgical trials. *Journal of Chronic Diseases, 40:* 513–522.

Rothman, D. J. (1987). Ethics and human experimentation: Henry Beecher revisited. *New England Journal of Medicine, 317:* 1195–1199.

Schneiderman, L. J. & Spragg, R. G. (1988). Ethical decisions in discontinuing mechanical ventilation. *New England Journal of Medicine, 318:* 984–988.

Society for the Right to Die. (1987). *Handbook of living will laws.* New York: Society for the Right to Die.

Steinbrook, R. & Lo, B. (1988). Artificial feeding: Solid ground not a slippery slope. *New England Journal of Medicine, 318:* 286.

Testa, A. & Simonson, D. C. (1988). Measuring quality of life in hypertensive patients with diabetes. *Postgraduate Medical Journal, 64:* 50–58.

Tomlinson, T. (1986). The physician's influence on patients' choices. *Theoretical Medicine, 7:* 105–122.

Wanzer, S. H. et al. (1989). The physician's responsibility toward hopelessly ill patients. *New England Journal of Medicine, 310:* 955.

Wu, W. C. & Pearlman, R. A. (1988). Consent in medical decision-making: The role of communication. *Journal of General Internal Medicine, 3:* 9–14.

Chapter 8

HEALING AS A VALUE

Wherever there is a heart and an intellect, the disease of the physical frame are tinged with the peculiarities of these.

Nathaniel Hawthorne, *The Scarlet Letter,* 1893

For many years, American medicine has been the envy of the world. It has gone from triumph to triumph in its fight with disease and its conquest of pain and suffering. The nature and circumstances of illnesses that cause death have changed dramatically over the last century. No longer are tuberculosis, scarlet fever, and gastroenteritis the major causes of death in the United States. These diseases, as well as most childhood illnesses, have been almost eliminated by medical science and modern health-care procedures. Now, the major causes of death in the United States are heart disease, cancer, and strokes. Thus, communicable diseases have been replaced by degenerative diseases.

American physicians have been pioneers in developing a myriad of surgical techniques that have prolonged life in an almost miraculous manner. And American pharmaceutical companies are responsible for devising hundreds of types of medication that are used by health care providers in their daily ministrations. For a long time in the United States, medical healers have enjoyed a status and income which has made them unique among the medical practitioners of all nations. However, never has there been a time in the last 150 years when so much controversy has surrounded the medical profession. One need only point to the record-breaking number of malpractice suits in the last ten years to show that the public's view of the healer has changed in a way that can only be harmful to medicine.

It is, therefore, time to reexamine the roles of the two principle members of the healing dyad: physicians and patients. The responsibility of the former is to make whole people who come to them seeking relief from disease and pain. Healing is obviously the highest value of medical and allied health professions, and health care providers are judged by their success, or lack of it, in freeing patients from various ills, insofar as that is possible. Thus, precisely because it is a value, healing involves ethical questions, some often so complex that even individuals trained in both medicine and philosophy disagree among themselves about the right course of action. It is no wonder then that the general public, both patients and mere observers, become confused as they face the moral issues pertaining to health care.

As if trying to resolve the ethical dilemmas which arise in the healing relationship were not task enough for health caregivers, they are now faced with the possibility that economic considerations may force them to adapt to a mode of health care delivery that, if not subversive of the value of healing, may be in conflict with it. Some health care practitioners, unable to accept the possible displacement of healing as the central value of medicine, have chosen to leave the profession altogether. It is quite possible that American physicians are now facing a crisis more serious than any they have ever faced before because it forces them to examine the basis of the healing relationship—the obligations, both medical and moral, they have to their patients.

But it is not physicians alone who have obligations in the healing relationship. Patients also have certain responsibilities to themselves and to the healer once they enter into an agreement to be treated. Does unwillingness on the patient's part to play an active role in decision making about the healing process reflect an attitude of moral abdication? Yes, it does. Can patients become truly "whole" or optimally "cured" if they have surrendered their autonomy to the healer? Probably not. It is important for us to understand the role of the healer and the patient, for there is much evidence that active participation by the patient in the decision making in the healing process actually helps that process along.

Values, Ethics, and Morals

When considering the professional dilemmas in the healing relationship, it is beneficial to distinguish between values, ethics, and morals. As noted in Chapter 1, these are the intangible principles that we employ to arrive at ethical decisions. *Values are the abstract, generalized concepts or beliefs that are often internalized from early social experiences.* They are prioritized according to what is of greatest worth or most desirable to us. A value must meet three criteria. It must be freely chosen, it must be

cherished and it must be acted upon (Reilly, 1989). Intrinsic values—
those we internalize—are usually ranked above extrinsic ones; and productive and fairly permanent values are preferred over those that are
less productive and less permanent. Generally, values are chosen on the
basis of our own ideals and life goals. Consequently, our values tend to
be consistent with each other and with the demands our life goals make
on us. When people are confronted with two negative situations, the less
negative one is usually selected. When behaviors do not match our
values, the result is personal and professional disequilibrium.

Ethics is the code of values of a person, profession, group or religion. Such
codes were formulated to guide our action, or to make possible the
application of our values in formal and informal situations. Pedagogically,
ethics consist of three subject areas: descriptive ethics, metaethics, and
normative ethics (Fowler, 1989). Descriptive ethics focuses on factual
descriptions such as are found in scientific research. It does not produce
moral judgments on behaviors or beliefs. Metaethics is more concerned
with theoretical issues of "meaning" and "justification," and with "logical
semantic questions." To be more precise, metaethics is concerned with
theories about ethics. Normative ethics, on the other hand, is concen-
trated in two major divisions: norms of values and norms of obligation.
Most of the current health care literature in ethics attempts to address
the normative issues in professional practice, education, and research in
order to formulate reasoned value positions in health care.

*Morals are related to decisions concerning "right or wrong" and "good and
evil" in matters of conduct and character.* They are principles sanctioned by,
or operative on, our conscience or judgment, and they relate to or act on
our mind, character, or will. Health care practitioners are beset by
conflicts in decision making that stem from a variety of interpretations of
morality in doing their jobs.

The earliest formal code of medical ethics, the Code of Hammurabi,
which dates back to about 2,000 B.C. was created by the Babylonians.
This was an extremely detailed document, but it was not flexible enough
to adapt to the rapid developments in medical practice or even to the
evolving complexity of cultural patterns of its time. Later, in the 5th
century B.C., a Greek physician and other medical practitioners developed
the Oath of Hippocrates (see Appendix A). This code protects the rights
of patients and instructs the healer by appealing to moral injunctions
rather than imposing penalties or sanctions. In 1803, Thomas Percival, a
British author, physician and philosopher, published a code of conduct

based on hospital situations. Most scholars agree that this was an outstanding contribution to medical ethics.

In 1847, the American Medical Association (AMA) met in Philadelphia and created a code of ethics that included minimum requirements for educating and training physicians. The code went unchallenged for many years, but, in the interest of stating the basic concepts in the clearest possible way, revisions were made in 1903, 1912, and 1947. In 1957, a drastic revision of the principles was accepted by the AMA House of Delegates — the code was reduced to a preamble and ten short sections. In 1977, another revision was made to respond to contemporary legal standards, and in 1980, at the request of the AMA Judicial Council, a revision was written that eliminated all reference to gender. This latter revision also provides medicolegal guidelines (see Appendix F). Spurred on by the various medical codes, nurses and other health care professionals have developed ethical codes and pledges of their own (see Appendices G & H).

The Role of the Healer

Physicians are usually defined as the dominant persons in the healing process. Parsons (1951) summarized this situation in the following way: "In many respects, relational nexus which generally becomes involved in health care resembles that of the family, with the physician or other agent of health care playing a quasi-parental role which emphasizes the adequate handling of the patient, and the latter playing a quasi-child role" (pp. 445–446). The parental metaphor used by Parsons is but one of his many views — albeit the predominant view — of the role of the healer.

Throughout the history of every nation, healers have been the object of veneration and awe, for they alone of all members of the community are believed to have the power to fend off disease and death with their special skills. Therefore it is not remarkable that in many rural cultures the individual regarded as a healer or medical force is often the equivalent of a priest or priestess in touch with the supernatural. How else can the masses account for the daily "miracles" these people perform? Certainly healers have never been seen as ordinary mortals in the thoughts of their followers, be they prehistoric, ancient, medieval, or modern peoples. At the same time, individuals so powerful can use their skills for either good or evil. Because healers have always held a kind of double-edged gift, their society has never let them stray, without retribution, from the twin paths of responsibility and beneficence. Surely, it is not without reason that the most admired physician in all history, Hippocrates, is not best remembered for medicinal or surgical innovations but for a code of ethics attributed to him—a code that affects those who would practice scientific medicine.

Still a moral beacon today is the Hippocratic Code of Medical Ethics that it is one of the very few secular guides to benevolent action that rank with the teachings of the great religious prophets. In its own way, perhaps, it too is primarily of a religious nature, for its creators were obviously convinced that the medical practitioner touched not only patients' bodies with their healing power but their souls as well, and the Hippocratic Code focuses on the burden of responsibility such powers bring with them. For this reason, if for no other, the practice of medicine can never be considered apart from the ideas of the "good" and the "holy." If medical scholars in 5th century B.C. Greece realized that the physician must be guided by moral precepts, it is certainly appropriate for us to wonder out loud how much more relevant today is this lesson for those who reap the vast rewards of modern medical technology.

It is fact that for the first time in history, there is the possibility that biomedical researchers will be able to push back the frontiers of death itself. Modern medicine requires an ethical system that is both complex and profound enough to make its new technology genuinely responsive to human values. Otherwise, its gifts to human beings will prove a mixed blessing at best and cataclysmic at worse. We must begin by asking: "Just what is it that the healer does for human beings?" "What is the major goal of medical science?" To say that physicians merely "cure" patients is to fail to appreciate their manifold responsibilities. Curing a disease is often but the first step in the healing process, for there are other times when curing a disease is not possible. Healing involves not only curing diseases, when possible, but it also involves returning sick individuals to a better state of health than they enjoyed before becoming ill. If health care providers allow patients to return to the style of life which brought on the sickness in the first place without at least warning them of the consequences, they can hardly be said to have accomplished an act of healing. Because healing is cumulative, it is the primary duty of health care providers to restore patients to the best possible condition, so far as that is within their power.

Certainly we always try to eliminate suffering and especially pain. But it is not the task of therapy merely to reduce mental and physical suffering. One may

be inclined to do this because one assumes that the elimination of suffering is
an essential or even *the* essential drive of man, as psychoanalysis proclaims in
the form of pleasure principle...One can achieve the right attitude toward
the problem of elimination of suffering in patients and in normal individuals
only if one considers the significance of self-realization and its value for
health. If the patient is able to make the choice we have mentioned he may still
suffer, but *no longer feel sick,* i.e., though somewhat disordered and stricken by a
certain anxiety, he is able to realize his essential capacities at least to a
considerable degree. (Goldstein, 1959, pp. 182–183)

When then does the practitioner heal but not cure? If patients are
suffering from a terminal illness, for example, it must be the goal of
healers to effect some compromise between what the disease allows and
the wishes of the patients. When patients learn that they are not going to
get well, it is the duty of practitioners to help them live as closely as
possible to optimum conditions. By helping patients to enjoy their
remaining time, insofar as they can, health care practitioners become
caretakers of the body and tutors to the soul, exemplifying the healer's
art at its highest level. One might say that it is at this level that medical
healers function as a bridge to eternity, for they, more than any other
human beings besides the clergy, have the privilege of touching the
boundaries of life and death.

In defining the relationship between health care providers and patients,
Agich (1983) maintains that it is marked by a three-step process: *explanation,*
prediction, and *control,* or, in other words, *diagnosis, prognosis,* and *therapy.*
Technical intervention based on scientific underpinnings is what differentiates medicine from other therapeutic occupations. Indeed, the medical practitioner is the possessor of particular technical skills as well as a
recognized social role. And these skills are crucial to the healer-patient
relationship. These skills are brought to bear on patients in an attempt to
ameliorate their condition. Competence is a necessary, but not a sufficient,
condition of healing. In health care, a balance is needed between *competence*
and *compassion* —the ability of the health professional to diagnose, treat,
and feel the illness. It is this balance that makes healing possible. Effective healing is shaped by the purposes of the healer and also by the
values of the patient.

Pellegrino (1982) suggested that health care professionals should begin
the healing process only when they have answered four questions overtly
or covertly asked by their patients: "What is wrong?" "What will it (the
disease or illness) do to me?" "What can be done for me?" "What should
be done for me?" The answers to these four questions should, in turn,

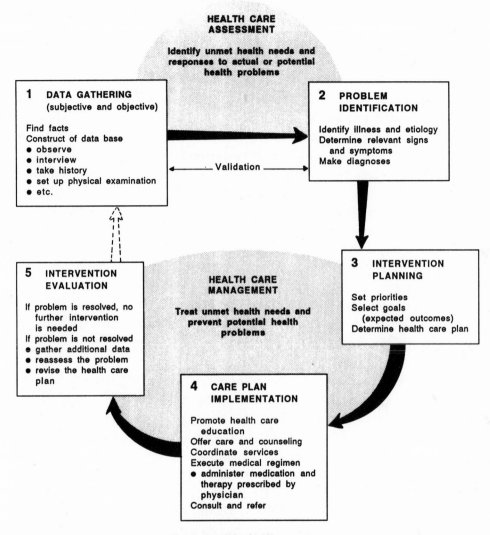

Figure 8-1. The healing process.

determine the choice of action. The proper healing intervention must meet three criteria. First, it should conform to the best available scientific information. It must make use of whatever data sources are relevant to the condition of the patient. Second, in order for the healer to be optimally effective, the information must be tailored to the particularities of the patient's illness. Special attention should be given to those things which make the patient a unique individual—age, gender, occupation, family relationships, race, etc. Third, the information must be adapted all along the way by the practitioner so that it will fit the goal of choosing the best interventions for the patient (see Fig. 8-1). Medicine is itself ultimately an exercise of practical values—a right way of acting in difficult and uncertain circumstances for a specific end, especially the good of a particular person who is ill" (Pellegrino & Thomasma, 1988).

The person who is ill, while needing to believe that the healer is a highly skilled practitioner, must also trust in him. Medicine is, after all, a science which deals with human beings, and sick human beings are very vulnerable. Most found that patients prefer emotional expressiveness and demonstration of affect by their health care providers to emotional neutrality (DiMatteo et al., 1985). So strong is this preference that patients often discontinue the therapeutic relationship with practitioners whom they believe do not show adequate emotional expressiveness. Peabody (1927) recognized this many years ago: "The treatment of a disease may be entirely impersonal; the care of a patient must be completely personal. The significance of the intimate personal relationship between physician and patient cannot be too strongly emphasized, for in an extraordinarily large number of cases both diagnosis and treatment are directly dependent on it. . . ." (p. 877).

So important to patients is emotional expressiveness on the part of care providers that their distress increases and trust decreases when healers are expressionless when interacting with them. Patient satisfaction with a medical regimen increases when practitioners communicate emotions through their faces and voices rather than assume a deadpan look and a monotonous way of speaking. Several studies verify the long-standing claim that the emotional needs of patients play a very important part in the interpersonal exchange between health care professionals and patients (Cousins, 1983; DiMatteo et al., 1985). Further, it should come as no surprise to learn that *reassurance* is the most valued of all emotions expressed by caregivers. Obviously, it is very important for patients to believe that not only can something be done to alleviate their suffering and fear, but that something will be done by skilled, sensitive healers.

It is the feeling of trust on the part of the patient that gives, to a great extent, the quality of holiness to the act of healing, for it has often been observed that the very presence of the healer has a placebo effect on the sufferer. There is no reason why a caregiver who is reassuring, warm, and concerned cannot also be medically skillful. To speak of competent *and* compassionate healers does not have to be a contradiction. Perhaps this is what many people mean when they refer to "the good old days" of medicine, the days when health care providers seemed to pay equal attention to the content of medicine as well as the process of healing. Although "the good old days" were really not so good for most of us, and returning to those earlier years would be impossible, when we speak of earlier years of medicine, we remember the doctor who came out to see us on a cold, rainy night. It meant that the healer was sincerely concerned about the patients' welfare. A doctor's presence at our bedside is still a tremendously reassuring experience when we are ill.

To counter the image of the "depersonalized" healer, Reiser and Rosen (1984) formulated what they call "four principles of medicine as a human experience." The first important principle for a medical practitioner to learn is *acceptance*. This term means that practitioners will take their patients as they are into their minds, their hearts, and their consciences. Acceptance is not an action; it is an encompassing attitude. Patients want and need to be received, embraced, taken in, and incorporated into a healing process. It is through acceptance that practitioners bond with patients. The basic reason for demonstrating acceptance is to build a relationship based upon trust and openness, to establish a situation that bolsters the patient's self-respect and, of course, to create an environment in which the patient can come to respect the practitioner. The essential ingredients involved in this aspect of healing are "caring" and "support" given through "respect." In a sense, many patients will perceive the health caregiver's attitude of acceptance as an either/or thing: either the health caregiver does or does not accept them. This may be an oversimplification, but patients who do not feel accepted will not be healed.

A second principle is *empathy*. This means the ability to comprehend and take part in another's feelings. The wise practitioner realizes that the patient's feelings are not identical to his or her own. It is the quality of empathy that enables practitioners to internally approximate what patients are actually experiencing. When internalized in correct proportion, empathy allows the healer to avoid breakdowns in communication and also to keep patient frustration and hostility to a minimum. Most people who seek help outside their families are reluctant to disclose to strangers their sense of failure about not being able to cope with their problems. A sensitive healer realizes that part of his or her job is to create a relationship in which patients tell their stories in a minimally defensive way.

Central to this process is empathic understanding. Human beings can no more survive psychologically with people who do not respond empathically to them, than they can survive physically in an atmosphere that contains no oxygen. The caregiver's behavior vis-a-vis a patient should be the expected average one—i.e., the behavior of a psychologically perceptive person vis-a-vis someone who is suffering and has come for help (Kohut, 1977).

A third principle in humanizing health care is *conceptualization*, which simply means knowing that healing as a human experience involves everyone concerned in it, especially health care professionals, patients, and patients' families. Conceptually, sensitive healers realize that they are a part of a vast network of human beings who have in common the quest for a cure or rehabilitation.

The fourth principle, *competence*, involves doing all that is medically possible to make the difference between life and death, recovery and degeneration, health and illness. Great medical skills and knowledge tend to be optimally effective when fused into a holistic cognitive, behavioral, and affective approach to healing.

It is particularly necessary for caregivers to bear the preceding four principles in mind as they go about their mission of healing since the almost miraculous technology which has allowed the saving and prolongation of life on a large scale, seemingly has, ironically, driven a wedge between healers and patients (Engelhardt, 1986). The vast knowledge required of present day health care providers has understandably given healers a feeling of eminence. In possession of temporary power over life and death, many practitioners have come to see themselves as holders of the keys to an earthly kingdom. Many of those who hold this view believe they are initiates into mysteries much too esoteric to be shared with patients. A certain amount of authoritarianism is necessary to deal with the emergencies that comprise health care professionals' jobs, but too often this authoritarianism leads to an attitude of "paternalism" toward patients.

In many cases, patients themselves perpetuate paternalism—they are dependent and childlike, insisting that health care professionals take over not only their case but their life as well (Bovbjerg et al., 1987). The healer's self-confidence and the patient's lack of it have led to the charge by many critics that paternalistic medical practitioners are a threat to the autonomy of patients. Paternalism refers to interference by physicians or other caregivers in the lives or decisions of individuals when that interference is independent of their wishes but is for their benefit (Perry & Applegate, 1985). It is precisely this attitude that has led to condemnation of medical practitioners in many quarters. No doubt, thousands of competent and caring professionals become defensive when they are told that their paternalism violates the autonomy of their patients. We are not talking about evil men or women, our subjects are basically good people who want to help others to get well.

It can be argued, and supported with considerable research data, that health care professionals have certain prima facie responsibilities to their patients (Gillon, 1986). They should give their patients at least what they believe is adequate information, and even more if they think it will help them make a good decision about their health care. The role of the healer does not include lying or otherwise deceiving patients—even when they want to be deceived. Practitioners have the right to advise patients, but they must also give patients the opportunity to choose whether to accept or reject the advice.

One of the major responsibilities of healers is to maintain effective, helpful communication with their patients. This kind of communication is never one-sided. It is imperative that healers respect their patients' autonomy by providing them with adequate information for informed decision making. Furthermore, healers must always remember to ask themselves whether their patients would wish them to do what they are doing or intend to do. Only through communication can they get this answer from their patients or their surrogates. Fewer problems would arise in the healer-patient relationship if practitioners would take the initiative in establishing and perpetuating communication. Nor should communication be one-sided. It should, therefore, be reciprocal. If it is not, it does not exist on a helpful basis. When the resolution for the healing is life or death, the only ethical course for the healer is to share both information and trust with patients. The most noticeable change in the conduct of doctors in the past two decades is that they are now usually rushed, so rushed that they are less accessible to patients and, relatedly, less communicative with them (Hawkins, 1989). Within our postmodern nation, the greatest hindrance to the doctor-patient relationship is the failure of the former to find time to listen or to explain to the latter.

The greatest irony is that the very success of health care providers and their wonder-working technology may also be responsible for the distorted view the public holds of the role of the healer. The average person believes that medicine can achieve much more than in reality is possible (Thomas, 1988). Medical researchers sometimes make exaggerated claims, and the news medias have certainly sensationalized medical discoveries— often extolling panaceas where none actually exist. Many people now believe that every disease can be effectively treated, even though this is not true. The healer is quite commonly regarded by the patient as someone who can solve all kinds of personal problems, ranging from anxiety to marital discord unhappiness. Perhaps the lesson is that if some practitioners, not content with their already exalted status, assume the role of chief priest, they must be prepared to produce miracles on every occasion or face cynically disappointed multitudes.

The Role of the Patient

Being a patient means learning to play what Parsons (1951) called the *sick role*. This role usually has four elements: first, patients are not responsible for their condition; second, patients are exempt from normal role obligations; third, patients recognize that being sick is undesirable in spite of benefits that come from being sick; and, fourth, patients have an obligation to try to get well. Hospitalized patients often feel helpless. They are separated from their significant other persons and become dependent on doctors and other members of the hospital staff. It can be very frightening to depend on others for visits, meals, medicine, and news. The sick person is expected to seek out and cooperate with medical practitioners, and most health care professionals legitimate the sick role. However, as long as patients continue trying to get well or to cope, they are considered to be behaving appropriately, even courageously, to their unfortunate life situations.

> We feel healthy when we are in a state of equilibrium between our already experienced shortcomings and our aspirations and thus have adjusted our goals to the gap between them. Health is a state of accommodation, defined in different terms by each person. Illness rudely upsets the equilibrium. It is an undesired, unsought, capricious interruption demanding a new equilibrium— one that may be drastically different. It may mean a loss of personal image, identity, or existence itself. The ill person becomes *homo patients*—a patient—a person *bearing* a burden of distress, pain, or anxiety; a person set apart; a person wounded in specific ways. (Pellegrino, 1982, p. 158)

In recent years, a great deal of emphasis in medicine has shifted from health caregivers to patients. For more than a century, the general philosophy of physicians was that of the Code of Medical Ethics, adopted at the founding of the American Medical Association in 1847. The general tenor of the code was heavily paternalistic, for it placed much greater stress on the obligation of patients to their doctors than on the duties of doctors to their patients. The key word for patients almost ever since that time has been "compliance"—what sick persons should do to carry out their doctor's and other health professionals' orders to the letter. Noncompliance on the part of patients has generally been thought of as indicative of some sort of character flaw, for traditionally there has been no question that the health care provider's role should be that of authority and dominance, and the patient's role that of meek dependence. Research literature about compliance, although offered apparently with the aim of improving medical services, is really literature about power and control.

In historical medical relationships, patients have been assumed to have certain traditional responsibilities, and even today few people would deny that they exist. No one doubts that patients should keep appointments promptly; at the same time, it is the health care provider's responsibility to arrange and keep to a regular schedule. Patients should also pay their bills as promptly as possible, with the understanding that the charges are reasonable and are made clear in advance. In other words, patients should at least treat health care professionals as courteously as they would anyone else who makes their living by their work.

However, if the patient's obligation in the medical relationship ended with simple courtesy, it is doubtful that very much healing would take place. Pellegrino and Thomasma (1988) put forth the virtues of a good patient: *truthfulness, probity* (compliance), *tolerance* of others, and *trust.* Patients must trust the care provider so that a valid medical history will be taken, and so that their health condition or complaint will not be misrepresented. At the same time, patients should be honest about the values and duties that determine their choices in the healing relationship. Probity is a necessity in the healing relationship because after entering into an agreement with a caregiver about a specific treatment plan, patients must be willing to take the required medication, exercise, and follow other health or diet recommendations.

Tolerance requires of patients that they realize health care professionals, though they have performed amazing things in the past fifty years, cannot cure all diseases or completely relieve all pain. Patients also must accept the fact that following a medical regimen has risk factors. Likewise, they must learn that illness may cause personality changes. And, of course, it is each patient's duty not to vent hostility about his or her illness on care providers. Finally, patients are expected to place their trust in health care professionals to the extent that they feel free to express reasonable disagreement as well as change their expectations and values during the relationship. No patient should be obliged to submerge either his personality or his judgments during the healing process. When healing takes place, the expression of gratitude in the spirit of friendship engendered by trust are perfectly appropriate responses.

However, the role of the patient does not end with the four virtues. All patients must do their best to articulate their illness to the healer, for, as Richard Baron (1985) noted, a great gulf still exists between the way health caregivers think about a disease and the way patients experience it. Frequently, patients weep in self-pity or rail in anger at their fate. But none of these behaviors can alter their illness. Understandably, on the one hand, health care practitioners think of a patient's illness almost exclusively in terms of scientific constructs and quantifiable data. On the other hand, patients think of their illness as they live it—in descriptive, subjective terms that have to do with everyday life and functioning.

The fact that patients may think about their illness in terms different from those of the practitioner does not make either definition less real. Rather, it means that patients live with their illness in its qualitative immediacy. No doubt, this is what makes health caregivers notoriously bad patients, for when ill, they soon become cognizant of the great gulf between their own personal experience of an illness and the scientific descriptions and explanations of it. Many physicians admit that as patients they have a difficult time discussing their condition with colleagues (Toombs, 1987). Simply because a patient does not use the same "illness language" that his or her health caregiver uses does not mean that the patient should refrain from giving voice to these thoughts. That is all the more reason why patients should let their healers know just how they feel.

Research Findings

For a number of years, the most controversial issue in medical literature concerning the physician-patient relationship has been that of patient autonomy. Many authorities believe that both members of the healing dyad should share in medical decision making, and some believe that the ultimate choice between options must rest with the patient. A seminal study by Reeder (1972) distinguished between the patient as "client" and the patient as "consumer," with the consumer assuming more bargaining power when interacting with health care professionals. From this perspective, clients come to professionals for advice and accept it, but consumers listen to the opinions of health care providers, or several providers, and then make their own decisions. The literature dealing with observational studies of patients' attitudes concerning medical decision making and information seeking establishes, at least tentatively, the conclusion that "clients" outnumber "consumers" by a large margin.

In a study of outpatients suffering from hypertension, Strull et al. (1984) found that in making a decision about medication 53 percent of the subjects told interviewers before the first visit with their physician that they desired to participate in the choice of options, while fewer than one-fourth wished to make a joint decision with their physician. However, when the actual visit took place, sixty-three percent of the subjects said that they left the decision completely up to the physician. While only 37 percent said that they had actually participated in the decision, physicians estimated that 80 percent of the patients had taken an active part. Interestingly, the majority of subjects in the study said that they wanted an extensive discussion of their medical decision, and 41 percent said that they preferred receiving additional information about their illness from their physician. However, the physicians underestimated their patients' desire for more discussion in 29 percent of the cases. It is likely that practitioners frequently underestimate patients' desire for information and discussion, and seriously overestimate their desire to make decisions.

In a study conducted by Beisecker (1988) of patients of various ages, the younger ones expressed "consumerist" attitudes much more often than did older patients, particularly when it came to challenging the authority of health care providers. Patients 60 years of age and older did not think it was a good idea to suggest alternative treatments to doctors or to challenge their authority, nor did most of them believe in the patient's right to make the decision concerning treatment. In fact, 19 of the 21 older patients placed the decision-making authority fully in the hands of their physician. Younger patients, while they wanted to give physicians more authority than themselves, were far more likely to favor joint decisions. Nearly all of the patients interviewed expressed a strong desire for information concerning a wide range of medical areas, although older patients did not want to use the information to make decisions. The most startling result was that when patients were actually interacting with a physician, most of the younger patients, as well as the older ones, exhibited nonassertive, passive behavior even though over 81 percent of them had said in the interview that they wanted some role in decision making. Thus, age apparently affects the attitudes or perceptions of acceptable patient behavior, but it does not affect actual patient behavior.

Age also proved to be a major factor in a study conducted by Ende and associates (1989) which showed that younger patients had more desire to be informed and to make decisions in their treatment. Stronger preferences for decision making were also associated with higher education levels, higher income, higher level of occupation, and divorced or separated marital status. But none of the age groups showed a strong inclination to make decisions, although many of them preferred to have the caregiver engage them in the decision-making process. The same study found that the more severe the illness, the more patients wanted health caregivers to take the major role as decision maker. Regardless of their views concerning decision making, however, all patient groups showed a strong desire for information. The study concluded that perhaps the most important predictors of patient preference for decision making and acquisition of information are socioeconomic characteristics. A similar study by Beisecker and Beisecker (1990) found much the same results, except that patient attitudes toward decision making seemed to be related to socially learned information-seeking communication behaviors and the length of interaction with doctors.

Subjects in two experimental groups of patients, one with diabetes and one with peptic ulcers, were coached by clinic assistants just before visiting their doctors (Greenfield et al., 1985; Greenfield et al., 1988). In the 20-minute session, the assistants reviewed diabetic patients' medical records with them, guided by a relevant disease algorithm. Using systematic prompts, the assistants suggested that patients utilize the knowledge acquired to negotiate personally appropriate medical decisions. A randomized control group in each study was given a standard educational session of equal length. The intervention with the experimental group increased patient involvement in the doctor-patient interaction. Compared to patients in the control group, patients in the experimental group also displayed improved blood sugar control and increased functioning in everyday life. The authors of the study concluded that patients who play a passive role when interacting with physicians lessen their ability to control the effects of their disease.

The companion study with patients suffering from peptic ulcers, which used the same type of intervention and disease algorithm as in the diabetes study, also displayed similar results. Compared to the control group of patients who were given a standard educational session of the same length over their disease, the experimental group showed a more active affect and opinion-sharing pattern of communication with their caregivers. The patients in this latter group, in spite of initially poorer health, reported more effective role and physical functioning than did those in the control group. The authors report that a change also occurred in the experimental group's general sense of well-being. They believe the study shows that a more active role by patients in the healing process will result in greater control over their illness.

Similar results linking patient interaction with disease control were found in a study conducted by Brody et al. (1989). The patients who played an active role displayed considerably lower postvisit levels of discomfort or dysfunction and more symptom improvement, or general improvements, in their medical condition than did patients who played a passive role in patient-physician interaction. The more active patients were in their health care, the more satisfied they were with their healers. A significant fact emerges from the medical literature dealing with the role of patient. A more active role in interaction with health caregivers appears to be beneficial for patients, yet most patients seem reluctant to play such a role. Many practitioners express a desire for patients to share in decision making, because they believe this improves the healing relationship.

Numerous professional health care organizations have called for more shared practitioner-patient decision making. It is evident that both practitioners and patients can facilitate positive health care. Even so, the fact that medical practitioners have mastered vast and difficult bodies of technical knowledge is so daunting to most patients that they are afraid to play an active role in the healing relationship. The psychological undertones of the healer-patient dyad are often an inhibiting factor for patients. Most patients in their encounter with professionals unconsciously act out the role of the submissive, dependent child they once played with their parents. Whatever factors underlie the behavior of patients in the healing relationship, it is clear that healers must be able to understand patients in their attempts to communicate their own values and preference (Forrow et al., 1988). Fortunately, greater emphasis on communication—verbal and nonverbal—is beginning to be made in medical and health professions schools curricula.

Changing Roles, Values, and Demographics

Over the past twenty-five years, physicians and other health care professionals have experienced a gradual decline in their autonomy, a lowering of their status, a questioning of their competence from a number of quarters and a threat to their professional life because of litigation. The decisions made by health care professionals now must be justified to a number of publics—patients and their families; the courts; local state and federal governments; insurance companies; health care corporations; and, of course, medical colleagues (Pellegrino, 1982). There are a number of reasons for the changed circumstances of healers, but most of them lead back to one basic fact. Since 1965, when Medicare was enacted, the yearly cost of health care in the United States has risen more than tenfold. In 1987, medical care accounted for $550 billion or 11.1 percent of the gross national product (Belkin, 1990). Patients, federal and state bureaucrats, insurance companies, and health care corporations have been arguing for a long time over the high cost of healing. And medical healers, moral agents by virtue of both skill and purpose, now find themselves in situations that seriously threaten their ethical status.

The single most destructive change in the role of medical healers has been their increasing involvement in an adversarial relationship with patients. Opinion polls show that a majority of physicians believe that they are losing the public's respect, that they believe patients have unrealistic expectations of what caregivers do, and that they believe patients are asking for more services than are necessary (Kolata, 1990). Seventy-two percent of American physicians in 1989 believed that the public had less esteem for them than it had ten years before (Altman & Rosenthal, 1990). This perception has been borne out by other studies in which respondents state that doctors are so intent on making money that they do not care about people as much as they used to. In follow-up-interviews, many patients complain that doctors have become more like aloof businesspersons. A growing minority of patients complain that they have to learn all they can about their disease and take charge of their own treatment (Kolata, 1990). The most shocking result is that nearly 40 percent of the doctors interviewed by Altman and Rosenthal (1990) said that based on what they now know about medicine as a career, they would definitely or probably not enter medical school if they had a career choice to make again. As Angell (1987) has pointed out, none of the traditional public responsibilities of medical practitioners has been in conflict with their primary role of serving the medical needs of their individual patients. However, this too is changing. With changing practitioner roles come changing health care values.

The number of physicians in the United States in 1990 was nearly double that in 1965: 586,000 vs. 298,000. The ratio of physicians for every 100,000 people rose to 237 in 1990, up from 148 in 1965 (Altman & Rosenthal, 1990). The number of other health care practitioners is also increasing faster than the American population. Where are they working? Because of competition, many young health care providers, and some older ones, are joining salaried group practices. In 1989, more health care providers were employees than were self-employed. Even more significant is the fact that in 1989 fewer than 40 percent of American physicians under 35 years of age were self-employed; the rest were salaried employees.

Some experts lament that the doctor-patient relationship changes for the worse when health care providers become salaried employees; they become increasingly impersonal. Individuals who were once regarded as patients are now treated very much as if they are customers. The independence of physicians is being destroyed as they become salaried employees. How long can the traditional values of medicine last in the corporate environments concerned mainly with profits? It is of little wonder that the image of medicine has largely become one of a gigantic business. The physician-patient relationship, once based on a covenant whereby the patient trusted the physician to do what was best for him or her, is becoming a contractual relationship in which the physician provides a specific measurable service at a negotiated price (Winkenwerder & Ball, 1988). Other caregivers are emulating physicians, but this change is not ipso facto bad.

In March, 1983, the U.S. Congress approved the Diagnosis Related Groups (DRG) Prospective Payment scheme of Medicare and, thereby, put great stress on physicians, the chief decision-makers in the health care system. It has been estimated that doctors control roughly 60 to 80 percent of all hospital costs through decisions about admissions, tests, length of stay, and ancillary services (Churchill, 1987). A hospital under DRG is reimbursed a fixed amount according to patient diagnosis, regardless of how much the patient's care actually costs. Thus, hospitals can lose money by providing too much care. On the one hand, most hospitals under the plan encourage physicians to provide less, rather than more, medical care to patients, and to discharge them as soon as possible. On the other hand, certain tests and procedures for patients with private insurance are handsomely paid for, so doctors are encouraged to order more of them (Angell, 1987). The two different situations illustrate the enormous pressure health care providers are under to simultaneously save money and to make it for a third party. It follows that such pressure will necessitate a reconsideration of medical ethics.

A few critics talk convincingly about the "deprofessionalization" of the medical profession. Believing that there is an obvious tie between autonomy and professionalism, these critics assert that health caregivers are being reduced to the status of technicians who simply obey the orders of their corporate and government supervisors. It is true that many health care professionals are pressured into competition to see who can provide service at the lowest price. We are witnessing, for the first time in the United States, the nonmedical management of medical treatment and care (Reed & Evans, 1987). Even so, the popular perception of American health care providers is of first-rate professionals whose primary concern is for their patients. How disillusioning must it be for physicians who agree with this perception to watch their colleagues—and themselves— scramble to control costs, particularly when it is not in the best interests of patients.

Whether health care providers wish to admit it or not, present conditions in American medicine are forcing them to become agents for rationing health care and treatment. A paradoxical situation has arisen in the last decade. Most medical practitioners deny that nonmedical professionals are capable of correctly allocating health resources, and thereby imply that they are the only ones qualified to do so. Yet, some doctors refuse to become health care rationing agents (Churchill, 1987). There is nothing inherently unethical about containing medical costs; in fact, such containment is a moral act when failure to do so would not be in the best interest of either patients or society as a whole. Nor do we doubt the right of physicians to withhold expensive treatment from terminally ill patients if they legally request that it be withheld. However, it is immoral for healers, in order to satisfy a hospital or some other medical system, to order unnecessary treatment or to withhold necessary treatment. Traditional medical ethics dictate that the healer is morally obligated to order tests and to utilize treatments that are beneficial for patients and not to restrict access for purely financial or economic reasons (Pellegrino & Thomasma, 1988).

When the healer primarily becomes the agent of someone other than the patient, the morality of the healing process comes into question. By choosing to be a financial gatekeeper for a health maintenance organization (HMO), hospital, insurance company or some state or federal review board, the healer frequently violates public trust and the assumption of beneficent care-giving which goes with it. Each time a health care provider unscrupulously withholds treatment or care, the sacred trust is broken. Indeed, the moral dilemma in which many physicians find themselves is a real one. The social costs of rationing health care are difficult to determine, but one thing is certain: in time it will rend the fabric of all our lives in some way. In the field of medical ethics, it is becoming ever more costly, personally and financially, for even the most morally dedicated professional to practice the altruism that beneficence-in-trust requires.

If all physicians could find a satisfactory solution to their moral dilemmas regarding their primary loyalty, they would encounter still another problem that poses as great a threat to their autonomy as any HMO. Practitioners are becoming overwhelmed with the paperwork required by insurance companies and government regulators. Some of them say that at least 40 percent of their time is taken up by routine paperwork. For those who are self-employed, hiring someone to handle the paperwork is often too expensive. A growing number of physicians no longer enjoy their profession because of the paperwork. Usually a computer merely makes the paperwork neater. The enormous amount of paperwork is demonstrated by the fact that while the number of physicians increased by 50 percent between 1970 and 1986, the number of health care administrators increased nearly fourfold (Belkin, 1990). Surely, the burdens of the business end of healing must be one major reason why so many practitioners are joining HMOs.

Another major way in which medicine is changing is in terms of race and gender. For the first time in history, the number of male applicants to medical schools has dropped—since the mid-1970s it has dropped almost 50 percent. In 1988–89, white males made up less than half of the first-year students in American medical schools. Females comprised nearly 40 percent. African-Americans, who make up about 12 percent of the nation's population, comprised only 8 percent of medical students and 4 percent of practicing professionals, but their numbers are growing. So too are the number of Hispanic Americans, American Indians, and other minorities entering medical schools. It is very clear to individuals who administer the admissions offices of medical schools that national demographics are changing. In terms of gender, the situation is greatly improving, if only because, in order to survive, medical schools can no longer afford to rely primarily on white male applications.

If white male dominance in American medicine is declining, the role of women in it is increasing. In 1988, one in six American doctors was female, but for doctors under the age of 35 years, the ratio of male to female in 1989 was 3 to 1. This is a significant change because, for doctors between the ages of 55 and 64, the ratio of male to female in 1989 was nearly 12 to 1 (*World Almanac*, 1990). Nevertheless, there is generally great inequity between the sexes in the matter of annual remuneration. Female physicians earn far less than their male counterparts of all ages and experience levels. For example, in 1987, male doctors practicing twenty years or more earned an average of $127,000, while comparable female doctors earned an average of $72,000. Among doctors practicing four years or less, men earned $110,600 and women earned $74,000 (Altman & Rosenthal, 1990). At the same time, female doctors often report that they are subjected to subtle, and not so subtle, discrimination because of their gender.

That there is an irreversible change in medical demographics is apparent from a statement by Arthur Reiman, editor-in-chief of *The New England Journal of Medicine:* "If recent trends continue, the medical profession in the United States, which not so long ago was composed almost entirely of white men, will soon have a majority consisting of men from racial minorities and women" (Altman & Rosenthal, 1990, p. A35). The inescapable conclusion is that there may also be a change in the ethics of health care. A broader representation of the American population among physicians is likely to make health care more responsive to the needs of greater segments of our society. Reinforced by a rigorous grounding in ethics while in medical school, this younger and more diverse generation of practitioners are reinvigorating the healing profession.

In Retrospect

In the healing process, physicians do more than merely "cure" patients. Their major objective is to restore them to the best possible condition. Where a cure is not possible, the practitioner may still perform healing by helping patients to accept the outcome of their illness and by making them as comfortable as possible. The healing relationship is marked by a three-step process: (1) explanation; (2) prediction; and (3) control, or, as stated earlier, diagnosis, prognosis, and therapy. The professional healer's interventions, unlike those of other therapeutic occupations, are based on scientific underpinnings. Further, these interventions must meet three criteria: conformity to the best available scientific information, while making use of whatever sources are relevant to the patient's condition; tailoring the information to the particularities of the patient's illness; and emotional expressiveness on the part of the healer, since the patient always needs genuine reassurance from the healer. The practitioner, if he or she is to be a successful healer, should bear in mind the four principles of medicine as a human experience: acceptance, empathy, conceptualization, and competence.

Patients must be helped to take an active role in making medical decisions. This is difficult because, whether they are young, middle-aged, or elderly, research data indicate that patients interact with doctors in a passive way. Such interaction is less likely to optimally utilize the professional skills of the healer. Realizing that many patients are reluctant to play a more active role in decision making, medical schools are beginning to place greater emphasis on practitioner communication skills. Effective communication is the key to effective healing.

Today, the traditional role of the healer is seriously threatened by the economic circumstances. This is becoming a tragedy as the primary obligation of doctors—caring for patients as fully as is possible—is being gradually overshadowed by the goals of cost reduction and conservation of medical resources. Whether they desire it or not, doctors are becoming rationing agents for federal and state bureaucrats, insurance companies, hospital administrators, and health care corporations. At the same time, they find themselves being placed in an adversarial relationship with patients. Accused by health care consumers of being interested in little more than the remuneration which their jobs can bring, a growing number of doctors wonder whether their profession is any longer worth the price they must pay to practice it.

On a positive note, as more females and ethnic minorities enter medicine, the healing process is beginning to become more humane. This is not to say that only these groups humanize medicine. There is a cadre of nonminorities who champion human rights, too. If more doctors and medical researchers become as concerned with the role of human emotions as they have become with the role of technology, both the human body and the human soul will greatly benefit. It must and, we believe, it will happen.

When physicians and other health care professionals respect patients' rights, responsibilities, emotional status, and religious beliefs—and do so with compassion—their behavior is ethical. A tremendous step toward high ethical standards is taken when health care professionals respect the patient's autonomy. A general, humane rule of thumb for health care professionals is to treat patients as they would want to be treated if they or members of their family were patients. This kind of respect and caring was illustrated in the behavior of a physician who, before examining a poverty-stricken patient, asked him, "Is your bed comfortable, and was your breakfast warm?" It is sometimes the seemingly small things that humanize both healers and patients. Where there is no compassion, there will be little, if any, effective healing.

REFERENCES

Agich, G. J. (1983). The scope of the therapeutic relationship, pp. 236–238. In E. P. Shelp (Ed.). *The clinical encounter: The moral fabric of the patient-physician relationship.* Holland: D. Reidel.

Altman, L. K. & Rosenthal, E. (1990). Changes in medicine bring pain to healing profession. *New York Times,* February 18: A1, A34 ff.

Angell, M. (1987). Medicine: The endangered patient-centered ethic. *Hastings Center Report, 17:* 12–13.

Baron, R. J. (1985). An introduction to medical phenomenology: I can't hear you while I'm listening. *Annals of Internal Medicine, 103:* 606–611.

Beisecker, A. E. (1988). Aging and the desire for information and input in medical decisions: Patient consumerism in medical encounters. *The Gerontologist, 28:* 330–335.

Beisecker, A. E. & Beisecker, T. D. (1990). Patient information-seeking behaviors when communicating with doctors. *Medical Care, 28:* 19–28.

Belkin, L. (1990). Many doctors see themselves drowning in a sea of paperwork. *New York Times,* February 19: A1, A13 ff.

Bovbjerg, R. R., Held, P. J. & Diamond, L. H. (1987). Provider-patient relations and treatment choice in the era of fiscal incentives: The case of the end-stage renal disease program. *The Milbank Quarterly, 65:* 177–203.

Brody, D. S., Miller, S. M., Lerman, C. E. et al. (1989). Patient perceptions of involvement in medical care: Relationship to illness attitudes and outcomes. *Journal of General Internal Medicine, 4:* 506–511.

Brody, D. S. (1980). The patient's role in clinical decision making. *Annals of Internal Medicine, 93:* 718–722.

Churchill, L. R. (1987). *Rationing health care in America.* Notre Dame, IN: University of Notre Dame Press.

Cousins, N. (1983). *The healing heart.* New York: Avon Books.

Davis, A. & Aroskar, M. A. (1983). *Professional ethical dilemmas in nursing.* Norwalk, CT: Appleton, Century, Crofts.

DiMatteo, M. R., Linn, L., Chang, B. L. & Cope, D. (1985). Affect and neutrality in physician behavior: A study of patients' values and satisfaction. *Journal of Behavioral Medicine, 8:* 396–398.

Ende, J., Kazis, L., Ash, A. & Moskowitz, M. A. (1989). Measuring patients' desire for autonomy: Decision making and information-seeking preferences among medical patients. *Journal of General Internal Medicine, 4:* 23–29.

Engelhardt, T. H., Jr. (1986). *The foundations of bioethics.* New York: Oxford University Press.

Forrow, L., Wartman, S. A. & Brock, D. W. (1988). Science, ethics, and making clinical decisions: Implications for risk factor intervention. *JAMA, 259:* 3161–3167.

Fowler, M. (1989). Ethical decision making in clinical practice. *Nursing Clinics of North America, 24:* 955–975.

Gillon, R. (1986). *Philosophical medical ethics.* New York: John Wiley & Sons.

Goldstein, K. (1959). Health as a value, pp. 178–188. In A. H. Maslow (Ed.), *New knowledge in human values.* Chicago: Henry Regnery.

Greenfield, S. Kaplan, S. & Ware, J. E. (1985). Expanding patient involvement in care: Effects on patient outcomes. *Annals of Internal Medicine, 102:* 520–528.

Greenfield, S., Kaplan, S., Ware, J. E. et al. (1988). Patients' participation in medical care: Effects on blood sugar control and quality of life in diabetes. *Journal of General Internal Medicine, 3:* 448–457.

Hawkins, C. (1989). Changing doctor-patient relationships: Part 1: The causes. *Contemporary Review, 255:* 146–151 ff.

Hawkins, C. (1989). Changing doctor-patient relationships: Part 2: The effects. *Contemporary Review, 255:* 184.

Kohut, H. (1977). *The restoration of self.* New York: International Universities Press.

Kolata, G. (1990). Wariness in replacing trust between healer and patient. *New York Times,* February 20: A1, A15 ff.

Munn, H. E., Jr. (1977). Communication between patients, nurses, physicians and surgeons. *Hospital Topics, 55:* 7.

Parsons, T. (1951) *The social system.* New York: Free Press.

Peabody, F. W. (1927). The care of the patient. *JAMA, 88:* 877–882.

Pellegrino, E. D. (1982). Being ill and being healed: Some reflections on the grounding of medical morality, 157–166. In V. Kestenbaum (Ed.). *The humanity of the ill: Phenomenological perspectives.* Knoxville: The University of Tennessee Press.

Pellegrino, E. D. & Thomasma, D. C. (1988). *For the patient's good: The restoration of beneficence in health care.* New York: Oxford University Press.

Perry, C. B. & Applegate, W. B. (1985). Medical paternalism and patient self-determination. *Journal of the American Geriatrics Society, 33:* 353–359.

Reed, R. R. & Evans, D. (1987). The deprofessionalization of medicine: Causes, effects, and responses. *JAMA, 258:* 3279–3282.

Reeder, L. G. (1972). The patient-client as a consumer: Some observations on the changing professional-client relationship. *Journal of Health and Social Behavior, 13:* 406–412.

Reilly, D. E. (1989). Ethics and values in nursing: Are we opening Pandora's box? *Nursing Health Care, 10:* 91–95.

Reiser, D. E. & Rosen, D. H. (1984). *Medicine as a human experience.* Baltimore: University Park Press.

Strull, W. M., Lo, B. & Charles, G. (1984). Do patients want to participate in medical decision making? *JAMA, 252:* 2990–2994.

Thomas, L. (1988). On science and technology in medicine. *Daedalus, 117:* 299–316.

Toombs, S. K. (1987). The meaning of illness: A phenomenological approach to the patient-physician relationship. *Journal of Medicine and Philosophy, 12:* 219–240.

Winkenwerder, W. & Ball, J. R. (1988). Transformation of American health care: The role of the medical profession. *New England Journal of Medicine, 318:* 317–319.

The world almanac and book of facts. (1990). New York: Pharos Books.

SUGGESTED READINGS

Benjamin, M. (1985). Lay obligations in professional relations. *Journal of Medicine and Philosophy, 10:* 85–103.

Berenson, R. A> (1989). A physician's reflections. *Hastings Center Reports, 19:* 12–15.

Cassell, E. (1986). The changing concept of the ideal physician. *Daedalus, 115:* 185–208.

Conrad, P. (1987). The noncompliant patient in search of autonomy. *Hastings Center Reports, 17:* 15–17.

Cousins, N. (1988). Intangibles in medicine: An attempt at a balancing perspective. *JAMA, 160:* 1610–12.

Culliton, B. J. (1986). Medicine as business: Are doctors entrepreneurs? *Science, 233:* 1032–1033.

Freidson, E. (1989). *Medical work in America: Essays on health care.* New Haven, CT: Yale University Press.

Gorovitz, S. (1982). *Doctor's dilemmas: Moral conflict and medical care.* New York: MacMillan.

Greene, J. G. et al. (1987). Psychosocial concerns in the medical encounter: A comparison of the interactions of doctors with their old and young patients. *The Gerontologist, 27:* 164–168.

Inglehart, J. K. (1986). The future supply of physicians. *New England Journal of Medicine, 314:* 860–864.

Kaplan, S. H. et al. (1986). Effects of patient attitudes on success of programs designed to expand patient involvement in care. *Clinical Research, 34:* 822.

Kapp, M. (1985). Medical discourse: Recent contributions on the patient's role. *Journal of Legal Medicine, 6:* 283–292.

Kassirer, J. P. et al. (1987). Decision analysis: A progress report. *Annals of Internal Medicine, 106:* 275–291.

Marzuk, P. M. (1985). The right kind of paternalism. *New England Journal of Medicine, 313:* 1474–1476.

Mechanic, D. (1985). Public perceptions of medicine. *New England Journal of Medicine, 312:* 181–183.

Merrill, J. M. et al. (1986). Measuring humanism in medical residents. *Southern Medical Journal, 79:* 141–144.

Nelson, A. R. (1989). Humanism and the art of medicine: Our commitment to care. *JAMA, 262:* 1228–1230.

Pauker, S. G. & Kassirer, J. P. (1987). Decision analysis. *New England Journal of Medicine, 316:* 250–258.

Putnam, D. (1988). Virtue and the practice of modern medicine. *Journal of Medicine and Philosophy, 13:* 433–443.

Reiser, S. J. (1985). Responsibility for personal health: A historical perspective. *Journal of Medicine and Philosophy, 10:* 7–17.

Rost, K. et al. (1989). Introduction of information during the initial medical visit: Consequences for patient follow-through with physician recommendations for medication. *Social Science and Medicine, 28:* 315–321.

Seeman, M. & Seeman, T. E. (1983). Health behavior and personal autonomy: A longitudinal study of the sense of control in illness. *Journal of Health and Social Behavior, 24:* 144–160.

Shelp, E. E. (1983). *The clinical encounter: The moral fabric of the patient-physician relationship.* Boston: D. Reidel.

Shelp, E. E. (1985). *Virtue and medicine.* Boston: D. Reidel.

Siegler, M. (1982). Decision making strategy for clinical-ethical problems in medicine. *Archives of Internal Medicine, 142:* 2178–2179.

Siegler, M. (1985). The progression of medicine: From physician paternalism to patient autonomy to bureaucratic parsimony. *Archives of Internal Medicine, 145:* 713–715.

Silverman, S. (1987). *Communication and medical practice: Social relations in the clinic.* New York: Sage, 1987.

Speeding, E. M. & Rose, D. N. (1985). Building an effective doctor-patient relationship: From patient satisfaction to patient participation. *Social Science and Medicine, 21:* 115–120.

Suchman, A. L. & Matthews, D. A. (1988). What makes the patient-doctor relationship therapeutic? Exploring the connexional dimension of medical care. *Annals of Internal Medicine, 108:* 125–130.

Waitzkin, H. (1984). Doctor-patient communication. *JAMA, 252:* 2441–2446.

Waitzkin, H. (1985). Information giving in medical care. *Journal of Health and Social Behavior, 26:* 81–101.

Wright, R. A. (1987). *Human values in health care: The practice of ethics.* New York: McGraw-Hill.

Chapter 9

HELPING AS A VALUE

What is usually called a "good" relationship is held to be so in that it provides the stimulus and nurture by which both persons involved feel sustained, loved, gratified, given to, helped, and freed to experience their selfhood and to realize their potential.

Helen Harris Perlman, *Relationship*, 1979

Physicians are the "healers" in health care, but they require many "helpers" to bring about an optimum outcome. The view of "helping" as subordinate to "healing," rather than coordinate to it, pervades health care delivery systems. Although health care helpers accommodate the wishes of physicians by submitting to the limits imposed by them, some of these imposed limitations have been challenged by nonphysicians. This can cause extremely difficult dilemmas for nurses, allied health professionals, and other health care personnel. Using nurses as an illustration, Bandman and Bandman (1985) observed that a growing number of medical helpers shun an intermediary role between physicians and patients. They prefer to be proactive—not just to follow orders, but to inform and educate patients regarding the options available to them.

The major objective of this chapter is to analyze some of the responsibilities, ethical dilemmas, and behaviors of individuals in health care helping professions. It is difficult for some helpers to carry out their professional responsibilities because they hold positions that are lacking in authority. Most helpers try to walk a finely drawn line between assisting physicians and being patient advocates. It is not surprising that some of them fail; it is surprising, however, that many of them succeed.

Prelude to Helping

Three major assumptions about the universality of helping should be remembered. First, all of us, at times, have physical or emotional prob-

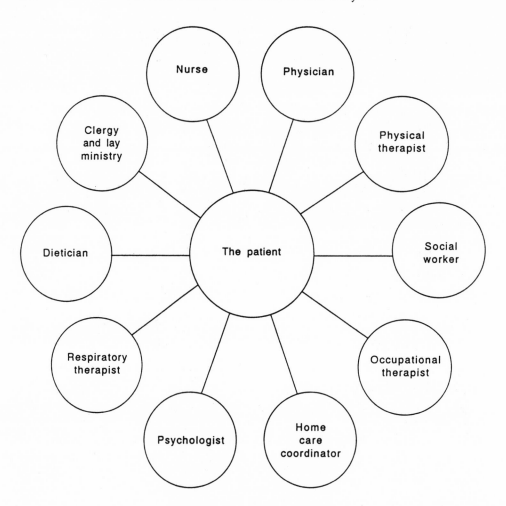

Figure 9-1. The health care team.

lems that we experience as unpleasant and painful. Second, all of us seek help for our personal problems. Third, all of us offer help to others who are experiencing physical or emotional difficulties. The help we seek and receive may come from a spouse, colleague, friend, or professional helper. A large portion of patients' needs is fulfilled by professional health care helpers.

Most definitions of help are based on subjective values—something tangible or intangible discovered in a relationship between a helper and the person receiving help in which the helper aids the recipient in achieving a measure of self-fulfillment. In actuality, help is something that a person discovers for himself or herself. Each of us should accept

Table 9-1. Differences between professional and social relationships

Characteristic	Professional Relationship	Social Relationship
Purpose	Systematic working-through of problematic thoughts, feelings and behaviors	Companionship, pleasure
Role delineation	Roles of caregiver and patient with explicit use of helping skills and interventions	Generally not present
Satisfaction of needs	Patient is encouraged to identify, develop and assess ways to meet own needs more effectively	Mutual sharing and satisfaction of personal and interpersonal needs
	Does not address personal needs of caregiver	

and act on helpful information with the knowledge that the ultimate responsibility belongs to us. In final analysis, help cannot be given to patients; it can only be offered. It is important that helpers do not try to rescue patients and make decisions for them.

The helping relationship has qualities that are the same whether it is between therapist and client, counselor and client, or nurse and patient. The psychological foundation supporting this relationship is much deeper and more complex than role descriptions. This is true for both the helper and the helpee. Numerous studies suggest that effective help is initiated not so much by technique or special knowledge, but by the positive attitudes of helpers. Furthermore, research findings suggest that experienced helpers have a better conception of what constitutes a helping relationship than do their colleagues who have mastered theoretical concepts but have spent little time as professional helpers (Henderson, 1989).

Contrary to popular notion, little empirical evidence supports the assumption that race or ethnic group per se is related to the level of understanding between caregivers and patients. Generalizations about race and cross-cultural helping should be made with care. At best, the literature on the subject is inconclusive. Several studies suggest that cultural barriers make the development of cross-cultural helping highly improbable. But other studies conclude that well-trained, empathic caregivers can establish a helping relationship with patients from other racial or ethnic backgrounds. In the end, ethnic similarity is not an adequate substitute for caregivers who are (1) linguistically compatible with patients, (2) empathic, and (3) well trained. This means that the initial edge held by caregivers of the same ethnic group as the patients will be lost if the caregivers are not sensitive and competent. Francis Peabody, one of the founders of medicine in the United States, stated that the secret of the care *of* the patient is the care *for* the patient.

Many health care professionals see the helping process as one in which they make intricate diagnoses of patients and then subject them to a wide variety of helping methods. Still other professionals define patients as being "sick" and themselves as being "well." These are not really helping relationships. On the contrary, they are *controlling* relationships. People who are ill are not "things" to be manipulated. They are often fragile people—frightened, confused, and defensive—but they are seldom "sick." When the patient becomes an object, rather than the subject, he or she is no longer the person who acts but, instead, becomes the person acted upon. Conceptually, a thin line separates wanting to help other persons and wanting to change them to conform with our expectations of them. Thus, practitioners must continually question their motives for helping others. The work of the medical professional is to help patients receive a service and otherwise solve or resolve a health-related problem.

In the various professions, there is an underlying assumption that trained persons can make a significant contribution to the lives of others if their training has instilled within them a commitment to effectively use themselves in the helping process. The primary technique in the helping relationship is the ability of the helper to offer him/herself as an instrument to be used by patients to achieve their health needs, and to do so with a measure of satisfaction. From the helper's point of view, this means that each patient will try to become more realistic and self-directing.

One depressing aspect of helping in health care settings is that some patients do not seem to want the help of health care professionals. Other patients who ask for help are afraid that, if offered, it will not be useful. There are many ways that patients ask for help: missing appointments, pretending that everything is fine, refusing to talk, etc. Health care practitioners must be aware of these pleas and be prepared to enter into a helpful relationship with patients. Patients learn to hide their feelings. They seldom openly or directly express their anger toward people on whom they depend; instead, they often agree to any request: "Yes, I will tell the truth." This is what the caregiver wants to hear. Most patients do not deliberately lie: It may be a response learned to protect him/herself. It could also be interpreted as passive aggression toward people in authority and an attempt to exercise some control over one's life (Robertson, 1969). Rogers (1958) defined the helping relationship as "a relationship in which at least one of the parties has the intent of promoting the growth, development, maturity, improved functioning, improved coping with life of the other" (p. 6). The characteristics that distinguish a positive helper-helpee relationship from a negative one are related primarily to the attitudes of the practitioner and the perceptions of the patient. Determining what is helpful and what is not depends, to a great extent, on cultural norms. For example, a white nurse may see an African American patient and two of her relatives arguing, with the patient receiving much verbal abuse. The nurse also may perceive that the helpful thing to do is to intervene and stop the argument. Yet, the patient might prefer to take the verbal abuse rather than later face her relatives, who, in all probability, will make fun of her for having had to be saved by a white person (Henderson & Primeaux, 1981).

Certain values in a helping relationship must be observed by professional helpers if, in the long run, it is to be productive. Doing a chore or making a decision for a patient may be helpful in the short run, but it will not help the patient to become more self-directing. Caregivers who try to do everything for their patients tend to do more harm than good. Ultimately, they cause patients to become unrealistically dependent on them. This chapter does not attempt to provide a how-to-do-it approach with clearly outlined steps to follow. Lists are presented, but they are used primarily to summarize various thoughts. Helping relationships do not allow a rigid structure. Therefore, this chapter presents a "be-it-yourself" approach, because health care professionals need an attitude of *being for* patients instead of *doing for* them. It is more important for a helper to be "aware" than to be an "expert." To be aware and to care about the world, values, and life styles of patients are significant aspects of the helping relationship, which can promote positive intrapersonal, interpersonal, and intergroup relationships.

Some of the skills involved in a professional role are listening, empathy, self-regulation, flexibility, and knowing when to refer the patient to another practitioner. Effective health care practitioners listen in such a way that they are able to understand what the patient is trying to say. This does not mean telling patients what to say. Being a good listener means identifying with the other person's point of view. Meaningful communication is impossible without empathy. Understanding and empathy can occur without losing one's identity and values. But, first, helpers must understand and accept themselves. Self-knowledge is a prerequisite to being an effective helper. And flexibility is important, too. Rarely is there only one effective treatment. That is why it is important to know when and where to refer patients for additional help.

This entire process evolves around cultural norms and values. Unless health care practitioners understand a patient's cultural norms and values, they are likely to intervene at the wrong time, i.e., before a patient has had an opportunity to talk with relatives or a folk healer. The task is to help patients blend orthodox and folk medical practices. This is best done with language and behaviors the patient understands. Help is meaningful only when it is perceived as such. This requires a nonjudgmental stance toward patients and their cultures.

Characteristics of a Helping Relationship

Rogers (1958) stated that a helping relationship is one in which the helper intends that there should come about more appreciation of, more expression of, more functional use of the latent inner resources of the helpee. We cannot change anyone else; we can change only ourselves, but only when we are aware of what needs to be done. And usually this occurs through interaction with someone else. This places the responsibility for health care where it belongs—with the patient. Thus, the job of the helper is to provide a medium, a situation, and an experience in which a health care choice is possible (Keith-Lucas, 1972). Ideally, the fears that restrain patients can, to some extent, be resolved through the helping relationship, and patients can find the courage to make a commitment to a health plan. To do this, they must learn some of the practical skills necessary to comply with a health plan. It is the helper's basic beliefs and values, rather than his or her grand schemes, methods, techniques, or years of training that are the real determiners of whether or not he or she will be effective or ineffective (Combs, 1969).

In a classic article entitled "The Characteristics of a Helping Relationship," Rogers (1958, pp. 12–14) asked a series of questions that he felt revealed the essential qualities of an effective helper. He believed that if practitioners can answer these questions concerning their interactions with patients affirmatively, it is likely that they are effective helpers.

Can I ... in some way be perceived by the other person as trustworthy, as dependable or consistent in some deep sense?

This question suggests that helpers must be more than rigidly consistent; they must be honest and congruent with their feelings. These helpers are unified, integrated persons.

Can I be expressive enough as a person that what I am will be communicated unambiguously?

If helpers are unaware of their own feelings, they will send patients double messages that will confuse the situation and cause the relationship to be marred. It is essential for helpers to avoid simultaneously affirming and denying their beliefs and intentions.

Can I let myself experience positive attitudes toward this other person—attitudes of warmth, caring, liking, interest, respect?

A professional attitude of aloofness is unhelpful; it creates a barrier or distance that protects scientific objectivity at the expense of establishing a helping relationship.

Can I receive him as he is? Can I communicate this attitude? Or can I only receive him conditionally, acceptant of some aspects of his feelings and silently or openly disapproving of other aspects?

Helpers are usually threatened when they cannot accept certain aspects of a patient's beliefs or behavior. Clearly, they must be able to accept those characteristics of other persons that they choose not to accept for themselves.

Can I act with sufficient sensitivity in the relationship that my behavior will not be perceived as a threat?

If patients are free from helper threats, they will be able to more easily experience and deal with their own threatening feelings. Patients who do not feel accepted and wanted will find it extremely difficult to relate to caregivers. Channels of communication are open when helpers uncritically accept the patient's efforts to "get well." Indifference, anger, impatience, and condescension, for example, are ineffective ways to help.

Can I let myself enter fully into the world of his feelings and personal meanings and see these as he does? Can I step into his private world so completely that I lose all desire to evaluate or judge it?

Evaluative comments are not always conducive to promoting personal growth, and they should be used with great care in a helping relationship. For example, positive evaluation can be threatening; it serves notice that the patient is being evaluated, and, conceivably, a negative evaluation could be forthcoming. Self-evaluation, instead of external evaluation, leaves the responsibility with the patient, where many practitioners believe it really belongs. Using nurses as the example, Ramaekers (1979) observed that rather than assisting patients in making their own decisions, some caregivers impose their opinions and solutions on them. These "helpers" give advice, moralize, intellectualize, and indirectly belittle patients' feelings. This behavior is not helpful.

There are four subtle attitudinal characteristics that are necessary for constructive change to occur. First, the practitioner must manifest empathic understanding of the patient. Second, the practitioner must manifest unconditional positive regard toward the patient. Third, the practitioner must be genuine or congruent—his or her words and feelings must match. Fourth, the practitioner's responses must match the patient's statements in intensity of affective expression. All of these things must be communicated to the patient. Professional helpers can convey genuineness, empathy, and unconditional positive regard through the following statements, including the feelings and actions that accompany them: "I know that it must hurt," "I am here to help you if you want me and can use me," and "You don't have to face this alone." These statements contain reality, empathy, and acceptance.

It should be emphasized that the words a helper uses are only one part of the communication process. As an old Indian once said about the treatment his people received from Anglos, "What you do speaks so loudly I cannot hear what you say!" To be effective, reality and empathy must be conveyed to the patient. Reality without empathy tends to be harsh and unhelpful. Empathy about something that is not important to the helpee is clearly meaningless and can only lead the helpee to what is sometimes called "non-choice." Reality and empathy need support, both material and psychological, if medical decisions are to be carried out. But support in carrying out unreal plans is a waste of time (Keith-Lucas, 1972). It is imperative that the helper focuses on problems he or she can help the patient think through. All people spend a portion of their lives in fantasy places. The fictitious world is a safe haven for persons who are ill, but this form of flight does not bring about a real world solution. Finally, the helper must have access to medical resources needed by the patient.

Now, let us look at three of the characteristics of a successful helping relationship—genuineness, empathy, and acceptance.

Genuineness

Lowell wrote, "Sincerity is impossible unless it pervades the whole character." To be genuine in a helping relationship requires practitioners to be aware of their own inner feelings. If our inner feelings are consistent with our behavior, it can be said that we are genuine and congruent. It is this quality of realness and honesty that encourages the patient to keep a steady focus on reality. To be genuine is to be transparent with our feelings. Basically, transparency is evident when we accept our own and other people's personalities. It is, in essence, the process of giving ourselves permission to be ourselves.

Life at its best is a process of sharing who we are at the moment and accompanying others in their search for physical and emotional equilibrium within themselves. To paraphrase a popular saying, health care professionals who are genuine with patients depict a "what you see is what you get" approach to helping. People who are physically or mentally ill need health care practitioners who can touch, smell, and smile at them. Above all else, they need helpers who are able to accept them as they are. Like effective teachers, health care professionals must acknowledge their humanity. To do is to know, as Menninger (1942) pointed out, that the world is made up of people, but the people of the world often forget this. It is hard for some caregivers to believe that, like themselves, patients are born of women, reared by parents, teased by friends, consoled by lovers, flattered by grandchildren, and buried by ministers and priests with the blessings of the church and the tears of those left behind.

Empathy

> "First of all," he said, "if you can learn a simple trick, Scout, you'll get along a lot better with all kinds of folks. You never really understand a person until you consider things from his point of view—"
> "Sir?"
> "—until you climb into his skin and walk around in it." (Lee, 1960, p. 34)

This passage from *To Kill a Mockingbird* accurately depicts the meaning of empathic understanding. It is literally an understanding of the emotions and feelings of another, not by cognitive processes but by a projection of one's personality into the personality of the other. It is a sort of vicarious experiencing of the feelings of the other to the degree that we actually simulate some of the pain the other person is suffering. While no person can ever feel the same as someone else, we can learn to experience feelings that are similar to those of others. Empathy requires us to temporarily leave our own life space and to think, act, and feel as if the life space of the other person is our own. Robertson (1969) captured the essence of this process for nurses:

> The nurse communicates empathy when she listens and relates to the patient's complaints with understanding responses. If the nurse is preoccupied with her own problems and feelings, her responses tend to be those of an efficient information-giver, a more comfortable role for the nurse but one which may cut off communication. Each of us needs the empathy of other people, and we are reassured when we feel that someone understands us. When positive emotions develop in the patient in response to the empathy of the nurse, they may provide the major motivating force in the patient. (p. 45)

Helpers must be able to maintain enough objectivity when they become empathic so that they can assist patients in overcoming medical problems. *Empathic understanding does no good unless it facilitates positive action.* This kind of understanding helps patients to make wise choices about their health care. One way of gaining this kind of understanding is through *active listening.* An effective helper listens to a patient's tone of voice, manner of speaking, and exact words. An effective helper also listens for what patients do not say. Often, this process involves long periods of silence. By being silent when appropriate, helpers give patients time to organize their thoughts. This can prevent helpers and patients from speaking too soon or jumping to erroneous conclusions. An effective helper listens in such a way that he or she is able to understand what the patient is trying to say. This does not mean telling the patient what to say, or how to feel. Listening is a tedious and, often, difficult art. Even when cure is not possible, helpers can ameliorate suffering by listening as patients discuss their thoughts and feelings.

The following points summarize empathic understanding: (1) It is seeing the situation in the way the patient sees it. (2) It is actively and imaginatively entering into the patient's situation and trying to understand his or her life conditions.

Acceptance

As noted earlier, if caregivers do not really accept patients, yet attempt to project acceptance, they will give a double message—acceptance and rejection. In such a case, the best that can happen is that patients will perceive these health care professionals to be phonies. The worst that can happen is that patients' self-esteem will be damaged. A helper's words may say, "I accept you and respect your feelings." But the nonverbal messages may be "I don't trust you," "Poor little insignificant you," "You are disgusting," "You are really sick." Deeply held nonverbal messages are difficult to hide—the owner does not have as much control over them as over verbal messages. We can run from people but, when in their presence, it is difficult to hide from them.

To the extent that health care professionals can be themselves as persons, expressing their real selves, hopefully with empathic understanding for other people, they will be able to accept their patients. It is important to note that practitioners who accept patients perceive them positively. In turn, this facilitates improved health care climates. It has been documented that if a helper communicates a positive perception of a patient, the patient will respond favorably to treatment. More specifically, it is extremely important for helpers to be aware of their patients' religious, racial, and ethnic beliefs. Some beliefs, such as religious ones, conflict with others. And the beliefs practitioners espouse are often different from those of their patients! Wrenn (1958) made five suggestions that can be considered basic principles of a humanistic helper:

1. I shall strive to see the positive in each patient and praise it at least as often as I notice that which is to be corrected.
2. If I am to correct or criticize patients' actions, I must be sure that this is seen by them as a criticism of specific behaviors and not as criticism of them as persons.
3. I shall assume that all patients can see some reasonableness in their behavior, that there is meaning in it for them if not for me.
4. When I contribute to patients' self-respect, I increase their positive feelings toward me.
5. To at least one patient, perhaps many, I am a person of significance, and he is affected vitally by my recognition of him and my good will toward him as a person.

With the preceding thoughts in mind, we will now briefly consider the complexity of the role of helper.

Roles of Helper

The helper is a central figure in health care. Historically, the helping professions arose out of the practice of wealthy persons hiring servant girls to care for their sick and to perform tasks that illness prevented them from accomplishing. Many practitioners complain that those early attitudes regarding the status of helpers have undergone little change.

Identified with the roles of females, especially mother-surrogate and nurturer roles, it has been difficult for nurses, physical therapists, and other professional helpers to shake the inferior status attached to their professions. Inadequate patient care is sometimes a result of role conflict and low status rather than a helper's technical skills. Much of the early day practitioner training was accomplished by apprenticeships that emphasized obedience to physician authority. Some of the current strains and unrest within the helping professions are triggered by physicians and health care administrators who demand that helpers give automatic, unquestioning response to their directives. Most helpers prefer situations where they can function on their own, responding directly to patients' needs and deciding when their intervention is appropriate.

How nonphysician practitioners administer a health care plan matters as much as its details. Under optimum conditions, each practitioner would carefully decide how best to maximize the health plan of each patient. It is useful to think of medical helpers as *guides*. They show patients the pathways to the various destinations of good health. As guides, the helpers monitor the pace and sequence of the trip; they often decide which route should be taken to achieve the desired end; and they are responsible for making the journey interesting and enriching for the patient traveler. The guide, with knowledge of a helping profession, must assist the physician in awakening and instilling in patient travelers, the desire and tenacity to complete the journey.

The helper is also a *model* for patients to emulate, an example they can follow. This is one of the greatest responsibilities of health professions helpers, and one from which they cannot escape. This part of the job is shaped by cultural sensitivity and professional knowledge. The impressions a helper makes remain forever in the minds of patients.

The helper as a *counselor* bears much responsibility for advising patients. Patients continually are faced with major problems, many of which are personal. During times of crisis, some patients turn to their professional helpers for guidance. In this capacity, a helper is able to bend and shape patients into many forms of behavior. Insensitive helpers make decisions for patients. Helpers who behave in this way do not provide optimum health care.

The helper is also an *actor*. She or he fits Shakespeare's definition:

> All the world's a stage
> And all the men and women are merely players.

They have their exits and entrances,
And one man in his time plays many parts.

An actor reads a script, decides he likes it, and studies it until he knows it. Then he goes on stage and portrays the character so that it is communicated to the audience, and they come to know the content of the character before they leave the theater. It is much the same with an effective helper. He learns the health care role, goes into a health care setting, acts as a care provider to patients and, before the performance ends, the patients come to know him as a good or bad helper.

When helpers guide patients, their chief work is assisting them to learn how to take better care of themselves. This means helping patients to define their own interests, needs, abilities, and problems. Furthermore, it is helping them to understand themselves and others. Out of this process emerges specific goals each patient will want to achieve. The helper's major role is to empower patients to formulate and evaluate health goals in terms of their own values and those of their community.

Beliefs That Harm

An important factor hindering a cooperative relationship between helpers and patients is the fact that many patients view themselves as uneducated and incapable of understanding the explanations given by professionals, whom they frequently describe as talking among themselves and using "big" words. Many patients feel excluded from their own illness. They are convinced that physicians and other health professionals deliberately and needlessly withhold information from them. Embarrassed by their ignorance, most patients do not ask their questions; instead, they act out their hostility at being pushed around and ignored as persons.

Confrontations with patients are distasteful for most practitioners. Only by coming to terms with the feelings that confrontational patients arouse in them will practitioners be able to appropriately handle such conflict. Even this insight may not be enough when dealing with undesirable or hateful patients. Because of the way they look, smell, talk, or behave, some patients frustrate or irritate care providers. Individuals who do not fit the constantly shifting and highly subjective normative characteristics of "good" patients are labeled "problems," "undesirable," and "hateful." When these persons get into trouble or become sick, some practitioners are not very empathic or forgiving.

Undesirable patients fit five categories: socially undesirable, attitudinally undesirable, physically undesirable, circumstantially undesirable, and incidentally undesirable (Papper, 1970). *Socially undesirable* patients include individuals who are alcoholics, members of ethnic minority (or majority) groups, and those who are crude in behavior. *Attitudinally undesirable* patients are individuals who are ungrateful or arrogant: those who think they "know it all." *Physically undesirable* patients include individuals who have identifiable physical illnesses, especially chronic illnesses. Some patients are *circumstantially undesirable* because of situations totally apart from them and beyond their control. An example of circumstantially undesirable persons includes individuals who replace a popular patient. Some patients behave like the persons Groves (1974) labeled "hateful." They fall into four classes: (1) dependent clingers, (2) entitled demanders, (3) manipulative help-rejecters, and (4) self-destructive deniers.

> Clingers escalate from mild and appropriate requests for reassurance to repeated perfervid, incarcerating cries for explanation, affection, analgesics, sedatives and all forms of attention imaginative.... Demanders resemble clingers in the profundity of their neediness, but they differ in that—rather than flattery and unconscious seduction—they use intimidation, devaluation and guilt-induction to place the doctor in the role of the inexhaustible supply depot....Help-rejecters, or "crocks," are familiar to every practicing physician. Like clingers and demanders, they appear to have a quenchless need for emotional supplies. Unlike clingers, they are not seductive and grateful; unlike demanders, they are not overtly hostile. They actually seem the opposite of entitled; they appear to feel that no regimen will help....Self-destructive deniers display unconsciously self-murderous behaviors, such as continued drinking of a patient with esophageal varices and hepatic failure. (p. 305)

The helper-patient relationship is also fractured by social class differences. The degree to which the qualities ideally defined as essential to the helping relationship, namely mutual trust, respect, and cooperation, will be present inversely with the amount of social distance. Conversely, the greater the social distance the less likely the participants will receive each other in terms of the ideal roles of professional and patient, and more likely they will interact with each other in terms of their social class status in the larger society (Simmons, 1958). A seminal study by Hollingshead and Redlich (1958) concluded that professional helpers tend to behave positively toward patients whose social class is comparable to or higher than their own, and negatively to patients from a lower class. Subsequent studies have corroborated this observation.

If caregivers are to be effective helping poor people, they must understand the meaning of poverty. Poverty is characterized by conditions of not enough—not enough money, food, clothes, adequate housing, or hope. Poverty has a familiar smell—a smell of rotting garbage and sour foods. It is the smell of children's and old people's urine and unwashed bodies. Above all else, it is the smell of people wasting away—physically, socially, and emotionally. Poverty does not respect race or ethnic background; no one is safe from it. Generally, when affluent people go without soap, hot water, lights, food, and medicine, it is because they elect to do so. When poverty-stricken people go without these things, it is because they have no choice. Therein lies the major difference between the poor and the affluent. The former are controlled by economic systems, and the latter control them.

Most of the poor are not recipients of welfare. Typical lower-class patients have less than an eighth-grade education and, if employed, are employed as unskilled or service workers. The family's income per person is often less than the minimum wage. They do not get their names in the news as outstanding representatives of their race or ethnic group; nor do they show up on welfare rolls or in the crime statistics. On the one hand, their children manage to keep out of trouble, and are not what might generally be conceived of as "uneducable." On the other hand, their children are likely to be overlooked when teachers want someone to pose for a picture, or to represent the school. These patients do not qualify for programs designed to help the poor and disadvantaged because they earn a few dollars more than program guidelines specify. Not all patients from lower-class families—welfare or nonwelfare—enter health care settings with a readiness to be combative or noncompliant.

There is a general agreement among medical researchers that low-status patients have a markedly lower chance of obtaining optimal care than the high-status patients. Several generalizations are given for this condition, including the following: low-status patients give less attention to medical symptoms, they are less willing to sacrifice immediate gratification for future health gains, and they display less initiative when seeking treatment. When taken at their face value, these reasons stereotype low-status persons as being shiftless and lazy. That is not our intention in this text. Social status is but one aspect of numerous factors that affect health care. A general guide applicable to patient care follows:

1. Health care providers cannot solve patients' problems, but they may be able to help them solve their own problems.

2. Every patient's problem has more than one possible solution.
3. The easiest, least creative response to helper-patient conflict is to pretend that it does not exist.
4. Every patient behaves according to unwritten family customs and traditions.
5. The most powerful factors in patient decision making are family precedents and community or religious norms.
6. Patient knowledge of scientific medicine can be alienating. Successful educational efforts by practitioners can alienate patients from relatives and friends who do not have such knowledge.
7. Humor can help practitioners and patients over rough spots; both parties must be able to laugh at themselves and with other people.
8. Previous experience is a valuable asset if it is used as a general guide. However, if viewed as offering *the* correct answer to every health care problem, experience (as well as the information in this book) will be a liability.

It is important to note that ethnic minority group patients need more (or a different kind of) attention than nonminority patients. Cultural understanding does not mean being "culture free" or "indifferent." It does mean being aware of cultural differences. There is nothing wrong with acknowledging cultural differences, as long as we do not misinterpret the differences in terms of inferiority or superiority. However, it is counterproductive to "treat all patients alike." People *are* different. Black Americans, as an illustration, are not white Americans; Catholics are not Protestants; women are not men; and physically handicapped are not physically able. A key to effective helping is knowing group similarities and differences. It is imperative that helpers be cognizant of health care barriers created by ethnic and social class differences. If a Hispanic patient is hesitant to trust an Anglo nurse, for example, it may be because she does not trust members of that particular ethnic group, or it may be because her nonverbal messages are "stay away." Rather than guess, it is better for helpers to ask patients what they think the difficulty may be. If this is done tactfully, it will get issues out in the open with a minimum of defensiveness. Often, patients are not aware of their own nontrusting behaviors. It is wise for helpers to examine perceived negative values, beliefs, and behaviors. This does not mean that the helper-patient relationship will always be nice and sweet.

Most patients' problems are rooted in their social environments.

Certainly, institutionalization or family therapy are alternatives. Another alternative is social action designed to change health care opportunities. If practitioners really want to be helpful, more of them will have to be active in community change. Frequently, a patient's rehabilitation depends not on his or her adjustment to an existing health facility, but instead, on being placed in one that does not yet exist. This kind of environmental change is not without a theoretical foundation. It is modeled after milieu therapy, preventive and community or social psychiatry. Too few community health resources are available to meet the needs of poverty-stricken people. There are many other community problems confronting professional helpers. Commitment to social change should lead to new order, not disorder. Those who do not feel comfortable being community change agents can at least try to improve the health care environment where they work. There are at least seven things practitioners can do to help patients become fully functioning persons:

1. Regard each patient as a vital part of the health care system.
2. View all patients positively. Whatever diminishes a patient's self — humiliation, degradation, or failure — should have no place in health care.
3. Provide for individual, cultural, and gender differences.
4. Apply the criteria of self-realization to every health care experience.
5. Learn how things are perceived by the patients.
6. Allow rich opportunities for patients to explore themselves and their health care environment.
7. Help patients to become interdependent.

Because sensitivity to our own feelings is a prerequisite to effective helping, it may be beneficial for all professional helpers to undergo some type of human relations training. People trained in such programs tend to be successful in helping others. Practitioners who are deficient in human relations skills are not able to effectively help patients from broad cultural groups.

Helping Terminally Ill Patients

It is a popular myth that we cannot successfully prepare for death. Explicit in this belief is the assumption that dying is something that merely happens and we have not control over it. An opposite view is that we can either live and die with dignity or grovel and whimper throughout these processes. Certainly, there are no universal rules to tell us how dying ought to be done. Each person must decide his or her own way of dying. Yet, it is commonplace for medical and allied health professionals to feel discomfort when talking about death with patients. As we noted in earlier chapters, caregivers are people who have doubts, fears, and uncertainties about death. Even so, they must be able to deal appropriately with dying patients, most of whom go through five psychological phases: denial, anger, bargaining, depression, and acceptance. These are overlapping states that can proceed progressively or skip or be delayed.

The first reaction to being diagnosed terminally ill is *denial:* "No, the doctors are wrong. I am not going to die." Denial is a general term to describe behavior that avoids facing reality, particularly an unpleasant reality. This phase differs with each patient in its intensity and manifestation. It may be momentary or lengthy. Even acceptance of an illness can be a form of denial. A patient may accept the basic fact of being ill, but deny that she is seriously ill. Or she may accept the fact that the illness is serious, but deny the diagnosis. She may accept the diagnosis, but deny that the condition is terminal. Or, if she accepts the condition, she may deny that it bothers her. Denial is almost always a temporary defense, and it will be replaced with at least partial acknowledgement of the inevitable. An empathic helper knows that denial is functional—it allows the patient to adjust to the shocking news and mobilize other defenses (Kubler-Ross, 1969; Simpson, 1979). Denial is a dimension of hope, and, as such, it is crucial to accepting therapy that often has humiliating and painful side effects. Skillful helpers permit patients the integrity of their denial.

Anger usually follows denial. The fantasy of being well is replaced with the reality of imminent death. The reaction "No," it can't be me" gives way to "Why me?" Then the patient feels rage, envy, and resentment —or some combination of these feelings. A once controlled, polite person may suddenly lash out in anger. During this phase, the patient believes that she has been dealt an unfair hand in the game of life. "Why me" sometimes gives way to "Why not you?" as the patient confronts caregivers and family members. This is probably the most difficult time for caregivers who desire reciprocal warmness from the patient. Helpers should not take personally the patient's anger, which is unfortunately directed toward the messenger rather than the message.

Next, anger gives way to *bargaining* —an attempt to negotiate the terms of the illness. During this phase, the patient tries to strike a bargain with

Table 9-2. Adaptive and maladaptive responses by phase of illness

Normal-Adaptive Behavior	Abnormal-Maladaptive Behavior
Prediagnostic Phase	
Constant or overconcern with the possibility of having cancer Denial of the disease's presence and delay in seeking treatment	Development of cancer's symptoms without having the disease
Diagnostic Phase	
Shock Disbelief Initial, partial denial Anxiety Anger, hostility, persecutory feelings Depression	Complete denial, with refusal of treatment Fatalistic refusal of treatment on the basis that death is inevitable Search for other opinions or unproved ("quack") cures
Initial Treatment Phase	
SURGERY Grief reaction to changes in body image Postponement of surgery Search for nonsurgical alternatives RADIOTHERAPY Fear of x-ray machine and side effects Fear of being abandoned CHEMOTHERAPY Fear of side effects Changes in body image Anxiety, isolation Altruistic feelings and desire to donate body or organs to science	Postoperative reactive depression Severe, prolonged grief reaction to changes in body image Psychotic-like delusions or hallucinations Residual drug-induced psychoses Severe isolation-induced psychotic disturbances Severe paranoia
Follow-up Phase	
Return to normal coping patterns Fear of recurrence	Mild depression and anxiety
Recurrence and Retreatment Phase	
Shock Disbelief Partial denial Anxiety Anger Depression	Reactive depression with insomnia, anorexia, restlessness, anxiety and irritability
At Point of Progressing Disease	
Frenzied search for new information, other consultants; quack cures begin	Depression
Terminal-Palliation Phase	
Fear of abandonment at death by others, pain, shortness of breath, and facing the unknown Personal mourning, with anticipation of death and a degree of acceptance	Depression Acute delirium

From Rainey, L.C., Wellisch, D.K., Fawzy, I., et al.: Training health professionals in psychosocial aspects of cancer: a continuing education model. *Journal of Psychosocial Oncology* 1:41-60, 1983.

caregivers or God: "If I do X, perhaps something heroic or altruistic, then I won't die as soon as projected." This is an effort to postpone what seems to be inevitable. But, alas, caregivers can neither honestly make these bargains nor keep them. The caregiver's primary obligation is to provide "safe conduct" for the dying patient. Medication can relieve the physical symptoms, especially pain or disfigurement, but only compassion and honesty can move the patient to the next phase.

When bargaining does not reverse the prognosis, the next phase, *depression,* is experienced. There are two types of depression a patient may experience—reaction depression and preparatory depression. Reaction depression is caused by losses of things such as financial security, possessions, or dreams. Preparatory depression manifests itself in a sadness for the impending loss of life. Professional helpers should be aware of the functional role of depression. It can facilitate transition to the next phase.

Acceptance is the final phase. The illness is no longer a condition to be denied or delayed, it is embraced. Now, the patient is able to go gently into the arms of death—rejecting Dylan Thomas' advice to "rage against the dying of the light." This is the time to tie loose social ends, to make tidy intimate relationships. Dying people need time to die, as sleepy people need to sleep, and there comes the time when it is wrong, as well as futile, to resist (Simpson, 1979). Succinctly, caregivers can do the following things to ease the dying process: (1) share the responsibility for the process with the patient so that he or she can deal with the impact of anxiety and bewilderment, (2) clarify and define the realities of the patient's day-to-day existence, (3) assist him or her to handle the loss of family, and, possibly body image, and (4) encourage the patient to devise a plan to live the remainder of his or her life with dignity and integrity (Wilcox & Sutton, 1977). There are no easy answers or foolproof tips on how to gracefully and inoffensively help people to die. The answers, if there are any, must come from the way we live with each other. The plaudits, questions, apologies, confessions, reprimands, anger, and joy are important aspects of terminal relationships.

Ethical Dilemmas

Similar to those of physicians, the basic responsibilities of nurses and allied health professionals are: (1) to promote health and prevent illness,

Table 9-3. The dying person's Bill of Rights

I have the right to be treated as a living human being until I die.	I have the right to have my questions answered honestly.
I have the right to maintain a sense of hopefulness however changing its focus may be.	I have the right not to be deceived.
I have the right to be cared for by those who can maintain a sense of hopefulness, however changing this might be.	I have the right to have help from and for my family in accepting my death.
	I have the right to die in peace and dignity.
I have the right to express my feelings and emotions about my approaching death in my own way.	I have the right to retain my individuality and not be judged for my decisions which may be contrary to beliefs of others.
I have the right to participate in decisions concerning my care.	I have the right to discuss and enlarge my religious and/or spiritual experiences, whatever these may mean to others.
I have the right to expect continuing medical and nursing attention even though "cure" goals must be changed to "comfort" goals.	I have the right to expect that the sanctity of the human body will be respected after death.
I have the right not to die alone.	I have the right to be cared for by caring, sensitive, knowledgeable people who will attempt to understand my needs and will be able to gain some satisfaction in helping me face my death.
I have the right to be free from pain.	

This Bill of Rights was created at a workshop on "The Terminally Ill Patient and the Helping Person," in Lansing, Mich., sponsored by the Southwestern Michigan Inservice Education Council.

(2) to restore health, and (3) to alleviate suffering. As they pursue these objectives, health care professionals may find themselves embroiled in ethical conflicts regarding the matter of allegiance. As an illustration, nurses are expected to carry out the orders of attending physicians; but according to their own professional code, they must safeguard patients when health care is threatened by the incompetent, unethical, or illegal action of any person (Cerrato, 1988; Berkowitz, 1986; Wright, 1987). What is the likely response of the nurse who needs her job and believes a physician is ordering an excessive amount of expensive tests that patients cannot afford? What will she do if a hospital administrator orders the premature release of a patient because his Medicare or insurance has been exhausted? These are the kinds of occurrences that force practitioners to seek clarification of their own values and determine the ethical options available for redressing such conflicts.

This is a very risky undertaking, for health professionals must weight their moral obligations to employers, supervisors, physicians, patients, and themselves. The quest for professional and moral excellence would be easier to pursue were clearer, unambiguous guidelines that spell out allegiance obligations established. Also helpful would be the availability of up-dated forms to forward to watchdog agencies for review. But most existing ethics guidelines are vague, and health care systems generate forms mainly to elicit payment, not criticism or ethics violations. Traditionally, the professional roles of nonphysician health care professionals have been inordinately shaped by physicians. However, the gentle winds of change are becoming tornados in some health professions.

Nonphysicians are expanding their public consciousness and echoing the desire for ethical behaviors that characterize the highest level of individual and community performances. Prompted by rebellion against abuses in government, health care professionals are challenging their professional associations' circumscribed roles in explicitly correcting unethical behaviors. A growing number of practitioners bemoan their own oppressions (McCloskey & Grace, 1982, pp. 590–591). Professional responsibilities and patient autonomy are the foremost issues around which ethical dilemmas evolve.

Professional Responsibilities

In recent years, nonphysicians have refined codes similar to the chronologically evolving codes of ethics for physicians that set forth responsibilities attending helping roles. As an illustration, the Code of Nurses was adopted by the American Nurse's Association in 1950. It has been periodically revised since that time in order to clearly specify, for both the nurse and society, the profession's expectations and requirements in ethical matters. The code is based on the belief that health care recipients and providers of nursing services have basic rights and responsibilities.

It is the responsibility of nurses to provide patient care with full regard for the dignity and uniqueness of every patient. Furthermore, they have the responsibility to safeguard the patient's right to privacy, and they must assume accountability for their professional actions. It is the nurse's responsibility to exercise the best professional judgment and to be professionally competent when giving consultation and delegating nursing activities to others. Also, it is the responsibility of each nurse to contribute to the development of the nursing profession. This includes contributing to the profession's body of knowledge, participating in efforts to implement and improve nursing standards, and establishing and maintaining high-quality conditions of nursing care. Finally, it is the responsibility of nurses to join together in efforts to protect the public from misinformation and misrepresentation that would reflect negatively on the integrity of nursing, and to collaborate with other health care providers to promote community and national health care needs.

While it is true such responsibilities are a great burden, several studies suggest that discontentment among nurses and allied health professionals involves more than working conditions and remuneration (Bandman & Bandman, 1985). Many practitioners believe they perform crucial functions but are not taken seriously as professional helpers. Hospital rules and medical traditions, they argue, deny them the authority to make even minor decisions, although many times they have the ethical responsibility to do so. They have little input into hospital procedures, yet they usually get to know patients better than do most physicians because of their proximity and continuity with patients. Some individuals and organizations have tried to promote the concept of joint practice — physicians and their helpers acting as equals; others ask that nurses become active in setting hospital policy. These proposals have received stiff resistance from physicians and hospital administrators.

Patient Autonomy

Helpers are surrogates and advocates for patients (Bandman & Bandman, 1985). They are surrogates who protect patients' right of self-determination, and they are advocates for institutional reforms that help patients. All health care practitioners, from time to time, mediate between patients' interests and those of other persons. This is a position of public trust. Ideally, as health resources, counselors, and community leaders, health caregivers foster patient health care rights. Competent patients should always be their own decision makers (Collopy et al., 1990). After all, it is patients who bear the risks, reap the benefits, and suffer the pain of treatment. In a perfect world, patient autonomy would outweigh physician beneficence, efficient management, cost-containment, and legal liability.

Gaul (1990) cites only three justifications for medical acts of paternalism: (1) a patient has diminished capacity for rational choice, (2) there is the potential for significant harm to the patient, and (3) there is reasonable assumption that the patient would, upon recovery, consent to the action taken by those who have spoken for him. As advocates, helpers are the patient's protector and friend; they take care of the patient's rights when he is unable to do so. Indeed, the helper performing as a patient advocate safeguards patients against abuse and violation of their health care rights. To do this job well, helpers must have compliant patients. And in order to protect patient autonomy and, at the same time, gain compliance, *rational persuasion* — instead of manipulation or coercion — seems to be the best approach. Here, too, helpers must recognize and respect the person-hood of all patients (Watson, 1990).

Manipulation tends to be unethical because it subverts the patient's rational beliefs, and *coercion* achieves only unwilling compliance. Both of these strategies violate a patient's right to self-determination (Krekeler, 1987). Coercion seldom produces a change of beliefs; instead, patients surrender to imposed force or intimidation without being convinced of its rightness. To contravene unethical practices that unduly influence patients and forestall their right of autonomy, the American Hospital Association approved a Patient's Bill of Rights in 1973. This bill states that patients shall have full information regarding their diagnosis, treatment, and prognosis. And it should be presented in language they can understand before signing informed consent forms.

The fact that hospitals and health clinics are places where patients are observed, monitored, checked, and recorded means that they are not places conducive to patient autonomy. By providing patients with as much privacy as possible and sensitively interacting with them, practitioners can minimize the feeling of helplessness that accompanies being sick. It is crucial for health care practitioners to question any medical order that appears to be unethical, and to refrain from implementing it if, in their judgment, it is unsafe (Benjamin & Curtis, 1986, p. 91).

Who Cares?

As our health care needs increase because of our nation's increasing aging population, it may be prudent to expand the capabilities and authority of key nonphysician health care providers. Our postmodern health care problems call into question old values, and new professional ethics must evolve if we are to meet the health needs of the 21st century (Bach, 1989; Beaton, 1987; Flight, 1987; Reilly, 1989). One thing seems certain: medical, nursing, and allied health academies must place a greater focus on the ethical and affective dimensions of health care.

A caring practitioner is able to reach past needles and tubes to elicit from patients their willingness to play a vital role in their own recovery. Practitioners of this kind are too few in medical institutions that have replaced tenderness with technology. Caring behavior is *direct or indirect nurturing, making decisions designed to help, maintaining an underlying moral commitment to help, exercising a will to help, and implementing helpful actions based on knowledge* (Kayser-Jones et al., 1989). The ethics of caring cause helpers to respect patients by keeping them informed and getting their consent when it is required. Caring mandates that practitioners not inflict harm; that they try to preserve the patients' quality of life by doing good for them; and that they minimize risks to themselves (Fowler, 1989; Vittetoe, 1990).

Caring is not a spectator sport; it requires active participation by all persons involved. Nor is it a garment that can be put on and taken off at will. The challenge to professional helpers is great. They must overcome their own negative behaviors, and also those of their patients. When measured in dollars, the rewards for this task may be few, but when measured in terms of professional and personal success, there are many rewards for being an effective helper. The most important things patients learn are not those that practitioners pontificate but, instead, the examples they set by being caring persons. The act of helping is simultaneously altruistic and egoistic. When we help other people, we help ourselves.

REFERENCES

Bach, J. S. (Ed.). (1989). *Biomedical ethics: Opposing viewpoints.* St. Paul, MN: Greenhaven Press.

Bandman, E. & Bandman, B. (1985). *Nursing ethics in the life span.* Norwalk, CT: Appleton-Century-Crofts.

Beaton, J. I. & Degner, L. F. (1987). *Life-death decisions in health care.* Washington, D. C.: Hemisphere.

Benjamin, M. & Curtis, J. (1986). *Ethics in nursing.* 2d ed. New York: Oxford University Press.

Bronowski, J. (1967). *The face of violence: An essay with a play.* Cleveland, Ohio: World.

Berkowitz, M. W. (1986). The role of discussion in ethics, pp. 193–208. In P. Chinn (Ed.), *Ethical issues in nursing.* Rockville, MD: Aspen.

Cerrato, P. (1988). What to do when you suspect incompetency. *RN, 56:* 36–41.

Collopy, B., Dubler, N. & Zuckerman, C. (1990). The ethics of home care: Autonomy and accommodation. *Hastings Center Report, 20:* 1–16.

Combs, A. W. (1969). *Florida studies in the helping professions.* Gainesville: University of Florida Press.

Flight, M. (1987). Medical ethics reach out and touch everyone. *The Professional Medical Assistant, 20:* 20–24.

Fowler, M. (1989). Ethical decision making in clinical practice. *Nursing Clinics of North America, 24:* 955–975.

Gaul, A. (1990). The ethics of clinical judgment in critical care. *Critical Care Nursing Quarterly, 10:* 24–28.

Groves, J. E. (1974). Taking care of the hateful patient. *New England Journal of Medicine, 291:* 301–306.

Henderson, G. (1989). *Understanding indigenous and foreign cultures.* Springfield, IL: Charles C Thomas.

Henderson, G. & Primeaux, M. (Eds.). (1981). *Transcultural health care.* Menlo Park, CA: Addison-Wesley.

Hollingshead, A. & Redlich, F. C. (1958). *Social class and mental illness.* New York: John Wiley & Sons.

Kayser-Jones, J. et al. (1989). An ethical analysis of an elder's treatment. *Nursing Outlook, 37:* 267–270.

Keith-Lucas, A. (1972). *Giving and taking help.* Chapel Hill: University of North Carolina Press.

Krekeler, K. (1987). Critical care nursing and moral development. *Critical Care Nursing Quarterly, 10:* 1–8.

Kubler-Ross, E. (1969). *On death and dying.* New York: Macmillan.

Lee, H. (1960). *To kill a mockingbird.* New York: Popular Library.

May, R. (1972). *Power and innocence.* New York: W. W. Norton.

McCloskey, J. & Grace, H. K. (1982). *Current issues in nursing.* Boston: Blackwell.

Menninger, K. (1942). *Love and hate.* New York: Harcourt, Brace & World.

Papper, S. (1970). The undesirable patient. *Journal of Chronic Diseases, 22:* 771–779.

Ramaekers, M. J. (1979). Communication blocks revisited. *American Journal of Nursing, 79:* 1080.

Reilly, D. E. (1989). Ethics and values in nursing: Are we opening a Pandora's box? *Nursing Health Care, 10:* 91–95.

Robertson, H. R. (1969). Removing barriers to health care. *Nursing Outlook, 17:* 40–45.

Rogers, C. R. (1958). The characteristics of a helping relationship. *Personnel Guidance Journal, 48:* 721–729.

Simmons, O. G. (1958). Implications of social class for public health. *Human Organizations, 16:* 16–18.

Simpson, M. R. (1979). *Facts of death.* Englewood Cliffs, NJ: Prentice-Hall.

Skinner, B. F. (1971). *Beyond freedom and dignity.* New York: Random House.

Vittetoe, M. C. (1990). Important ethical issues. *Clinical Laboratory Science, 3:* 25–28.

Watson, J. (1990). The modern failure of the patriarchy. *Nursing Outlook, 38:* 62–66.

Wilcox, S. G. & Sutton, M. (1977). *Understanding death and dying: An interdisciplinary approach.* Dominquez Hills, CA: California State College.

Wrenn, G. C. (1958). Psychology, religion and values for the counselor. *Personnel Guidance Journal, 36:* 40–43.

Wright, R. A. (1987). *Values in health care.* New York: McGraw-Hill.

SUGGESTED READINGS

Anderson, G. R. et al. (1987). Ethical thinking and decision making for health care supervisors. *Health Care Supervisor, 5:* 1–12.

Arbeiter, J. S. (1988). Are you merely a witness to the patient's consent? *RN, 51:* 53–57.

Archer-Duste, H. (1988). Clinical ethics: A mandate for nursing. *Journal of Perinatal and Neonatal Nursing, 1:* 49–56.

Aroskar, J. A. (1987). The interface of ethics and politics in nursing. *Nursing Outlook, 35:* 268–72.

Auerbach, V. et al. (1989). Neurorehabilitation and HIV infection: Clinical and ethical dilemmas. *Journal of Head Trauma Rehabilitation, 4:* 23–31.

Botter, M. L. et al. (1987). Allocation of resources: Nurses, the key decision makers. *Holistic Nursing Practice, 4:* 44–51.

Bresnahan, J. F. (1987). Suffering and dying under intensive care: Ethical disputes before the courts. *Critical Care Nursing Quarterly, 10:* 11–16.

Brooke, P. (1988). Informed consent: An ethical dilemma having life/death and legal implications. *Clinical Nurse Specialist, 2:* 157–161.

Brown, M. L. AIDS and ethics: Concerns and considerations. *Oncological Nursing Forum, 14:* 69–73.

Bruckner, J. (1987). Physical therapists as double agents: Ethical dilemmas of divided loyalties. *Physical Therapy, 67:* 383–87.

Clough, J. (1988). Making life and death decisions you can live with. *RN, 51:* 28 ff.

Cole, J. (1989). Moral dilemmas: To kill or allow to die? *Death Studies, 13:* 393–406.

Fall, J. M. et al. (1988). Bioethical decision making for the health care professional. *Nursing Connections, 1:* 19–28.

Glantz, L. H. (1987). Withholding and withdrawing treatment: The role of the criminal law. *Law, Medicine, and Health Care, 15:* 231–241.

Kirk, W. R. (1987). Professional ethics and practice . . . health services administration. *Journal of the American Medical Record Association, 58:* 39–42.

Lawrence, J. A. et al. (1987). Consistencies and inconsistencies in nurses' ethical reasoning. *Journal of Moral Education, 16:* 167–176.

Patterson, J. B. (1989). Ethics and rehabilitation supervision. *Journal of Rehabilitation, 55:* 44–49.

Rainey, N. B. (1988). Ethical principles and liability risks in providing drug information. *Medical Reference Services Quarterly, 7:* 59–67.

Ross, J. W. (1989). AIDS, rationing of care, and ethics. *Family and Community Health, 12:* 24–33.

Sciegaj, M. et al. (1987). A framework for applying ethical theory to public health practices. *Family and Community Health, 10:* 15–23.

Tomlinson, T. & Brody, H. (1988). Ethics and communication in do-not-resuscitate orders. *New England Journal of Medicine, 318:* 43 ff.

Welles, C. (1988). Ethical and professional liability considerations for the administrator: Incidents and principles. *Occupational Therapy in Health Care, 5:* 119–34.

Chapter 10

TRUTH-TELLING AS A VALUE

Some shrewd old doctors have a few phrases always on hand for patients that will insist on knowing the pathology of their complaints without the slightest capacity of understanding the scientific explanation.

Oliver Wendell Holmes

Truth-telling can affect every aspect of an individual's illness. At its best, truth-telling can be empathic communication that stimulates patients to put forward their own best effort to get well or to cope with their illness. At its worst, it can be psychologically or physically destructive. Truth-telling has this facility because honesty is the foundation upon which motivation is built in the health caregivers-patient relationship. Specifically, truth-telling reinforces the subjective dimension of our psychological constitution that activates self-regulation and self-healing potentialities (Cousins, 1983). Because words have the power to hamper or to heal, seemingly insignificant negative verbal messages can activate a disease mechanism (e.g., stressing the heart). Examples of the restorative power of positive messages, and the ability of optimism to slow or reverse a down-spiral in an illness, are amply documented in medical research. Since patient attitudes are both responsive and vulnerable to the authority of the healer, great care should be taken by the healer to satisfy the patient's legal and moral rights "to know."

It is an unfortunate fact that health care practitioners tend to score higher in veracity on psychological tests when they enter medical and allied health schools than after they graduate. The professional schools' curricula tend to encourage deception over shared power and emphasize technology instead of human rights. Most health care providers are students of science who concentrate on accumulating and analyzing hard, factual data. "While science may explain how a virus multiplies, it leaves unanswered why a tear is shed" (Cousins, 1983, p. 24). Correct diagnosis is a good test of medical science, but the ability to tell patients what they have to know in a sensitive and helpful way is a good test of

277

medical artistry. Whether truth-telling is done in an authoritarian or a participative relationship, the major question we will explore is: "Under what circumstances is a health care professional justified in using lies, deception, and nondisclosure?" The answer to this question begins with an understanding of the art of truth-telling.

The Art of Truth-Telling

Despite the focus on contemporary economic issues in health care, the art of medicine requires health caregivers to remember always the complex elements that exist in their relationships with patients. Among the activities that should engage the practitioner's attention, truth-telling is primary in the practice of good medicine. It is a difficult art to master, however, because it must be exercised in professions that are scientifically based but full of uncertainties. Truth-telling requires the ability to be honest and lucid and, in a gradual and sensitive way, to convey the meaning of an illness or infirmity to an apprehensive patient. Those individuals who tell the truth would be wise to heed Smith (1984): "Truth-telling, by relating all of the cold, hard facts in a blunt manner, betrays the compassion and respect inherent in the art of medical practice. The truth can be frightening, leading to depression or sometimes suicide. At times the truth may be so veiled in language that it becomes unintelligible" (p. 10). Also important is Smith's advice that health care professionals should not tell more than they know.

Medical practitioners continually debate whether or not patients should be told the truth about their health conditions. Like all sciences, medicine is based on probability (Katz, 1984). A health caregiver may be able to predict that the chances are 99 out of 100 that a patient will experience certain physiological outcomes. In this instance, the uncertainty and imprecision of medicine as science is evident. The health caregiver is not able to say with certainty that a particular patient will be the one who is the exception to the rule. Furthermore, because human conditions are not static, change is possible. Consequently, today's truth may become tomorrow's lie. This, too, must be communicated to the patient.

There are countless stories of ill persons whose health care providers gave them deceptive and incomplete disclosure of medical information. Often, these patients become real life versions of Ivan Ilych, the fictional character in Leon Tolstoy's book, *The Death of Ivan Ilych* (1960):

What troubled Ivan Ilych most was the deception, the lie, which for some reason that all accepted, that he was not dying but was simply ill, and that he only need keep quiet and undergo a treatment and then something very good would result. He however knew that do what they would nothing would come of it, only still more agonizing suffering and death. This deception tortured him—their not wishing to admit what they all knew and what he knew, but wanting to lie to him concerning his terrible condition, and wishing and forcing him to participate in that lie. Those lies . . . were a terrible agony for Ivan Ilych. (p. 137)

Like Ivan Ilych, they begin to discern the essence of their life only in their dying moments, and then only because they realize the truth of their mortality. Also like Ivan Ilych, in light of their imminent death, they begin to reorder their priorities in hope of giving more value to what life remains. And, finally, like Ivan Ilych, if they had been robbed of the opportunity to recreate their lives, a human tragedy would have been exacerbated. We all must make choices about how to best spend the time we have to live. The fact that health care practitioners, in general, and physicians, in particular, cannot say with certainty whether or when we will die from an illness does not relieve them of the moral obligation to provide the best information available. No one has a medical license to deceive patients.

There are many reasons some health care professionals distort or conceal the truth, including the desire to leave patients with hope, the reluctance to confuse them, and the wish to improve the chance for a cure by adding optimism. In the art of truth-telling, these professionals try to use information as a therapeutic tool—employing it in the amounts, admixtures, and timing they believe are in the best interest of their patients. For professionals who adopt this perspective, strict adherence to truth-telling is of lesser consideration (Todd & Still, 1984). With what is undoubtedly the best of motives, patients, relatives, and professional helpers often try to create an illusion of hope even where none exists (Bok, 1978; Duff & Campbell, 1980). This kind of humble heroism is carried out to a great extent because there is no written source of patient-centered ethics for the profession of medicine. Nowhere is this deficiency more glaring than in the care of severely handicapped persons and of those who are dying (Chapman, 1979). Organized medicine has joined most religions and the state in opposition to a formalized policy of living as one wishes at the end of life (McCormick, 1989). Thus, decisions of this kind lack coherent policies.

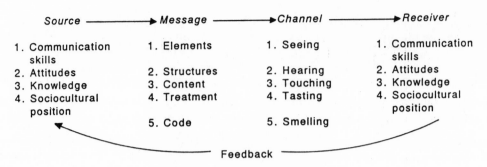

Figure 10-1. A communication model.

Communicating truth to patients and their families is fraught with other problems. Effective communication is comprised of a sender, a message, channel of transmission, a receiver, and a response (Fig. 10-1). It is difficult to achieve accurate communication, as was penned by an anonymous writer: "I know that you believe you understood what I said, but I'm not sure you realize that what you heard is not what I said." People attach different meanings to the same words. This is especially true of words associated with sickness—"cancer," "heart attack," and "physical disability" are three of many words that have negative connotations to most lay persons. Using the most helpful and the least frightening words is an art that few persons of any profession have mastered. Yet, it is clear that the patient and his or her family has the right to know something about the illness. The question is: "What do they have the right to know?"

Fiore (1979) encouraged health care providers to give patients all the information they need to know, but not without first understanding how each person might interpret the information. To many of us "cancer," for example, means a terminal illness and a protracted, painful death with no hope of escaping either the disease or the treatment. Specific, concrete descriptions of the illness (i.e., its stages and the treatments available) are less likely to be misunderstood or to leave us to our fantasies about what the doctor really means. Comaroff's study (1976) of general practitioners in South Wales provides a glimpse of a common rule many physicians still use for giving information to patients: Those who ask about their symptoms or treatment are given simple explanations. A corollary to this is that those who ask no questions receive little information. This strategy of communication reflects the power dynamics in the health care professional-patient interactions. A further elaboration of this strategy is that professional healers tend to provide more information to patients they believe to be highly intelligent or socially powerful.

Some patients are reluctant to discuss their illness. This is frequently true of individuals who are scheduled for surgery or inpatient psychiatric treatment. It is important that they be given information about routine hospital procedures. Most people want to be told that they will be well after their operation or treatment, but the health care professional must not set patients' expectations too high. This is easier said than done. Of course, any explanation should be tailored according to the capacity of patients and their relatives to grasp the complexities of the illness. If the information would alarm patients and, possibly, impede rather than facilitate their return to health, should they be told the truth?

The more effective health care professionals recognize that their words can wound as deeply as a scalpel. What they say can be as therapeutically important as what they do. Individuals who argue that disclosure of negative information should be the rule instead of the exception must also bear the responsibility to master the art of effective communication. Succinctly, they must learn how to humanely communicate both verbal and nonverbal messages. But their responsibility does not end there. They must be able to emotionally sustain patients once the bad news is out. The psychological difficulties that accompany disclosure must never be overlooked. This, then, is the art of negating or minimizing the harm implicit in communicating bad news and maximizing the benefits to the patient of learning the truth (Reiser, 1980).

The assumption that there is one simple, magical answer to truth-telling is incorrect. This assumption should be replaced by the intention to create an on-going dialogue with each patient. Guidelines for truth-telling in biomedical sciences can be optimally effective only when health care professionals *know* their patients and *understand* the implications of a medical event or procedure for each patient. This is a challenging task. Health care professionals walk a thin line, which they all fall from at some time. The public expects—and frequently gets—medical science miracles. The communication task is formidable: patients must be given the best chance of getting well and the least chance of disillusionment. This, of course, is the perennial problem of humanely managing the living, consoling the dying, and giving dignity to the dead. Clearly, considerable human relations skills are needed to perform these tasks. The care provider's role in the therapeutic relationship evolves around technical skills, impartiality, and the ability to communicate with patients. In our imperfect world, patients tend to expect perfection from individuals to whom they entrust their lives.

Our ability to use words is what makes us human; their value is transcendent. At the same time, words are full of human relations traps. Their meanings can be distorted and, when this occurs, a patient may experience physical pain and psychological misery beyond all reason. In summary, patients' distortion of health care professionals' words have cost them their health and, in some cases, their lives. There is no escape from this problem. Words are helpful, harmful, or neutral in their effect. To use an analogy, words are like a sharp ax—invaluable for cutting through barriers but also capable of injuring the people behind the barriers. For this reason, numerous writers have advised health care providers that words and their meanings will, to a great extent, determine how successful or unsuccessful they will be in relating to the patients. Indeed, the art of medicine centers on communication.

Deception, Lies, and Nondisclosure

In the nineteenth century, Percival (1803) stated that the first and foremost role of the physician is to be a minister of hope and comfort. In response to "How far is it justified to violate truth for the supposed benefit of the patient?" he concluded that physicians do not actually lie when using actions of deception and falsehood, as long as the objective is to give hope to a dejected or sick patient. Even when truth is required, deception or incomplete disclosure of medical information is sometimes "justified" by health care providers as a "therapeutic privilege" (Childress, 1982). Those who claim such a privilege often do so under the rubric of their duty to "do as little harm as possible" and to "do what is best for the patient." This was vividly illustrated by Lael Wertenbaker (1957) when her husband, Charles (Wert), had exploratory intestinal surgery. She had promised to tell him the truth about the result of the surgery, but his physician, Jim, forced her to weigh the relative merits of dignity and hope:

> "Now," said Jim gently, "what shall we tell Wert?"
> "Tell him the truth," I said
> "You can't," said Jim. "You can't take hope away from a human being."
> "Is there no hope?" I asked Jim.
> "No" said Jim. . . .

"Then," I said, "that's that."

"... Lael, I tell you, it is better if they hope. It is one thing to take a brave chance on dying and another to know that you are going to die—soon. You cannot take that hope away from Wert."

"I cannot lie to this man," I said. "That would take his dignity away from him. He would rather have dignity than hope."

"You cannot know *any* man that well," said Jim. (pp. 55–56)

Only by coming to terms with their own fears and feeling of omnipotence will health care providers be optimally responsive to the needs of patients. Nowhere is this more evident than when dealing with patients who are dying. Most patients and medical practitioners fight the thought of death. Some practitioners believe that they must save every patient—even those labeled "terminal." Without being aware of how much they demand of themselves, caregivers can experience a disturbing sense of personal discomfort when they face dying patients. Death is a painful reminder of the limits of the science of medicine and the skills of the health professionals, as well as a reminder of human mortality (Mumford & Skipper, 1967). An anonymous dying patient left this poem for medical personnel to read after her death:

> I huddle warm inside my corner bed,
> Watching the other patients sipping tea.
> I wonder why I'm so long getting well,
> And why it is no one will talk to me.
> The nurses are so kind. They brush my hair
> On days I feel too ill to read or sew.
> I smile and chat, try not to show my fear,
> They cannot tell me what I want to know.
> The visitors come in. I see their eyes,
> Become embarrassed as they pass my bed.
> "What lovely flowers!" they say, then hurry on,
> In case their faces show what can't be said.
> The chaplain passes on his weekly round,
> With friendly smile and calm, untroubled brow.
> He speaks with deep sincerity of life,
> I'd like to speak of death, but don't know how.
> The surgeon comes, with student retinue,
> Mutters to sister, deaf to my pleas.
> I want to tell this dread I feel inside,
> But they are all too kind to talk to me.

Whatever their situation, patients have the right to know the truth. Yet, as we have noted, there is often a collaboration among health care professionals and the patient's family and friends in the deception or withholding of information in order to make the illness easier. This behavior has ample precedent. The physician-patient relationship—the epitome of health care—was not founded on the duty of truthfulness. Indeed, the duty of truthfulness is not in the Hippocratic Oath or in the 1948 Declaration of Geneva by the World Medical Association. For many years, in fact, the Principles of Medical Ethics of the American Medical Association gave physicians discretion about what to disclose to patients. From this foundation, the use of truth depends on its projected utility in health care. And disclosure, or nondisclosure, of information becomes a part of the "art of medicine." The typical moral advice given medical school students in the early 1900s was: When you are thinking about telling the patient a lie, ask yourself whether it is simply and solely for the patient's benefit. If you are acting for the patient's good and not for your own benefit, you can go ahead with a clear conscience (Cabot, 1903).

Novack et al. (1989) offered a cogent perspective of deception in medicine. It is useful to discuss decisions to deceive in terms of who is being deceived and who will benefit from the deception. Health care professionals may deceive patients, patients' families, insurance agencies, and themselves. And one or more of these parties may benefit from the deception. Health care providers may deceive terminally ill patients in an attempt to avoid creating additional psychological distress in the patients and their family members. Insurance carriers may be deceived, too, in order for practitioners to get money for medical tests that would benefit patients and themselves. Of course, caregivers can benefit from self-deception, as in believing the truth is too uncomfortable for patients, when it is really too uncomfortable for themselves.

Practitioners who decide to deceive patients usually adopt a *consequentialist approach*. That is, they justify their behavior in terms of the good consequences produced by the deception and the bad consequences avoided as a result of it. While such altruistic motives are most often described as an overriding concern for patients' welfare, they actually relegate the right of patients to be told the truth to a lower priority. Of equal importance is the determination of how much of the truth should be told. It could be argued that under some circumstances health care professionals should not tell the whole truth. Generally, this argument for discretion about disclosure of information is based on the presumption that particular information may be harmful to the patient's psyche. From this perspective, the art of patient care is the ability of a professional healer to know what psychological approach would be best for each patient. This argument is flawed because few health care professionals are well trained in psychological diagnosis and prognostication.

The moral presumption against deception, lies, and nondisclosure of information is grounded in the principle of respect for other persons as independent, choosing beings who require truthfulness. There is no general duty for caregivers to disclose information to patients, but there is a general duty not to lie when they request information. At issue is the application of the principle of veracity in diagnosis, prognosis, and treatment. Childress (1982) focused on two principles of medical veracity: (1) dissemination of information about diagnosis and prognosis where consent is not required and (2) dissemination of information about diagnosis and therapeutic procedures to which consent is required.

Withholding information in accordance with a patient's wish is, in general, not morally wrong as long as other people are not adversely affected. While this may be personally unacceptable, the health care professional has no duty or right to force patients to know the reality of their situation. Sometimes, this will render vital health resources inaccessible to a patient, especially if an agency's treatment requires informed patients. In some instances, when a patient requests nondisclosure of information, there may be a moral and legal duty to disclose it, even though no other person will be directly harmed by the nondisclosure. An example would be an individual who volunteers to test an experimental prosthesis. In this instance, it would be prudent to insist upon informed consent. This would not prevent patients from leaving treatment choices to the clinician as long as they are aware of the implications of that decision. If the clinician is willing to accept the responsibility, the process does not insult or disrespect patients' rights (Lynn, 1986).

Sometimes it may seem that reality is too brutal for patients. Granted, the truth is not always painless; as the old saying goes, "The truth shall make ye free—but first it shall make ye miserable." It is important to repeat our injunction that being open and honest is not a license to be brutal. Helpful, as opposed to destructive, disclosure is very much like the difference between a fatal and a therapeutic dose of a painkiller—it is only a matter of degree. It is wise for health care providers to evaluate their reasons for being less than truthful with patients.

To protect people from the truth about their health or skills is to make a very serious judgment about them. It is to say that they are not capable of facing their real problems. Conversely, if health care providers only gave truth in the relationship, it probably would not be very helpful. Empathic understanding is also needed. On the one hand, reality without empathy is likely to be harsh and unhelpful. On the other hand, empathy about medical conditions that are not real is clearly meaningless and can only lead the patient to frustration and failure. Reality and empathy together need support, both medical and psychological, if health decisions are to be successfully carried out.

Informed consent

At the end of his narrative, *The Plague*, Camus (1983) observed of those who fought against the terror and relentless onslaught of disease in the 1940s that, although they were unable to be saints, they did not bow down to pestilences; instead, they tried their utmost to be healers. No law or professional ethic requires health care professionals to be saints or martyrs, but laws do set minimum standards of conduct below which practitioners cannot fall without risking lawsuits and loss of license. Physicians, nurses, and other health professionals would be wise to know their legal obligations when treating patients.

The rule of consent to diagnostic and therapeutic procedures is grounded in the case laws of torts as negligence and battery, especially battery which involves touching an individual who has not consented to the contact. Consequently, health care professionals have no legal right to touch patients who are capable of consent without first getting their consent. By its very nature, Western medicine is violent—practitioners often poke patients, give injections, take x-rays, and prescribe drugs. These and many other procedures can be a source of harm or pain. Relatedly, health care professionals have a legal, and moral, duty to get each patient's consent to diagnostic and therapeutic procedures. In *Schloendorff v. New York Hospital* (1914), Judge Cardozo wrote: "Every human being of adult years and sound mind has the right to determine what shall be done with his or her own body." In order for consent to diagnostic or therapeutic procedures to be valid, a patient must (1) be *competent* to consent, (2) *understand* the procedures, and (3) *voluntarily* give his or her consent.

Informed consent is a modern American legal principle. Specifically, it is a hybrid legal concept based on battery and negligence in medical malpractice litigation (Katz, 1972). When forced to choose between providing hope and comfort or not paying legal judgments, most health care professionals choose the latter. Until the 1960s, relatively few patients' rights existed in American law. The movement for patients' rights was a reaction to custodialism among mental health professionals (Brown, 1984). However, truth-telling and consent-seeking for specific medical interventions—particularly surgical invasion—are part of a long medical tradition (Pernick, 1982). While the patient's right of prior consent has long been protected under the laws of assault and battery, as Silverman (1988) points out, only recently has the doctrine been very narrowly defined. Historically, physicians were obliged only to disclose the *nature* of a proposed procedure; the patient had the right of refusal. In *Slater v. Baker and Stapleton* (1767), a British judge ruled that "a patient should be told what is about to be done to him, that he may take courage and put himself in such a situation as to enable him to undergo the operation."

The competency of a patient is a primary concern because only a competent person can give the informed consent required to initiate a course of treatment recommended by a health care professional. When patients are incompetent, decisions should be based on their previously expressed wishes. If these are unknown, the patients' best interest should be the guiding principle. For example, alcoholism is an area that involves decisions of competency. Chemically dependent persons may make medical demands that are clinically contraindicated. In these cases, the health care provider may feel the need to compromise in truth-telling in order to act rationally on behalf of patients whose judgment is, at best, questionable (Doyal, 1987). The most common standards of judgment used are the typical professional standard, the reasonable person standard, and the subjective standard. The test of the professional standard is whether a *typical* professional would behave as the individual whose judgment is at issue. The *reasonable person* standard examines whether a hypothetical reasonable person would reach the same conclusions as the practitioner in question. The *subjective standard* takes into account whether the patient's informational needs are unique because of some personal characteristic or quality. If so, the health care provider must take this uniqueness under consideration when deciding what to tell and how much to tell.

It is important for the health care professional to explain the technical aspects of disease and illness in terms that will make treatment procedures understandable to lay persons. Research data show that in order for patients to willingly participate and accurately follow medical regimens, they must understand and accept the physician's diagnoses and treatment plans. *Individuals affected by a health plan must understand it if optimum compliance is to occur.* In the United States, health care professionals are required by law to get *written consent* before entering patients into a treatment program. Explicit in such a written document is the admission that all medical decisions are characterized by degrees of uncertainty (Fox, 1984). Included in this uncertainty are the treatment outcome, patient response to therapy, and side effects. Along with informed consent has come renewed questioning of each professional's specialized knowledge. Practitioners are obliged to tell patients that they do not know which treatment will be most effective in a particular case. Some writers lament that the mystique of the health care professional is undermined by the consent process (Taylor & Kelner, 1987). Indeed, the consent form does call into question whether health care professionals will always strive to act in the best interest of their patients.

While the legal requirement for patient consent has a long history in the United States, research focusing on the *quality* of that consent is a recent development. Of particular interest to us is the case of *Nathanson v. Kline* (1960), in which the court stated that the physician administering treatment had a duty to inform the patient of the nature of the treatment and the possible risks. Failure to disclose information about risks means that the patient did not give informed consent to the treatment, thus, making the health care provider negligent, regardless of how skillfully the treatment was administered. The notion of disclosing to patients information about risks and alternatives is foreign to traditional medical practice (Kaufman, 1983).

Few people know exactly what is ailing them until they have received sufficient data from a physician or other medical personnel. To be told by medical personnel what is wrong is in itself a relief for many patients. But being told is not enough. Cure or rehabilitation must follow. This is likely to occur when a patient has answers to the following questions: "What is wrong with me?" "Am I normal?" "What caused it?" "What's going to happen to me?" "What can I do to help?" Schoene-Seifert and Childress (1986) put this issue into sharper focus in an article entitled "How much should the cancer patient know and decide?" After exploring the question on two levels—first, "How much information should professionals disclose to patients?" and, second, "Should the professional, patient or the patient's family be the primary decision-maker?"—they concluded that competent patients have the right to know and decide. In short, the patient is the primary decision-maker. The right of patients to know and to decide are not absolute and do have limits. If patients cannot make autonomous choices, it is the health care professional's duty to protect them from their nonautonomous choices. But there is no moral justification to accede to the family's request. As transmitters of choices to patients, practitioners should:

1. Use simple, accurate words to describe diagnoses and treatment plans.
2. Provide patients with enough information so that they can put their choices into proper perspective.
3. Secure validation of what patients understand.
4. Clarify the nature of their statements so that facts, beliefs, opinions, and assumptions are clearly delineated.

It has been extensively documented that physicians tend to withhold information from patients contrary to informed consent laws (Taylor & Kelner, 1987). When given information, patients often are not told very much about their treatment (Lidz et al., 1984), and they frequently do not understand very much of what they were told. Other studies document that much of the information patients receive is communicated to them in such a way as to be almost incomprehensible (Grunder, 1980; Morrow, 1980). Equally important is the finding of some researchers that middle-class patients are more likely to receive answers to their questions than are patients of lower socioeconomic status (Kaufman, 1983).

Truth-Telling to Cancer Patients

As a whole, health care providers pay little attention to dying patients. They spend less time with terminally ill patients and, when visiting them, seem to have even less to say. Medical science has provided little room in its activities for dying or the natural and inevitable process of death. Consequently, practitioners are much more at ease postponing death or relieving physical pain than treating a dying person in psychological distress. This is not surprising. Individuals whose major concerns are therapy and cure have great difficulty discussing death with patients. This is vividly seen in the commonplace treatment of AIDS patients. Yet, in their more lucid moments, most practitioners acknowledge that death is not a tragedy for individuals such as the man whose stroke leaves him with a live body but a dead brain. His relatives feel both grief and relief when he is finally pronounced dead and all life support systems are removed. Although death is a universal human phenomenon, few practitioners seem to grasp the essential psychological verities of the experience. And considerably fewer practitioners can sensitively tell patients about it.

Since the early 1960s, sociomedical literature which emphasizes the importance of communication between medical personnel and dying patients, has emerged. In answer to a questionnaire administered to physicians in 1961, 90 percent of the respondents expressed a preference for not telling cancer patients their diagnosis (Armstrong, 1987). Three-fourths of the respondents cited clinical experience as the major factor determining their preference, but many of the respondents showed inconsistent attitudes, personal bias, and resistance to change or further research. Some authorities (e.g., Novack et al., 1989) speculate that a priori personal judgment is the major determinant of physician truth-telling decisions, and they are undergirded by feelings of futility and pessimism about cancer.

While problems in truth-telling are not unique to oncology patients, much attention has been focused on this specialty. There are many claims and counter claims by clinicians faced with ethical dilemmas of truth-telling in this area. Goldberg (1984) noted that many health care providers believe that withholding information at times turns out to be the most humane approach. Other problems that consistently recur are those that arise when patients want to know more than the health care professional feels required to tell them, when the family adds stress to the situation by not wanting the patient to be told, and when patients behave as if they were unaware of the truth that has been communicated. Unfortunately, too often, clinicians must make judgments on these issues without the benefit of a lot of time for personal reflection.

Some health care providers personally defend their right to furnish only as much information as makes sense for a particular patient at a particular time. Others contend that all patients have the right to know as much as possible. This apparent conflict in the truth-telling obligation, which includes informing patients and protecting them, creates an ongoing tension for a practitioner who has moral integrity. The strain created by a lack of truth-telling can isolate patients and create an atmosphere of perplexing communication and mistrust.

Gautam and Nijhawan (1987) studied a sample population in Jaipur, India, to determine whether the diagnosis of cancer should be communicated to patients and their relatives; why the diagnosis of cancer should, or should not, be revealed to patients and relatives; what the emotional reaction of patients and their relatives is when they know the diagnosis is cancer; whether patients perceive any changes in their own behavior after they know the diagnosis; whether there are changes in the attitude of relatives toward cancer patients once they have knowledge of the diagnosis; and whether the knowledge of having cancer has an effect on patients' expectations of the course of their illness.

Results of the study showed that only 48 percent of 100 cancer patients knew about their diagnosis and its outcome. The immediate emotional reaction of most of the patients after they were told the truth concerning their diagnosis was "anxiety." This was followed by feelings of "dejection" in 42 percent of the respondents. Emotional reactions were *not* related to the location of the cancer, but instead appeared to be related to age. The older age group—60–80 years of age—reported "anxiety," while "dejection" was the predominant emotion in the 30–50 year age group. Concerning whether there were changes in patient behavior after being told the truth about their illness, 57 percent said "yes." Specific changes included a preoccupation with the illness, loss of interest in daily routines, irritability and changes in the intensity of involvement in family affairs. Concerning attitudes of relatives toward the patients, 46 percent reported "no change," while 54 percent believed their relatives were "more empathetic" and "paid more attention to them."

Based on the Gautam and Nijhawan study, it is reasonable to hypothesize that the truth-telling responsibility should rest with someone close to patients; that adequate time should be allocated for the facts to be absorbed and questions to be raised; that patients should not be told there is nothing more that can be done for them; and that the way the truth-telling is done should take into account the patient's personality, intelligence, religion, and any other relevant factors the care provider can ascertain.

A related study was conducted in Israel by Amir (1987) who sampled 104 general surgeons, with the objective of examining the guidelines they used when informing cancer patients about their diagnosis and prognosis. She concluded that if patients do not want to be told about their illness, they should not ask about it. The truth is of greatest benefit to patients who are intelligent enough to comprehend the information and initiate the inquiry. Amir also concluded that the age of the physician is important in determining the extent of truth telling that will occur. If the physician is a young person, patients will probably be given a more realistic prognosis than if he or she is an older practitioner with many years experience. When physicians of all age groups are uncertain about a diagnosis or prognosis, they are least likely to engage in truth-telling—it is embarrassing not to know what is the truth. It is also the case that the better the prognosis, the more likely patients will receive correct information. Generally, physicians respond best to patients they perceive as "intelligent" persons because they identify with them. Finally, truth-telling is not an all-or-nothing situation. There are different degrees of choice concerning giving information to patients.

In another study, Newall et al. (1987) compared the views of cancer patients in the United Kingdom (U.K.) with those in the United States. They administered a questionnaire to determine the nature and source of information patients received about their illness. There were similarities between the patients in the two countries, but differences were noted in the way the diagnosis was confirmed. There were also differences in the patients' desire for complete information and the persons who conveyed the information. Twenty percent of the U.K. patients, but no American patients, reported that the confirmation of their diagnosis had been delegated to a junior staff member; 30 percent of the U.K. patients and 14 percent of the American patients believed their doctors had sufficient time to engage in profound communication; 70 percent of the U.K. patients and 24 percent of American patients stated that they relied on nonmedical sources for information about their cancer. The data suggest there is a cultural difference in attitudes between British and American patients. American patients tend to show a greater desire for more information about their condition and they also place more overt emphasis on the importance of religious beliefs.

A similar study focused on the quality of breast cancer information given to 944 patients in 62 Italian general hospitals (GIVO, 1986). Physicians were asked to report what they told cancer patients about their diagnosis and treatment. The completeness of such communication was then assessed to measure precision and lack of ambiguity. Specifically, a three-level category was used—"thorough," "partial," and "no information" —to categorize the information given. The research showed that although 37 percent of the patients received thorough information, only 18 percent of them complained about the lack of complete truth-telling. Physicians, by contrast, considered their information to be thorough for

69 percent of the patients. This disparity suggests a lack of understanding and differences in perspective between physicians and patients.

The studies we have cited support the notion that both the sick and the well want to know their medical diagnoses and would feel more helped than harmed by news of their terminal illnesses. Relatedly, a 1977 study of 264 physicians concluded that 98 percent of them supported being totally frank with patients who have cancer, and all of the respondents said they would want to be told if they had cancer (Novack et al., 1979). This brings us back to the issue of certainty. It is impossible to make a knowledgeable prediction about a patient's chance of recovering without knowing how he or she compares with the norm and also what his or her physical and psychological resources are. In blunt terms, no practitioner knows exactly how long a specific patient will live. Nothing is gained and much may be lost by announcing borderline findings to a patient. Imagine the confusion aroused by informing a patient, "I don't think you have much to worry about. Your tests seem O.K., but we want to watch your pancreas because it looks a bit abnormal."

Frequently, health care professionals provide family members with the least important—from the family's perspective—information. Relatives of critically ill patients in Molter's study (1979) stated that they preferred: (1) to know the prognosis, (2) to have their questions answered honestly, (3) to know specific facts concerning the patient's progress, (4) to receive information about the patient once a day, and (5) to have explanations given in terms that are understandable. The least helpful, but most frequent, messages they actually received: (1) talked about negative feelings such as guilt or anger, (2) encouraged them to cry, (3) told them about someone to help with family problems, and (4) told about other people who could help with nonfamily problems.

The data are conflicting. Butcher (1979) described the special needs of relatives of patients with brain death. Succinctly, their needs were to be gently told about the illness in order to avoid false hope and to be introduced to other professionals who may be able to offer spiritual and concrete support. Clearly, these needs differ from those outlined by Molter. And these differences dramatize the need to know what is helpful to both patients and their relatives.

Truth-Telling in Rehabilitation

Rehabilitation counseling in health care basically consists of a one-to-one relationship between an individual counselor and an individual patient. One of the most fundamental aspects of this relationship is the attitude the health care provider and the patient have toward each other. Rehabilitation efforts may fail dramatically if the primary parties involved are unable to establish a cooperative relationship. A necessary element in cooperation is establishing effective communication, which is strongly facilitated by truth telling.

One of the first areas where there may be trouble in establishing trust is in reaching a mutual decision about what the primary problems and goals of the patient are. Differing perceptions account for the frequent complaints by health care practitioners that their patients are "unmotivated" (Makas, 1980). If this is not true, but the attitude is held by a rehabilitation counselor, it is unlikely he or she will provide optimum care to the patient. Members of a rehabilitation staff are most helpful when they familiarize themselves with the communities and cultures that are native to their patients. And, certainly, familiarity with various disability groups and knowledge of their specific disabilities will result in a more favorable attitude about patients.

A study was undertaken in Israel by Ben-Sira (1986) to examine the factors that contribute to promoting or impeding physical rehabilitation. He found that it is not the severity of the impairment, but the rehabilitation counselor's subjective assessment of its implications that has stress-inducing consequences. *The essence of rehabilitation is to enhance the disabled person's chance of returning to social life as an integral member of society.* This integration can be characterized as the counselor's enhancement of the disabled person's ability to successfully cope with the demands of life, including assuming meaningful social roles and receiving esteem-enhancing rewards from his or her significant others.

One of the most difficult tasks in rehabilitation is the practitioner's role in delivering negative information to parents who have given birth to a mentally or physically disabled child. Here, truth-telling is put to a strenuous test. To guard against communicating less than helpful information, health care providers should examine their own reactions to the diagnosis and not distort the information to fit their own needs. They should also determine whether they have sufficient information to answer questions, and, whether the information is current and reliable. It is advisable for rehabilitation counselors to become familiar with any family characteristics that would be negative factors in the patient's ability to assimilate and adjust to the disability. Some of these characteristics include extremely limited financial and emotional resources, destructive modes of coping among family members, lack of experience with the disability, and unrealistic parental expectations (Olson et al., 1987).

In the delicate act of truth-telling to parents of a disabled child, the practitioner should schedule consultation meetings in a private, comfortable place and have available well-written materials that will give a comprehensive, but not confusing, explanation of the disabling condition. The most immediate parental response to a mentally disabled child is often profound sorrow and pity for themselves and the child; and parents of mildly disabled children are usually disappointed. Too often, rehabilitation counselors overestimate the negative impact of a disabled child on the family unit, and they underestimate the ability of the family to cope with the situation. When this happens, a negative prophecy fulfills itself. Parental reactions to a disabled child are influenced by how, when, and where they are given the diagnosis; the degree of the family's social isolation; the severity and kind of disability; the family's income; the gender of the care providing parent; the attitudes of members of the family; and the attitude of the rehabilitation counselor. When conveying information about a retarded child, practitioners are prone to give a pessimistic prognosis. This can precipitate grief and impede parental bonding with the child. Careful truth-telling, taking into account the vulnerability of the family, can ease the shock and help the family to adjust to the disability.

To facilitate rehabilitation, all health care professionals are advised to avoid jargon and to give explanations that are easy to understand. Furthermore, punctuating truth-telling with silence can often be effective as this gives the family time to absorb the news before responding. It is imperative for professionals to review their diagnosis with the family with the end goal of correcting any misinformation. Also, if possible, the rehabilitation counselor should initiate follow-up contact with parents to see whether they have any additional questions. Although truth-telling cannot lessen the impairment of a disabled person, it can facilitate the healing process.

Gross et al. (1982) measured the effectiveness of training parents of physically disabled children to perform physical therapy at home. The children in his study received three physical therapy treatments a week from the school therapy staff but no gains in motion were observed until treatment incorporated their parents into the rehabilitation regimen. The parents were taught how to perform physical therapy in two 20-minute sessions. Gross concluded that parent participation in therapy for physically disabled children is a crucial variable in obtaining cost effective motor function improvement. Other studies encourage a holistic approach to working with disabled patients (Evenson, et al. 1986). This approach is based on the premise that a disability affects the whole family. Common sense tells us that family responses to a disabled member—child or adult—can be positive and supportive or negative and disruptive. Negative and disruptive behaviors may be triggered by overprotection, which leads to dependency, neglect, and denial of the truth of the diagnosis. Family rehabilitation programs that concentrate on the family unit as a whole are becoming widespread.

When Little Help Can Be Provided

Few diseases are more disabling or incapacitating than Alzheimer's disease. For these patients, the health care provider can offer little help—no medication can slow the disease or stop it. In time, the patient will not be able to drive a car or find his way when he is walking outside the house. Ultimately, he will not be able to dress or bathe himself, and, at some point, he will stop using the toilet. He may even stop talking. Yes, he will become like a newborn baby—wearing an adult diaper, unable to feed himself. After awhile, he will die. Should a person diagnosed as having Alzheimer's disease be told about the possibility of developing these symptoms?

Of 214 adult Alzheimer's disease patients surveyed by Erde et al. (1988), 90 percent wanted to know the complete truth of their diagnosis. The reasons they stated for wanting to be told the truth included the wish to make plans for their health care and to settle family matters. Even though several patients indicated that learning about the prognosis of the disease made them feel suicidal, this did not outweigh their need to know the truth. When placed in the position of making difficult ethical choices, many of the health care providers in the studies reviewed for this book engaged in some form of deception. Their justifications varied, including the belief that negative consequences might ensue.

Still others placed higher value on their patients' welfare and their need for hope than on the truth for its own sake.

But how can practitioners be sure their messages will be understood when the truth is told? Munn (1977) provided a practical approach to determining whether a patient and his or her family members understand the diagnosis, prognosis, and the projected medical procedure: "Doctors and nurses should never ask patients, 'Do you understand?' In a sense this is calling for a predisposed answer and all the weight is on the patient to answer yes. Rather, we should explain the procedure and then ask, 'What do you understand?'" (p. 7).

In Retrospect

Truth-telling is one of the most significant aspects in the relationship between health care professionals and patients. It is the foundation for trust which, in turn, can motivate patients to participate actively and positively in their own healing. However, truth-telling is difficult because it is the art of sharing information that will foster the autonomy and uniqueness of each individual person. As such, it is an art that requires commitment, caring, compassion, honesty, empathy, patience, and loyalty —all qualities that tax our humanness. Health care providers have varying opinions about how much truth their patients can assimilate.

Some practitioners believe they are the best judge of what information will benefit patients and what will harm them. Critics of this view argue that lying or withholding information completely compromises truth-telling. Yet, many practitioners do it because they are uncertain about medical outcomes, fearful of blame from patients and their families, and they do not wish to remove the element of optimism, which may activate a patient's will to live, from patients. The problems of practitioner-patient communication often are the result of inadequate training. Few caregivers are taught to elicit information—how to talk, to listen, and to provide helpful feedback. But this is not to suggest that there are no practitioners who can effectively communicate with patients. There are many who possess this skill. Sadly, most of them are self-taught. Something as important as communication should not be left to intuition or chance; it should be part of health professions education.

Nor should the patient's understanding of his or her illness be left to chance. Numerous studies conclude that a large number of patients receive insufficient information about their conditions and treatment. Specifically, many patients are released from treatment without ever having understood what their health care provider diagnosed as their illness, why certain procedures were followed and, if operated upon, what their operation consisted of and the reasons for the related preparations. A patient's rights include the right to courteous, prompt, and accurate information. We could build a case of patient ignorance being a by-product of the medical mystique. That is, scientific medicine is commonly perceived as being administered by men and women whose training and predilections place them in a special service category. There is a tendency for patients to be in awe of health care professionals. But beyond this intangible dimension of the health caregiver-patient relationship, practitioners remain divided over what information should be given to patients and how that information should be given.

As we noted earlier, there are many reasons for failure to communicate pertinent information to patients. Since human communication is a two-way process, both practitioners and patients distort messages. Some patients forget medical information that is clearly communicated to them. This sheds doubt on the validity of patients' dissatisfaction with the medical information they have received. Research that demonstrates that patients who understand their illness get well faster than those who do not is sparse. From this narrow perspective, we could conclude that patients' understanding of their illness is unimportant if adequate histories can be obtained and patients follow prescribed treatment. But, if the goals of medicine and health care include relieving, reassuring, and restoring patients, it is important for patients to understand their illness. It is each person's right to be told the truth about his or her medical condition.

The dynamics of health care are threefold. First, the facts that constitute health problems must be understood. Facts frequently consist of objective reality and subjective interpretation. Second, the facts must be thought through. They must be probed into, reorganized, and turned over in the patient's mind in order for him or her to grasp as much of the total configuration as possible. Third, a plan must be devised that will result in resolving or alleviating the problem. Central to all of this is the truth. The basic ingredient for effective health care is confidence in and reliance upon medical and other health professionals who respect the principle of veracity. The duty of veracity is an overt expression of fidelity or promise-keeping. By entering into a relationship in the biomedical context of therapy or research, the patient or subject has a right to the truth regarding his or her diagnosis, prognosis, and medical procedures. Lies and other forms of deception, however benevolent, are wrong.

REFERENCES

Amir, M. (1987). Considerations guiding physicians when informing cancer patients. *Social Science and Medicine, 24:* 741–748.

Armstrong, D. (1987). Silence and truth in death and dying. *Social Science and Medicine, 24:* 651–657.

Anderson, D. (1988). Death and dying: Ethics at the end of life. *RN, 51:* 42–51.

Ben-Sira, Z. (1986). Disability stress and readjustment: The function of the professional's latent goals and affective behavior in rehabilitation. *Social Science and Medicine, 23:* 43–55.

Bok, S. (1978). *Lying: Moral choice in public and private life.* New York: Pantheon Books.

Butcher, P. H. (1979). Management of relatives of patients with brain death. *Anesthesiology Clinic, 17:* 327–332.

Cabot, R. (1903). The use of truth and falsehood in medicine: An experimental study. *American Medicine, 5:* 344–349.

Calloway, S. D. (1986). *Nursing ethics and the law.* Eau Claire, WI.: Professional Education Systems.

Camus, A. (1983). *The plague,* trans. by S. Gilbert. New York: Alfred A. Knopf.

Chapman, C. B. (1979). On the definition and teaching of the medical ethics. *New England Journal of Medicine, 301:* 630–634.

Childress, J. F. (1982). *Who should decide?* New York: Oxford University Press.

Comaroff, J. (1976). Communicating information about non-fatal illness: The strategies of a group of general practitioners. *Sociological Review, 24:* 79–96.

Cousins, N. (1983). *The healing heart.* New York: Avon Books.

Doyal, L. & Hurwitz, B. (1987). Respecting autonomy and telling the truth in general practice. *The Practitioner, 231:* 775–779.

Erde, E. L., Nadal, E. C. & Scholl, T. D. (1988). On truth telling and the diagnosis of Alzheimer's disease. *Journal of Family Practice, 26:* 401–406.

Evenson, T., Evenson, M. L. & Fish, D. E. (1986). Family enrichment: A rehabilitation opportunity. *Rehabilitation Literature, 47:* 274–280.

Fiore, N. (1979). Fighting cancer: One patient's perspective. *New England Journal of Medicine, 300:* 287.

Fox, R. (1984). The evolution of medical uncertainty. *Milbank Memorial Fund Quarterly, 58:* 1–10.

Gautam, S. & Nijhawan, M. (1987). Communicating with cancer patients. *British Journal of Psychiatry, 150:* 760–764.

GIVO. (1986). What doctors tell patients with breast cancer about diagnosis and treatment: Findings from a study of general hospitals. *British Journal of Cancer, 54:* 319–326.

Goldberg, R. J. (1984). Disclosure of information to adult cancer patients: Issues and update. *Journal of Clinical Medicine, 8:* 948.

Gross, A. M., Eudy, C. & Drabman, R. S. (1982). Training parents to be physical therapists with the physically handicapped child. *Journal of Behavioral Medicine, 5:* 321–327.

Grunder, T. M. (1980). On the reliability of surgical consent forms. *New England Journal of Medicine, 302:* 900–902.

Katz, J. (1972). *Experimentation with human beings.* New York: Russell Sage Foundation.

Katz, J. (1984). Why doctors don't disclose uncertainty. *Hastings Center Report, 14:* 35–44.

Kaufman, C. L. (1983). Informed consent and patient decision making: Two decades of research. *Social Science and Medicine, 17:* 1657–1664.

Lidz, C. W. et al. (1984). *Informed consent: A study of decision making in psychiatry.* New York: Guilford.

Lynn, J. (1986). *By no extraordinary means: The choice to forgo life-sustaining treatment.* Bloomington, IN: Indiana University Press.

Makas, E. (1980). Increasing counselor-client communication. *Rehabilitation Literature, 41:* 235–239.

McCormick, R. A. (1989). *Theology and bioethics. Hastings Center Report, 19:* 5–10.

Minogue, B. P. & Taraszewski, R. (1988). The whole truth and nothing but the truth? *Hastings Center Report, 14:* 35–44.

Molter, N. C. (1979). Needs of relatives of critically ill patients: A descriptive study. *Heart and Lung, 8:* 330–334.

Morrow, G. (1980). How readable are subject consent forms? *JAMA, 224:* 56–58.

Mumford, E. & Skipper, J. K. (1967). *Sociology in hospital care.* New York: Harper & Row.

Munn, H. E., Jr. (1977). Communication between patients, nurses, physicians and surgeons. *Hospital Topics, 55:* 7.

Nathanson v. Kline. (1960). 186 Kan., 393, 350 P.2d 1093, 1104 (1960).

Newall, D. J., Gadd, E. M. & Priestman, T. J. (1987). Presentation of information to cancer patients: A comparison of two centres in the UK and USA. *British Journal of Medical Psychology, 60:* 120–127.

Novack, D. H., Plumer, R., Smith, R. L. et al. (1989). Physicians' attitudes toward using deception to resolve difficult ethical problems. *JAMA, 261:* 2980–2985.

Olson, J., Edwards, M. & Hunter, J. A. (1987). The physician's role in delivering sensitive information to families of handicapped infants. *Clinical Pediatrics, 26:* 231–234.

Percival, T. (1803). *Medical ethics: Or code of institutes and precepts, adopted to the professional conduct of physicians and surgeons.* Manchester, England: S. Russell.

Pernick, M. S. (1982). *The patient's role in medical decision making: A social history of informed consent. Making health policy decisions.* Washington, DC: Government Printing Office.

Reiser, S. J. (1980). Words as scalpels: Transmitting evidence in clinical dialogue. *Annals of Internal Medicine, 92:* 840–841.

Schloendorff v. New York Hospital. 211 N.Y. 125, 127, 129, 105; N.E., 92, 93 (1914).

Silverman, W. A. (1988). Consent for experimentation involving neonates. *American Journal of Medical Sciences, 296:* 354–359.

Slater v. Baker and Stapleton. 95 Eng. Rep. 860 (1767).

Smith, D. A. (1984). Telling the truth in medical practice. *Pennsylvania Medicine, 87:* 10.

Taylor, K. M. & Kelner, M. (1987). Informed consent: The physician's perspective. *Social Science and Medicine, 24:* 135–143.

Todd, C. J. & Still, A. W. (1984). Communication between general practitioners and patients dying at home. *Social Science and Medicine, 18:* 668–672.

Tolstoy, L. (1960). *The death of Ivan Ilych.* New York: New American Library.

Viswanathan, R., Clark, J. J. & Viswanathan, K. (1986). Physicians' and the public's attitudes on communication about death. *Archives of Internal Medicine, 146:* 2029–2033.

Wertenbaker, L. T. (1957). *Death of a man.* New York: Random House.

SUGGESTED READINGS

Barton, E. H., Jr. (1972). Don't talk down to me, at me, around me . . . Talk *with* me! *Journal of Rehabilitation, 38:* 33.

Blumenfield, M., Levy, N. B. & Kaufman, D. (1979). Current attitudes of medical students and house staff toward terminal illness. *General Hospital Psychiatry, 1:* 306–310.

Boreham, P. & Gipson, D. (1978). The informative process in private medicine consultations: A preliminary investigation. *Social Science and Medicine, 12:* 409–416.

Brody, H. (1982). Deception in the teaching hospital. *Programs in Clinical Biological Research, 139:* 81–86.

Cartwright, A., Hockey, L. & Anderson, J. L. (1973). *Life before death.* London: Routledge & Kegan Paul.

Dayringer, R., Paiva, R. E. A. & Davidson, G. W. (1983). Ethical decision-making by family physicians. *Journal of Family Practice, 17:* 267–272.

Faden, R. R., Becker, C., Lewis, C. et al. (1981). Disclosure of information to patients in medical care. *Medical Care, 19:* 718–733.

Farber, B. & Ryckman, D. B. (1965). Effects of severely mentally retarded children on family relationships. *Mentally Retarded Abstracts, 2:* 1–17.

Gadow, S. (1981). Truth: Treatment of choice, scarce resource, or patient's right? *Journal of Family Practice, 13:* 857–860.

Ganos, D. (1983). Deception in the teaching hospital, pp. 77–97. In D. Ganos, R. E. Lipson et al. (Eds.), *Difficult decisions in medical ethics.* New York: Alan R. Liss.

Gilhooly, M. L. M., Berkely, J. S., McCann, K. et al. (1988). Truth telling with dying cancer patients. *Palliative Medicine, 12:* 64–71.

Goldberg, R. J. (1984). Disclosure of information to adult cancer patients: Issues and update. *Journal of Clinical Oncology, 2:* 948–955.

Greenwald, H. P. & Nevitt, M. C. (1982). Physician attitudes toward communication with cancer patients. *Social Science and Medicine, 16:* 591–594.

Hagman, D. G. (1970). The medical patient's right to know: Report on a medical-legal, empirical study. *UCLA Law Review, 17:* 758–816.

Hardy, R. E., Green, D. R., Jordan, H. W. et al. (1980). Communication between cancer patients and physicians. *Southern Medical Journal, 73:* 755–757.

Hinton, J. (1980). Whom do dying patients tell? *British Medical Journal, 281:* 1328–1330.

Jonsen, A. B., Siegler, M. & Winslade, W. J. (1982). *Clinical ethics: A practical approach to ethical decisions in clinical medicine.* New York: Macmillan.

Kroth, R., Olson, J. J. & Kroth, J. (1986). Delivering sensitive information (or, please don't kill the messenger!). *Counseling and Human Development, 18:* 9.

Light, D., Jr. (1979). Uncertainty and control in professional training. *Journal of Health and Social Behavior, 310:* 320–325.

McIntosh, J. (1976). Patients' awareness and desire for information about diagnosed but undisclosed malignant disease. *Lancet, 2:* 300–303.

Mitchell, G. W. & Glicksman, A. S. (1977). Cancer patients: Knowledge and attitudes. *Cancer, 40:* 61–66.

Munson, R. (1983). *Intervention and reflection: Basic issues in medical ethics.* Belmont, CA: Wadsworth.

Murphy, M. A. (1982). The family with a handicapped child: A review of the literature. *Journal of Developmental and Behavioral Pediatrics, 2:* 73–82.

Standard, S. & Nathan, H. (1955). *Should the patient know the truth?* New York: Springer.

Vogel, J. & Delgado, R. (1980). To tell the truth: Physicians' duty to disclose medical mistakes. *UCLA Law Review, 28:* 52–94.

Weir, R. (1980). Truth telling in medicine. *Perspectives in Biology and Medicine, 24:* 95–112.

Willner, S. K. & Crane, R. A. (1979). A parental dilemma: The child with a marginal handicap. *Social Casework, 60:* 30–35.

Chapter 11

VALUES AND ETHICS IN CONFLICT

This above all: to thine own self be true.

William Shakespeare
Hamlet, 1600

Everybody has a little bit of Watergate in him.

Rev. Billy Graham
February 3, 1974

E very major social change in a society forces a confrontation with its
values. In its power to change the conditions of birth and death, to
alter behavior, to impose dilemmas about the relationship between individual and social good, medical research forces a new confrontation with
some of the oldest human questions. What is the relationship between
"happiness" and health? What should medicine's role be in bringing
happiness about? What is a "good life" and a "healthy life?" What is a
"good death" and what are medicine's responsibilities and limitations in
the care of the dying? Questions of this kind are ethical and laden with
the values of society and individuals (Callahan, 1977).

It is painful to deal in a rational way with ethical issues, but it must be
done. If not confronted and resolved, these issues become even more
entangled in the complexity of rapid change. It may be necessary to
develop new values to manage modern health care, modify old moral
standards, and, perhaps, reaffirm some traditional values in adapting to
social change. Basic moral choices will have to be made as all of the
alternatives will not be possible.

Key Values

Values arise in response to society's need, so values change. The same
value can reappear at different points in the history of a society as the
need dictates. For example, ecology and environmental preservation,
which were popular among the young in our society during the 1960s,

303

were forgotten in the 1970s, only to reappear in the 1980s. By process of selection, those values that have survival value for a culture are maintained and strengthened, while less important values are forgotten or de-emphasized. Two values that are considered to be fundamental to a value system are individual dignity and autonomy (Brody, 1981). These are especially key values involved in some of the ethical dilemmas in health care. Autonomy is a key rationale underlying the American Hospital Association's Patient's Bill of Rights. Patient's autonomy is protected by informed consent and confidentiality. The autonomy of the health professional is protected by a professional code of ethics, but there are limits to autonomy, especially when it threatens the well-being of others. Beneficence and nonmaleficence are two other key values in health care, i.e., to try to do good and not do harm. Finally, how people are treated, or justice, is an essential value in health care (Anderson & Glenes-Anderson, 1987). Ethical dilemmas in the health professions involve a complex interplay between several factors, including statutory law, the individual values of the health care provider and of the patient, and the ethical principles relating to autonomy, beneficence, nonmaleficence, and justice (see Fig. 11-1).

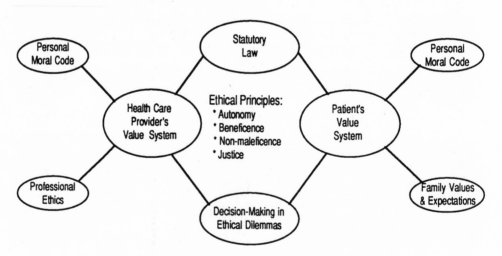

Figure 11-1. Factors involved in deciding ethical dilemmas.

In a dilemma, one is faced with alternative choices, neither of which seems a satisfactory solution to a problem. Dilemmas arise in situations of ambiguity and uncertainty, when it is difficult to predict the consequences of one's actions, and when the general principles upon which one normally relies either offer no help or seem to contradict one another. There are many apparent moral dilemmas for which solutions can be found. In the case of terminal illness, great advances have been made in developing methods of pain control which do not endanger the life of the patient. Had these new methods been available earlier, physicians would not have had to make choices between maintaining life and preventing suffering. As the techniques and treatments available to physicians have increased, many of the old problems of choice between unsatisfactory alternatives have been solved. Unfortunately, new techniques bring fresh moral problems. The development of organ transplantation, for example, has eliminated some problems connected with the care of patients suffering from kidney or heart disorders, only to replace them with new dilemmas concerning the permission of donors or their relatives, the life expectancy of recipients, and the definition of death. Moral dilemmas will continue to occur in health care as long as choices, which involve pitting one set of values against another, must be made (Campbell, 1984).

The purpose of this chapter is to examine current examples of conflicts that exist between ethics, values, and making medical choices. A process of resolving conflicts will be proposed so that old and new values can be examined and tentative directions chosen that will be in harmony with our culture, our politics, and our individual rights.

A logical place to begin an examination of moral choices is with the concept of "health," the dilemmas surrounding the right to health, and the value of health.

The Right to Health and the Value of Health

Most definitions of health are so broad and idealistic that health is considered an unattainable goal by society, medicine, and individuals. We often speak of "health problems" in a broad sense when we intend to lump together several interrelated problems in a community, which affect the physical, mental, or social well-being of residents. "Health problems" can include drug abuse, human abuse, pollution, teenage pregnancy, and accidents. On the individual level, when we do not wish to specify the exact nature for the reason for a visit to the doctor, we say we have a "health problem." Despite our vagueness about health, the World Health Organization (1976) has declared that everyone has a "right to health" and a "right to health care." The right to health might mean that a society has an obligation to guarantee the health of its members. But medicine cannot guarantee that a person will always be healthy. One might say the right implies the obligation to make the attempt. It can reasonably be said that citizens have an obligation not to jeopardize the health of others, but it is an enormous step to claim that the good health of all is the responsibility of all (Callahan, 1977). The concept of a "right to health" does not provide a firm basis for a policy regarding health care.

Some industrialized societies have converted the moral claim to a "right to health" into legal rights. The British and some other European governments have extensive "cradle to grave" health plans. This notion of a "right to health" or a "right to health care" has not been converted into law and practice in the United States. National health insurance legislation would have to require our government to guarantee a minimum level of health insurance coverage for *all* citizens. While we have not enacted such a comprehensive plan, new groups have been added to the list of guaranteed health insurance coverage, e.g., Medicare and Medicaid (Harron, Burnside & Beauchamp, 1983).

The Value of Health

Part of the difference in how societies have regarded the "right to health" is due to the fact that societies differ in the value they place on health compared to other values. Since the definition of health is broad, health may be given lip-service as an important value, but when economic and other resources are allocated, health-related facilities, activities, and personnel may end up with fewer resources than, for example, the military (Susser, 1974).

The conflict between advocating health as a right and valuing health enough to promote it is apparent in some of the contradictory behaviors in which we engage. We warn people about the health risks of smoking tobacco, yet the government subsidizes tobacco growers. We know the high speed on highways is related to the number of accidents and fatalities, yet there has been a gradual raising of, or ignoring of, the speed limit in many states. One of the reasons for the inconsistencies between the ethics of health and the value of health is that health has been considered a responsibility of the individual in our society. Individuals vary greatly in how they define health for themselves and the degree to which they think they are responsible for their health. Each person assesses his/her own risks for losing health and puts a value, whether monetary, social, or spiritual, on his/her own life. Indeed, many people do not recognize their personal responsibility for maintaining, promoting, or enhancing their health (Knowles, 1977). While there is evidence that Americans are "conscious about their health" and many are engaging in healthy activities, it is not clear that this social movement is affecting national health policy.

The phrase "quality of life" often is tied to the "right to health" and the "right to health care" by their advocates. Traditionally, a desirable level of quality has been proposed to promote happiness. It was derived by first determining what was "human essence," from which one could know what was required to obtain happiness, and thus a desirable "quality of life." The focus has changed from the Socratic to the Anglo-American tradition, away from "the good life" to the quality necessary to live a "human" or moral existence (Aiken, 1982).

With the concern for liberty as a prerequisite for maintaining a human quality of life came the recognition of the universal equality of human beings and their universal entitlement to liberty. Yet, liberty alone is insufficient to ensure an equal minimal human quality of life. The emphasis on the minimal necessary conditions is inherently egalitarian, that is, it stresses the insurance of minimal goods or resources for all human beings. The declaration of the equal entitlement of all humans to liberty and to a minimal level of well-being is much like the declaration of the "right to health." Yet, we have not determined what the desirable level of quality of life is, nor discovered the means for attaining or maintaining it. Harron, Burnside & Beauchamp (1983) have summarized our dilemmas as follows: "If we are tempted to believe that each person is entitled to health care and protection, we must realize . . . that under the present circumstances, we probably cannot afford to provide it for at least many services. . . . We feel ourselves forced to decide how much health care we shall administer, to whom, and according to what criteria. We make these choices knowing that they will determine who enjoys what level of health and even who shall live and who shall die. We are in the position of having to establish public policy in matters of health, life, and death on the basis of our moral values (pg. 129)."

The Right to Self-determination and the Value of Personal Control

A second common dilemma health professionals face is the professional's and client's respective rights to self-determination (autonomy) and the value each places on controlling the content and outcome of his/her encounter. Probably the most common current criticism of the medical profession is that doctors too often violate their patient's personal autonomy. One of the major complaints has been that physicians do not provide sufficient information to their patients: often they do not fully (or at all) explain what is wrong with them, they do not inform patients of the risks involved in the treatment they recommend, they do not adequately explain the advantages and disadvantages of alternative treatments. Without such information, it becomes impossible for patients to exercise the right of self-determination (Bassford, 1983).

Barnard (1985) has noted that, since patients must place themselves under the authority and judgment of a professional expert for care, patients are placed in a dependent position where, historically, they have followed physician's orders. Patients have been viewed as incapable or unwilling to take responsibility for their own medical treatment. Barnard refers to this as the "benevolent authoritarian" approach. Physicians often assume that if patients desire information, they will ask for it. It has been shown that information exchange in the physician-patient relationship is inversely related to socioeconomic status. Lower class patients report a desire for information equal to that of higher classes. Lower class patients, however, ask fewer questions than upper class patients and tend to be less verbal, in general, in the physician-patient interaction. As a result, physicians tend to judge lower class patients to be less linguistically competent and, hence, to have less desire for information, as well as lower comprehension (Waitzkin & Stoeckle, 1972).

Health professionals should not assume that the lack of assertiveness or inquisitiveness on the part of patients is a failure or shortcoming. Indeed, some patients may be reserved or silent because they do not want to look foolish by asking simple questions or they may fear the answer to some questions, so they do not ask them. Some patients do not elect to ask information and place decisions in the hands of their doctors. Yet, the results of the few studies that have been conducted indicate that patients who are informed appreciate the information and have fewer difficulties (including a lower complication rate) than patients who are not informed. Self-respect and a sense of dignity require that people have control over how their lives are conducted. When people are ill, their sense of control over their lives is lost and with it is lost much of their sense of dignity. But with the provision of information about risks and alternative treatment, some degree of control is reestablished and anxiety is reduced.

Both health professionals and patients have their own methods for asserting control when they meet. Patients can withhold information, not follow the presented therapeutic regimen, fail to keep appointments, or file litigation. Health professionals practice paternalism, which they justify because they want to prevent someone from harming themselves. Paternalism implies unequal status, such as exists in the parent-child relationship. Paternalistic practices by health professionals have been viewed by ethicists as illegitimate exercises of power, which are only justified when illness removes autonomy (Brown, 1985). There are instances, however, which involve dangers that are either not understood or appreciated by the person involved such as the dangers of smoking cigarettes. Wasserstrom (1971) suggests that we would be more likely to consent to paternalism in those instances in which it preserves and enhances the individual's ability to rationally consider and carry out his/her own decisions.

The autonomy of health professionals and patients should be mutually respected. It is consistent with the responsibility often overlooked in health care: the responsibility to educate (Tormey & Brody, 1978). Skilled clinicians should be able to relate to patients in a way that combines decisiveness and support with disclosure of relevant facts and an openness to further discussion.

The Value of Life

Though we do not consciously consider it, the value of life is involved in decisions we make every day. We decide to fly or drive to another city on the basis of our evaluation of different risks to our life. Some people rarely, if ever, fly, despite the fact that flying is less risky than driving. Some people also make decisions that place a value on the life of others, such as allocating resources to health care or deciding on locating a chemical plant near water and food sources.

The conviction that one should always choose life lies at the heart of the practice of medicine. The immorality of choosing death as an end is founded upon our religious faith that life is a gift. To choose death is to reject this gift. So also religious faith affirms that life is a trust and not to accept life as a trust is to abandon trusteeship. We are stewards and not owners of our lives (Ramsey, 1978). In this respect there is no such concept as a right to die. Indeed, we will all die. However, we can influence how and when we die by our actions or inactions. We can take our life by suicide, or flagrantly engage in habits and activities that we have been told will shorten our life, or hasten our death by assuming no responsibility for the maintenance of our health, or merely "give up" on our desire to live. These are life choices. Many people die prematurely. "Normal" death results from a harmonious wearing out of the body at a different genetic rate in each of us. It is suspected that there is a biological limit to the length of time the machine can go on running, but we know that a majority of people seldom approach this limit. Medicine is only beginning to understand why healthy people die too soon (Dempsey, 1975).

Quality-of-life judgments are problematic. Inevitably one person's judgment of another's quality of life is filtered through one's values. Indeed, we each value life differently. An example is the legal concept of "wrongful life." The suits for tort for wrongful life raise the issue not only when it would be preferable not to have been born, but also when it would be wrong to cause a person to be born. This implies that someone should have judged that it would have been preferable for a child never to have had existence under certain circumstances. Further, it implies that the person's existence under those circumstances should have been prevented and that, not having been prevented, life was not a gift but an injury.

The idea of responsibility for acts that sustain or prolong life is key to the notion that one should not under certain circumstances prolong the life of a child. Unlike adults, children cannot decide with regard to euthanasia. The difficulty for parents and health professionals lies in determining what makes life not worth living for a child (Munson, 1988).

Adults make decisions, consciously or unconsciously, about how and when they will die by the way they live. The right of persons to control their own bodies is a basic societal concept. Yet, we place a value on each other's lives and make judgments about the rightness or wrongness of how an individual dies. We are uncomfortable with individuals who value life differently than we value our own life and attempt to intervene in an individual's process of dying. Since we expect each person's life to have value, we feel a responsibility to ensure that each person "dies well" (Ramsey, 1978).

The Value of Death

Amazing technological advances in medicine have made it possible for life today to be sustained by artificial support mechanisms. Death can be postponed and programmed to coincide with the needs of survivors as well as the patient. As Morison (1977) has asked, "Is death a process or event?"

The status of assisted suicide as public policy in the U.S. is unsettled and reminiscent of the legal status of abortion in the years preceding the 1973 decision in Roe v. Wade. The call for legalized suicide has been increasing in several quarters, from suicide advocacy organizations like the Hemlock Society, the Society for the Right to Die, and Americans Against Human Suffering. The attitude of Americans toward assisted suicide is ambivalent. An Associated Press poll in 1985 found that 68 percent of the respondents believed that incurable patients ought to be permitted to end their lives by active means. Conflicting legal decisions have added to the confusion. The rising incidence of suicide contributes to this turmoil. In 1985, 28,500 Americans committed suicide, making suicide the nation's eighth leading cause of death (Rosenblum & Forsythe, 1990).

Anecdotal evidence suggests that assisted suicide in the U.S. is increasingly being performed, particularly by patients with AIDS (New York Times, May 24, 1989, A1). In addition, public opinion polls indicate that the majority of Americans believe that assisted suicide should be permitted (New York Times, May 24, 1989, A1). Advocates of assisted suicide suggest that it is a natural extension of the principle that hopelessly ill patients may refuse life-prolonging medical care (Orentlicher, 1989).

Currently, twenty-six states prohibit the assistance of suicide. No states expressly legalize suicide through legislation or constitution. Only the California Court of Appeals in the Bouvia case has gone so far as to permit suicide through the refusal of food and fluids by a competent, nonterminally ill patient (*Bouvia v. Superior Court*, 1986). The court held in Bouvia that a competent patient with cerebral palsy and quadriplegia, who was neither terminally ill nor imminently dying, had a right to refuse food and fluids through a nasogastric tube in order to bring about her death. Several courts have allowed the withdrawal of food and fluids from incompetent patients through substituted judgement. The decision of the New York Supreme Court in Delio v. Westchester County Medical Center abandoned the distinction between extraordinary and ordinary treatment. Delio addressed the issue of the withdrawal of food and water through both a gastrostomy and jejunostomy tube from Delio who was in a chronic vegetative state. Likewise, the Massachusetts Supreme Court in the Brophy case allowed the withdrawal of fluid and food through a gastrostomy tube from a patient in a persistent vegetative state, but not terminally ill or imminently dying. Dissent from these decisions has revolved around whether food and water are basic human needs versus the view that food and water should be viewed as medical treatment.

Gratton (1990) argues that there is no morally relevant distinction between letting and making death happen, and between withholding and withdrawing life-support. Dagi (1990) counters, saying that while . there may be no inherent moral distinction between withholding and withdrawing care, the two decisions have been traditionally perceived differently, the courts treat them differently, and they appear different to many clinicians. They are morally linked to other considerations which are not separable. In that sense, and with the realities of clinical practice, withholding and withdrawing care are not the same.

The engagement of physicians in the introduction of assisted suicide would change the role of the physician from that of a healer. Legalized suicide would introduce two further problems: (1) an inability to limit "rational suicide" to "hard cases," and (2) the inability to enforce these limits that are imposed. Legalized assisted suicide would also pressure persons with disabilities to forgo care, and could be applied to a wide class of disabled persons. Finally, assisted suicide implicates the rights of conscience of medical personnel and could open up "wrongful living" suits against them just as Roe v. Wade caused "wrongful birth" and "wrongful life" suits (Rosenblum & Forsythe, 1990).

Should a physician be able to assist the suicide of a hopelessly ill patient? A panel of distinguished physicians, brought together by the Society for the Right to Die, says yes (Wanzer et al., 1989). Deeply rooted traditions and guiding principles of medical practice say no. According to 10 of the panel's 12 members, if a hopelessly ill patient believes his or her condition is intolerable, then it should be permissable for a physician to provide the patient with the medical means and the medical knowledge to commit suicide. For example, the physician could prescribe sleeping pills for the patient and indicate how many pills there are in a lethal dose (Angell, 1988). Assisted suicide, then, differs from euthanasia in the extent to which the physician participates in the process (Orentlicher, 1989).

Ordinarily, a physician provides medical care to sustain life and to relieve suffering. A long-standing rejection of assisted suicide by the American Medical Association's Council on Judicial and Ethical Affairs, rests with undermining a patient's trust in the physician. There is a felt distinction between acting to hasten death and refraining from delaying death. Kass (1989) argues that physicians serve the needs of patients because they are sick. What the sick need and are entitled to from the physician is health. Treatment designed to bring on death, therefore, is inconsistent with the physician's role. Orentlicher (1989) points out, however, that withdrawal of life support does not violate the nature of the physician-patient relationship. While the physician has a duty to care for those who want to be healed, there should not be an obligation to impose treatment on those who don't want it. Kantor (1979) argues that an independent adult's decision to refuse life-saving treatment must be respected by the judiciary no matter what the reason for refusal. Hegland (1979), on the other hand, argues that because of society's interest in the life of an individual, and because of the law's traditional view of the sanctity of human life, the law should not protect an individual's decision to choose death.

It could be argued that death can have value. We usually think of death as a negative event and, as noted earlier in this book, negative things and events are not usually valued. However, some religions see death as entering a new life. One that is free from human problems and, therefore, is a desired state, especially if one's current life is burdensome and painful. If illness further limits the meaningfulness and satisfaction of living, death may seem preferable to life. As noted previously, all social value is reduced to the personal value of one's own life. Only each individual can determine the relative advantages of living or dying, and the advantages and disadvantages change as one ages and encounters life's problems.

To speak of the value of a person's life is ambiguous. We must specify to whom it is valuable. The *personal value* of a life is its value to the person whose life it is. The *social value* of a person's life is its value to other people. The *total value* of a person's life is the sum of its personal and social value, its value to everyone (Bayles, 1987).

In considering the personal value of life, we have to determine what makes a life valuable to the person who lives it. The principle that physicians should always prolong life assumes that biological life is valuable, but if one is comatose, one's biological life is not of value to anyone. Therefore, consciousness, at some level, is a necessary condition for life having a personal value. Bayles (1987) argues that personal value could be based on the number of years of conscious life. The longer one is consciously alive, the more valuable life is. But life can have both a positive and a negative value. Consciousness makes it possible for life to have value, but it does not necessarily make life good. Some people who are seriously injured or dying might not label their life as good, and might prefer an early death. Any theory of the value of life must allow it to be both positive and negative.

If the value of conscious life can vary, then it must depend on some qualities of life, besides consciousness, that can vary. Some have suggested that the capacity to think, or to give or receive love, or to feel pleasure or pain pertain to the capability of life having value. These factors do not make life good or bad. The personal value of life depends on the characteristics of the *experiences* one has. Some people value life even if they are unhappy and some people do not seem to value life even if they are successful. At least two different factors affect the personal value of life—the happiness it involves and the pursuit or accomplishment of one's goals. In medicine, judgments of the potential quality or value of a person's life are often made on the basis of physical and mental capacity and pain. While these factors can limit happiness and accomplishments, capacities only set limits to possible value. Bayles (1987) suggests that the personal value of life is a function of the length and quality of conscious life.

The social value of a person's life is somewhat easier to conceptualize than its personal value. Social value can be divided into three aspects. One is its emotional or psychological value. People are often emotionally involved with a particular individual who is seen as irreplaceable. A second aspect is personal services—the special things that only a particular person can do. The third element is the economic value of a person's life to others. A person's life can also be an economic liability or cost to others. The distinction between personal and social value is a relative one depending on whose life one considers. In the final analysis, all social value reduces to the personal value of other persons' lives.

Personhood

Closely tied to the value of life is the question, "What is a person?" (see Fig. 11-2) The Oxford English Dictionary defines "person" as a self-conscious or rational being. There is wide disagreement over the meaning of "person," but it is acknowledged to be a value-laden concept (Donovan, 1983). The concept of person is only partly biological. Genetic individuality is a biological component and is established during fertilization at the single cell level. Multicellularity comes next, but singleness at this level is not established for perhaps two weeks, closely associated with fusion of the developing offspring with the tissues of the mother. The offspring now develops within the fusion zone as an embryo, with rudiments of a central nervous system and brain. As this system matures, behavior begins. Integrated behavior, such as we associate with persons, appears midway in the third trimester, along with maturational changes in the upper brain. Professional behavioral observers have described this as a rudimentary awareness, possibly the first appearance of a consciousness of self (Grobstein, 1983).

The question of personhood enters into the abortion debate in a

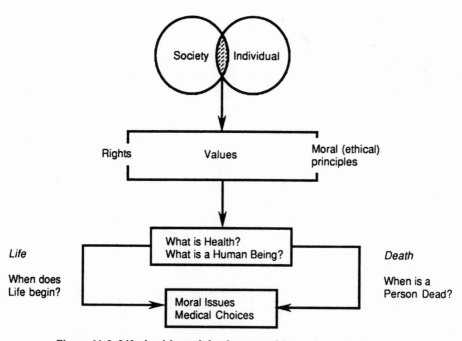

Figure 11-2. Life, health, and death as moral issues in medical choices.

familiar way: anti-abortion activists argue that abortion, which ordinarily involves killing the fetus, is wrong because fetuses are persons. Pro-choice advocates call attention to the pregnant woman's right to privacy, but often their argument involves the claim that abortion can be justified because fetuses are not persons. The range of developmental milestones to mark the beginning of personhood—conception, onset of brain function, viability, birth—is evidence of conceptual disarray. Philosophers also vary widely in their choice of criteria. Some view all products of conception as persons; others deny this status to fetuses but extend it to some animals. One philosopher has denied that there are any persons at all (Unger, 1979).

Personhood is an important concept in ethics because we ordinarily afford special consideration to organisms called persons. But the concept of personhood does not offer a promising avenue for resolution of the abortion debate (Wikler, 1983). As Callahan (1972) has observed, "abortion does not seem like the kind of moral issue which is just 'solved' once and for all; it can only be coped with."

Macklin (1983) notes four issues regarding personhood, on which writers in the field of bioethics disagree.

1. Equivalence of meaning between "human" and "person." Some writers distinguish between these two concepts, while others consider them synonomous.
2. Indeterminancy of the status of the fetus as a person. The sharpest disagreement is between those who offer criteria for personhood and those who deny the feasibility of such a definition.
3. The importance of personhood for efforts to resolve moral debates surrounding abortion. Since the majority of writings on personhood occur within the context of the abortion debate, it is not surprising to find the widest variation of claims made about the relevance and importance of defining personhood.

- Settling the abortion issue depends on coming to some agreement about whether the fetus is a person and, if so, when, in its development, personhood begins.
- Settling the abortion issue has little or nothing to do with when personhood begins since abortion may be morally justified even if it is acknowledged that the fetus is a person from the moment of conception.
- Since it is impossible to provide a set of necessary and sufficient

conditions for personhood and, therefore, impossible to secure agreement on the criteria for personhood, that issue must be seen as irrelevant to arriving at a solution to the abortion controversy.

4. The importance of personhood linked to the need to ascribe rights. Most writers accept without question a strong link between being a person and being the bearer of rights, especially the right to life.

The most obvious point of disagreement on personhood is the dispute about the properties an entity must have to satisfy the criteria of personhood (Macklin, 1983). Personhood is not a useful concept for resolving dilemmas in bioethics. Much of the literature discusses personhood solely in the context of abortion. A variety of biomedical phenomena and clinical conditions have become foci of questions concerning personhood, and of the bearing of personhood on issues that involve medical judgment, decision-making, and action (Fox & Willis, 1983). These include fetal development and abortion, human genetics, *in vitro* fertilization and other forms of reproductive technology, organ transplantation, mental retardation, brain disease, and certain chronic and progressive neurological disorders, states of senility, dementia, as well as coma, terminal illness, and "brain death." Within this framework, the beginning and end of life, particularly in connection with abortion on the one hand, and terminating life-sustaining treatment on the other, have elicited the most deeply felt consideration of personhood. The womb and the brain are important symbolic, as well as anatomic, loci of these personhood discussions.

However varied the form and content of the many different considerations of personhood, they are unified around one predominant theme: individualism (Fox & Willis, 1983). The autonomous self-awareness of the individual and his/her self-reliance, independence, and freedom are consistently emphasized, along with the uniqueness, worth, and dignity of each person. These attributes are not only presented as virtues, but as entitlements. They are frequently expressed in "rights" language: the right to autonomy, the right to privacy, the right to decide for one's self, the right to control one's own body and psyche, the right to life, and the right to death. Whole categories of persons (infants, women, patients, the mentally ill, the retarded, the impaired, the comatose) and also incipient persons (fetuses) and the dying are separately treated in terms of their own, distinctive, self-oriented, individual rights.

A second theme that permeates discussions of personhood concerns the interrelationship and the interdependence of individuals and groups. Authors stress the obligations we have to others and the willingness to care for others and to allow others to care for us. Underlying personhood is a conception of community and society.

Why is the American tradition of individualism and its relationship to community and personhood now so problematic? Why has this problem led to such questions as: What is life? What is death? When does life begin, and when does it end? Some authors suggest it is due to the secularization of matters of collective conscience. The scientific and technological aspects of medicine and their impact on the human condition have acquired greater societal significance. Medicine is one arena in which our society is struggling with basic questions of value and belief. Fletcher (1954) has said that problems of conscience in medicine are created by four phases of medical growth: (1) changes in technology; (2) professional experience; (3) scientific advances; and (4) cultural changes. The moral problems of medicine are almost always a mixture of several of these developments.

Attempts to resolve conflicts over medicine-related issues of personhood through public discussion, legislatures, commissions, and the courts, have generated two opposing types of difficulties. On one hand, attempts to bring about a consensus through legal statements about personhood have stirred up more controversy than they have settled. For example, U.S. Senate Bill 158, introduced by Senator Jesse Helms on January 19, 1981, declared that "the Congress finds that present-day scientific evidence indicates a significant likelihood that actual human life exists from conception . . . ", and goes on to reinterpret the Fourteenth Amendment to cover all human life including the fetus *in utero*. The bill elicited passionate disagreement over its constitutionality. On the other hand, the consensus about personhood reached by more diplomatic and intellectual means is also problematic because it tends to play down issues. Sometimes consensus avoids many of the questions that caused the examination of personhood in the first place (see Roe v. Wade, Appendix C). (A chronology of the abortion issue from 1973 to 1990 is shown in Appendix D.)

When questions like those of personhood go to courts or commissions, the problem usually is narrowed and its aspects are relegated to technical categories. For example, the President's Commission for the Study of Ethical Problems in Medicine and Biomedical and Behavioral Research tackled the definition of death in 1981. The report focused almost exclusively on the use of heart-lung and brain criteria for the determination of death with a detailed consideration of the role that the law and medicine might play in enacting a definition of death. The report did not deal with the broader social, cultural, religious or ethical significance of death, despite the fact that members on the commission represented these areas.

Veatch (1983) has asked the question, "Can death help define life? He suggests that the definition of the beginning of life requires a determination of features of human life that give moral standing to an individual. The critical issue to be decided is what essential feature signals the beginning of moral standing. He reviewed several criteria that could be used: a unique genetic code, circulatory and respiratory activity, a functioning nervous system, and a capacity for consciousness. Veatch (1983) pointed out that the development of a fixed unique genetic code, which occurs about two weeks after fertilization, is never considered in the debate over when death occurs; death traditionally has been associated with the cessation of heart and lung activity. If cardiac function or a working nervous system are determined to be the essential feature for moral standing, Veatch (1983) said, the issue focuses on when such activity begins in the fetus. The answer will depend upon whether one attributes significance to mere cellular level activity or to organic functioning. Most experts today believe that it is the latter that is important.

In order to know when one should be treated as having moral standing, one must know whether the essential feature being searched for is *capacity* or *potential.* Veatch (1983) suggests that the definition of death could finesse the issue that is critical to the definition of the beginning of life, that is, when one irreversibly loses the critical capacity—circulatory, integrative, or mental—one simultaneously loses any *potential* for that capacity. It will never return again. What cannot be agreed upon is whether capacity or potential is critical. On that question, the definition of death can tell us nothing. We are forced to live with the uncertainty this creates, just as we live with uncertainty over when we should treat people as dead.

The Right to Health Care and the Value of Social Justice

A fourth common dilemma of ethics and values in our country has to do with the right to health care and distributive justice. Indeed, whether health care is a right is itself a subject of debate. Slade (1971) argues that the right to health care is immoral because it denies the most fundamental of all rights, that of a person to his/her own life and the freedom of action to support it. In Slade's view, health care is neither a right nor a privilege; it is a service that is provided by health professionals to people who wish to purchase it. It is the provision of this service that physicians and others depend upon for their livelihood, and is a means of supporting their own lives. Slade specifies several fallacies that have been perpetuated by the basic fallacy that health care is a right. He notes that one of these fallacies is that health is primarily a community or social rather than an individual concern. More than one-half of all deaths in the United States are due to diseases known to be caused or exacerbated by alcohol, tobacco, overeating, or accidents. Each of these factors is largely correctable by individual actions. Other fallacies have to do with the form and structure of delivering health care, especially the fallacy that state medicine has worked better than free enterprise medicine.

Perhaps, one of the problems in the concept of the right to health care is that it has focused on the individual or micro level of moral decision making. Who should receive liver transplants or open heart surgery? Should a hydrocephalic newborn with spina bifida be treated at all? There is also a macro or social level of decision making that has been much less discussed, even though it has a greater impact on our health. The macro level concerns basic health care institutions. This includes our high technology hospitals and clinics, academic health science centers, research institutions, and public health agencies concerned with the control of infectious disease, drug and food protection, consumer product safety, health hazards in the environment, and programs concerned with prevention. Health care also includes institutions that provide services to the mentally and physically disabled.

Health Care: The Larger Picture

Macro decisions determine what kinds of health care services will exist in a society, who will get them and on what basis, who will deliver them, and how the burdens of financing them will be distributed (Daniels, 1987). These decisions affect the level and distribution of the risks of getting sick, the likelihood of being cured, and the degree to which others will help if we become impaired. Because macro decisions affect the level and distribution of our well-being (health), they involve issues of social justice. The rules for the distribution of health care resources in any society are related to its system of values.

Daniels (1987) raises several questions about how to consider the issue of health care services. Should health services be viewed as are other commodities in our society? Should we allow inequalities in the access to health services to vary with whatever economic inequalities are permissible according to the principles of distributive justice? Or is health care "special" and not to be treated like other commodities? Issues of distributive justice lie at the center of the debate about health care delivery. They underlie demands for more equal access to personal health services, for more planning of health care resources, and for more effective regulation of health care providers to ensure cost control and quality control.

The issue of access to health care is really two issues: access for whom? and access to what? To many, access should be for anyone in need of medical services. Sometimes this point is asserted as a right, but, minimally, what is demanded is that certain nonmedical barriers, such as the ability to pay, should be eliminated. To support this view, some offer the argument of function, that is, the function of medical services is to meet health needs. Yet, we do not offer this argument for nonmedical commodities. If there is a right to health care, is it because it meets *special* needs?

Historically, access to health care was less important than it is today. Medical care had little effect on health (Daniels, 1987). Increased scientific and technological bases for health services increased the cost of care and made access more difficult. Insurance plans grew to replace a system of direct payments, but gaps occurred in insurance coverage and, thus, in access. Medicare and Medicaid were established to guarantee health care financing to the poor and elderly, two of the largest groups without insurance coverage. Coverage gaps remain for those who are temporarily out of work or who fail to meet state eligibility requirements for Medicaid. Twenty-five million Americans have no insurance coverage at all. Efforts to bring providers to medically underserved areas have had an impact on reducing some inequalities in access to care.

As public policy has moved in the direction of reducing barriers to health care it has had to face the question, "access to what?" Health care services are not homogeneous. Should we guarantee access to *all* the services provided anywhere in our health care system? Is there a social obligation to provide access to all services or to a minimum? Many critics have argued that our health care system is biased in favor of acute care and ignores prevention. Others complain that there is a bias in favor of acute care over other kinds of personal health care, e.g., social services, home health care.

Just as there is no free lunch, whatever health care is provided must be paid for by someone and staffed by someone. Guaranteed access to care has an impact on resource allocation and on the roles and responsibilities of health care providers. If society insists that certain services have to be provided in certain areas, health care providers will have to be available. There are obvious conflicts between traditional liberties, privileges, and responsibilities of providers and the requirements of justice. Some of the controversy reflects a simple conflict of interest between consumers and providers. Providers have a vested interest in a system that guarantees them power, autonomy, and healthy incomes. Considerations of justice and social controls threaten those interests. Much of the controversy also revolves around conflicting views of health care as a social good. The "specialness" of health care centers around needs. To specify health needs, we need a clear definition of health and disease. The basic idea is that health is not only the absence of disease, but an ideal level of well-being, and disease is a deviation from natural (or normal) functioning. Health care needs are those things we need to maintain normal functioning.

Daniels (1987) introduces the concept of *normal opportunity range* which is a range of key features of society that are available to individuals. The share of normal range open to an individual is determined to a significant degree by his/her talents and abilities. So impairment of normal functioning through disease and disability constitutes a restriction on individual opportunity relative to the range of skills and talents that would have been available to him/her. Daniels proposes that the impairment of the normal opportunity range could be used as a crude measure of the relative importance of health care needs at the societal level. Impairment of normal functioning at the societal level can also decrease satisfaction or happiness at the individual level. Thus, health care has a direct impact on the opportunity enjoyed by individuals. Health care institutions help provide the framework of liberties and opportunities within which individuals can pursue the satisfaction of their own health needs.

Theories of Justice

Harron, Burnside, and Beauchamp (1983) discuss three theories of distributive justice: libertarian, egalitarian, and utilitarian. The *libertarian* sees the physician as someone who, by hard work, has earned the right to offer health services. This is a right that should not be violated by society's priorities for the distribution of health resources. Similarly, the right of the patient to seek whatever care he/she wants, and can afford, is an inviolate right. It follows naturally for the libertarian that, because abilities, opportunities, and wealth are distributed unevenly in society, access to health care will also be distributed unevenly. Any plan to redistribute health care resources more equitably is not an excuse for violating the rights of physicians or patients to enter into private fee-for-service agreements. The *egalitarian* concept is rooted in deontological moral justifications and emphasizes, as does the libertarian, the status and claims of individual persons. The egalitarian position deduces that all human beings are entitled to equal access to health care resources. Each of us has a claim to, and society has an obligation to provide, a certain level of health care, which should be available to everyone, irrespective of circumstances. Beyond the decent minimum differences, additional levels of care would be allocated according to education, wealth, and social status. The *utilitarian* concept of distributive justice argues that we ought to allocate limited health resources according to the principle of providing the greatest good for the greatest number of people. The focus always is on the aggregate health of the total population. Utilitarians favor preventive medicine, the use of cost/benefit analysis, and public health programs over acute care medicine.

There are strengths and weaknesses in each of the positions of distributive justice discussed above. Many criticisms are linked to the moral claims by which they have been justified. The libertarian concept values maximizing an individual's freedom, the egalitarian concept deals with the problems of unequal access, and the utilitarian concept favors adequate health care for the statistical majority. Perhaps the only hope for consensus lies in the debate over underlying moral assumptions.

The Right to Know and to Decide and the Value of Honesty

Truth-telling is intimately linked with problems of autonomy. Persons who hold autonomy to be an absolute principle will, under all circumstances, tell their patients the absolute truth. Paternalists, on the other hand, are apt to judge what is, in their view, to the patient's benefit to know and not to know, and act accordingly. Always telling the truth can become an end in itself instead of a means to a moral end (Loewy, 1989). Following principles, in this way, severely limits moral agency and its choices. Not telling the truth may be the best choice from a range of poor options. Patients may not wish to know the truth. The patient's desire not to know is as autonomous a decision as is the opposite. When truth-telling succeeds in removing all hope from dying patients, moral duty extracts a heavy price. Ethics need to be tempered by compassion and understanding (Higgs, 1985).

The physician's assessment of the patient's perceived needs and interests is becoming less dominant over the patient's perspective, often expressed as patient's rights. The patient is now seen as an active, participating member of the decision-making team. Information about the patient, though not a possession in law, is seen as something to which the patient has a right of access.

The *Patient's Bill of Rights* (Annas, 1976) (See Appendix E) states that the patient has the right to informed participation in all decisions involving his/her health care program, a right to know what research or experimental protocols are being used and what alternatives are available, a right to a clear concise explanation of all proposed procedures in laymen's terms, including the possibilities of any risk of mortality or serious side effects, problems relating to recuperation, and probability of success, and a right to know the identity and professional status of all those providing service. In a strange way, patient's rights have confused the issue between knowledge and truthfulness. Some physicians have provided facts instead of honest communication. It raises the issue of how much information, and what kind, a professional can expect or demand to be told by a patient. What are the limits to patients' autonomy and right to know?

Arguments for Lying

Some have suggested that health professionals have a special exemption from being truthful because of the nature of their work. One of the arguments used to defend lying to patients is that it is difficult to put across a technical subject to those with little information and understanding. Can the patient understand the effects of a treatment? What future symptoms might occur are important questions for the patient, but may only be informed guesses for the physician. Yet to say that we do not know is not an honest answer. We can make informed guesses. To deprive a patient of honest communication because we do not know everything is depriving the patient of the ability to choose and to plan.

Sontag (1978) has discussed how we use illness, especially cancer, as a metaphor. She contends that as long as cancer is treated as an evil predator, and not just a disease, most people with cancer will be demoralized by learning what disease they have. The solution is not to stop telling cancer patients the truth, but to rectify the conception of the disease, to demythicize it.

Sontag notes that someone who has had a heart attack is as likely to die of another one as someone with cancer is likely to die from cancer. But no one thinks of concealing the truth from a cardiac patient; there is nothing shameful about a heart attack. She states that cancer patients are lied to, not just because the disease is a death sentence, but because it is felt to be obscene and repugnant. The metaphors surrounding cancer refer to topography (cancer "spreads," or is "diffused"), whereas cardiac disease implies a weakness or failure, with no disgrace. As Sontag (1978) notes, "the cancer metaphor will be made obsolete, long before the problems it has reflected so persuasively will be resolved" (p. 88).

Another argument for not telling patients the truth is that no one likes hearing bad news. Most surveys have found a preference for openness among patients and only a small group who do not wish to be informed. Health professionals do not like to be bearers of bad news as they like helping people and derive much satisfaction from the feeling that the patient is benefited. When the question of whether to tell a patient certain information arises, the professional should ask "For whose benefit are you going to tell it?" and "For whose good are you acting, the professional's or the patient's?" The answer to these questions will help the professional act in good conscience.

A third argument for not telling the truth is that truthfulness can actually do harm. However, harm is a personal concept. Certainly, bare facts, given with no follow-up or knowledge of whether social support is available to the patient, are cruel. Some socially isolated patients may become severely depressed or resort to desperate measures, such as suicide. What these examples point out, however, rather than reasons not

THE CHOICE: LIVE A LIE OR LOSE A JOB
Mary Flood

The Houston Post Staff

Two 44-year-old grandmothers fired this week from their jobs driving Houston school buses said Thursday they lied about their prison records on employment forms because getting a job was more important than telling the truth.

Constance Flagg, who worked for the Houston Independent School District for eight years, and Thressie Maxie, who had driven for HISD for only a year, were fired this week for lying about criminal records discovered in a Houston Post investigation.

Both women contacted The Post Thursday to say they wanted to regain their jobs and tell their story.

"I want to know: When a person does time and gets rehabilitated and seeks work and gets it and does a good job, how long do they have to pay?" asked Flagg, a Houston native who passed a high school equivalency exam in prison.

She acknowledged that she went to prison for felony theft in 1976, that she was on parole when she applied at HISD and that she had been sentenced for other felony theft charges before. All the charges resulted from shoplifting clothes, she said. Her record also shows prostitution and robbery convictions, but she said she was never convicted of those charges.

Flagg, who lost a post-prison job as a seamstress before trying HISD in 1980, said she knows lying on the application was wrong and agrees that HISD had every right to fire her for that.

"But if I'd said 'yes,' they wouldn't have hired me because of my conviction," she said. "And I was a good employee, did a good job."

"I loved my job, but it was rough sometimes. I've been threatened on the bus by a kid with a knife. Bus drivers have been beaten up. We get the raw end of the deal," said Flagg, who worked about 30 hours a week at HISD.

She and Maxie said they are annoyed because they were fired while others they think are doing drugs on the job were not.

Maxie, who left school in the 11th grade, acknowledged she went to prison in 1980 on two drug convictions for possessing synthetic heroin, but she said she does not remember the misdemeanor welfare fraud and weapons sentences that also appear on her Harris County record.

"My reason for lying about my convictions is that I only thought they'd check back five years. I didn't think something that happened as far back as 1979 would matter," she said, noting she thought she could not have gotten the job if she disclosed her drug sentences.

"Since my conviction was drugs, why didn't they just drug-test me? I look at Ann Richards, she has her problems but is running for governor. Another man was in prison for murder and changed to a woman, and he's running for office.

"But when you get down to the little poor people who work 25 hours a week it's different," said Maxie, a Houston native who worked some fast-food jobs before becoming a bus driver in March 1989.

Maxie and Flagg said HISD and other employers need to look at a person's work record and rehabilitation, understanding that felons are "between a rock and a hard place" when seeking employment.

"I need my job, I liked my job and I had no problem with the kids. But now I know the parents would think, " 'Oh, she's an ex-felon.' Well, that really has nothing to do with it," Maxie said.

Flagg said she has no paycheck now and she doesn't know what she'll do.

"My record is clear for 10 years. If I were stupid and foolish, I'd probably resort to crime right now. That's where this puts you. But I won't," she said.

Friday, March 30, 1990, *The Houston Post*

to tell the truth, are reasons for sensitivity and caring in determining how much the patient wants to know and for providing full support.

While there are many other arguments why health professionals should not tell patients the truth, knowledge is power. Health professionals should not let the fear or discomfort of confrontation keep them from telling patients the truth. Patients do eventually find out information they want to know if they are unsuccessful in getting the information from their direct caregivers. This leads to the erosion of trust between the patient and his/her caregivers. The preservation of the patient's autonomy should be an important guiding principle. Whether or not knowing the truth is essential to the patient's health, telling the truth is essential to the health of the physician—patient relationship (Higgs, 1985).

Approaches to Ethical Problem Solving

There is no formula for solving problems in medical ethics. Problem solving in ethics requires facts and a consideration of values. Solutions, however, cannot be "final" or absolute since situations change (Loewy, 1989). Fletcher (1966) has stated that there are three approaches to making moral decisions: (1) the legalistic approach; (2) antinomian (undisciplined approach); and (3) the situational approach. Situation ethics would judge each situation purely on its own merits, aiming for the most "loving" solution. Fletcher considers love and justice synonomous. Love is the ruling norm of situation ethics. Situations must be considered in a general framework of rules of thumb. The rules must conform to some prior insight of the "good" or of "love." Such insight is either the product of "truth" or will be seen to vary from society to society in its definition. Fletcher's situation ethics breaks down when one considers that what is "right" is not merely determined by the "goodness" of the outcome.

Medical ethics has tried to establish moral principles and apply these to medicine. Medicine deals with individuals in specific situations. Thomasma (1984) argues that answers to moral quandaries in medicine do not rest on principles alone and that the medical context itself functions as a moral rule in the resolution of ethical dilemmas. He proposes a bridge between abstract principles and concrete cases using a contextual grid (see Table 11-1). The grid is a means by which to locate a moral problem and the likely values and principles at issue within that locus. The context having been established by such a grid, the discussion can proceed to the means for resolving the problem by protecting the interests and values of those affected by it (Thomasma, 1984).

The grid (Table 11-1) rests on a two-fold distinction: its coordinators. The first is the distinction between primary, secondary, and tertiary care. Its importance for moral justification lies in the seriousness of the medical problem. The second distinction or coordinate of the grid is the number of persons affected by the problem. The moral significance of this distinction is based on the increased complexity of moral values, the more different persons are affected, and our tendency to protect the whole rather than personal freedom when large numbers of persons are affected. The purpose of the grid is to describe the variable context rules and identify the moral principles most likely to be given weight in formulating moral policy or an indicated course of action. The example of population ethics is used in Table 11-1 to illustrate how the grid can be applied to a moral problem. The grid can be helpful for any number of broadly conceived ethical problems.

Self (1979) asserts that the first step in solving a medical-ethical dilemma is to identify a central moral issue. But, Pinkus (1981), elaborating upon

Table 11-1. Thomasma's Contextual Grid of Moral Rules

Example: Population ethics

<table>
<tr>
<td rowspan="3" style="writing-mode: vertical-rl;">Intensity of Medical Problems</td>
<td>A married. pregnant woman contracts leukemia necessitating a therapeutic abortion because of radiotherapy and chemotherapy.

Moral rule: values of patient hard to obtain and individual rights are protected only if there are presumptions for a value of continued life.</td>
<td>A nuclear accident occurs in which five women and their fetuses are exposed to damaging amounts of radiation.

Moral rule: Despite individual values this level of seriousness of the danger to life and fetal damage might require terminating the pregnancy.</td>
<td>Enforced sterilization of a population in a poor country without sufficient food.

Moral rule: Individual rights are superceded not only by the social crisis of overpopulation but also by the common good of decent economic development.</td>
</tr>
<tr>
<td>A married patient with a chronic illness requests sterilization without which a pregnancy may threaten her life. It is medically indicated.

Moral rule: Both the principles of self-determination and beneficence must be weighed in the disposition.</td>
<td>A retarded. unmarried adult is considered a candidate for sterilization but objections from family members might override a request from the retarded person.

Moral rule: Family may override individual rights.</td>
<td>A retarded child is sexually active and parents request sterilization.

Moral rule: Society values in eugenic laws. class interests of the retarded. or an absence of laws may override individual rights.</td>
</tr>
<tr>
<td>An unmarried adult requests sterilization. The request is not medically indicated.

Moral rule: Patient's right to self-determination.</td>
<td>A married adult requests sterilization. The request is not medically indicated. Family obligations and economic factors demonstrate a reasonable cause.

Moral rule: Patient's right of self-determinatioln must be balanced with the physician's obligation to do no harm and the current situation and values of the family.</td>
<td>A married adult requests sterilization. The request is not medically indicated. The married partner or some member of the health care team objects or hospital policy does not permit it.

Moral rule: Social values and institutional values predominate.</td>
</tr>
</table>

Number of persons affected

(from Thomasma. D.C.. 1984) Reproduced with permission

Self's approach, suggests that a medical-ethical question should be replaced with a direct, practical question "Will the type of treatment or intervention planned improve the quality of the patient's life?" She feels that medical choices are guided by diagnostic possibilities and the therapeutic modalities available. These factors are what should be discussed with the patient and his/her relatives in resolving the dilemma.

Health professionals cannot ignore moral dilemmas in health care. When a conflict in values exists between a health professional and a patient, the professional is faced with several options: (1) provide care he/she regards as wrong; (2) refer the patient to another professional who will provide the care; (3) refuse to provide the care and not refer; or (4) attempt to resolve the conflict in values (Christie and Hoffmaster, 1986). The health professional possesses the power to "win" value conflicts, but health professionals should not pursue their own values at the patient's expense. The principle of autonomy entails the fundamental requirement of benefiting patients, but with the qualification that benefit be defined by patients *with* their physicians rather than by physicians *for* their patients. Determining "benefit" involves choosing a path that makes us least anxious; we balance a host of values according to the scale of our conscience. As Hundert (1987) notes, "We typically go through this process unconsciously, and it is quite difficult to articulate the pattern of balancing of values that we have achieved. It is, in fact, difficult to list all of the relevant values that stand in need of balancing" (p. 839). The "balancing equations" that are our moral principles are more complicated than the moral actions we take as a result of the balancing, e.g., the abortion, the unplugging of a respirator. It is no small matter that the demand for consistency applies at the level of principles, not actions. Veatch (1981) has concluded that although individual judgments and actions will be required, we need a general theory of how case by case decision-making relates to more general ethical rules and principles. Aristotle struggled with the question of whether it is better to be governed by law or by the judgments of good individuals. His answer was that, "a feast to which all guests contribute is better than a banquet furnished by a single man."

In Retrospect

More and more health care professionals must decide not only what is legally and professionally right, but what is ethically right. Health care professionals often experience dilemmas when they try to separate their personal values from professional responsibilities. And, health care professionals must often make ethical decisions without clear-cut standards to guide them.

Ethics, or in the present book, bioethics or biomedical ethics, is the study of what constitutes good and bad human conduct in the context of health care. Values are assessments of worth. We behave differently when we are confronted with situations, people, or things that have a great deal of value to us. When our strongest values are challenged, we defend them, as they are part of us. But others have equally strong values and have the right to defend them. When our values clash with those of someone else, it may be easy to turn away from a resolution. But, in the case of health care, when one person is a health care professional and the other person is a patient, it is not possible to avoid confrontation and a decision. Indeed, time may be an enemy to the opportunity for reflection and consultation.

Health care is no longer limited to the restoration of health and return to normality. Health care professionals providing care at all levels, primary, secondary, or tertiary, are confronted with making clinical decisions which involve values. The AIDS epidemic is an example of a disease which involves conflicts between values and ethics at all phases from prevention, to diagnosis and treatment, and finally death. Health care professionals, even if they are not providing direct patient care, cannot escape dealing with ethical and value-laden issues. Ethical decision making involves everyone and is not limited to catastrophic situations. It involves decisions and policy making about such issues as gene manipulation, human experimentation, the allocation of resources to health, and rationing health care. Health professionals are the content experts and will be increasingly looked to by the public to provide leadership in developing a more affordable and equitable system of health care.

REFERENCES

Aiken, W. (1982). The quality of life. *Applied Philosophy, 1,* 26–36.

Anderson, G.R. & Glenes-Anderson, V.A. (Eds.). (1987). *Health care ethics: A guide for decision makers.* Rockville, MD: Aspen.

Angell, M. (1988). Euthanasia. *The New England Journal of Medicine, 319,* 1348–1350.

Annas, G.J. (1976). *The rights of hospital patients: The basic ACLU guide to a hospital patient's rights.* New York: Avon Books.

Barnard, D. (1985). Unsung questions of medical ethics. *Social Science and Medicine, 21,* 243–249.

Bassford, H.A. (1983). Processes in the formulation and legitimization of professional ethics in a changing world. *Social Science and Medicine, 17,* 1191–1197.

Bayles, M.D. (1987). The value of life. In D. Van De Veer & T. Regan (Eds.), *Health care ethics: An introduction* (pp. 265–289). Philadelphia, PA: Temple University Press.

Bouvia v. Superior Court: 179 Cal. App. 3d. 1127, 225 Cal Rptr. 297, (1986).

Brody, H. (1981). *Ethical decisions in medicine* (2nd ed.). Boston: Little, Brown.

Brown, K. (1985). Can medical paternalism be justified? *Canadian Medical Association Journal, 133,* 678–680.

Callahan, D. (1972). *Abortion: Law, choice and morality.* New York: Collier-Macmillan.

Callahan, D. (1977). Health and society: Some ethical imperatives. In J.H. Knowles (Ed.). *Doing better and feeling worse: Health in the United States* (pp. 23–33). New York: W. W. Norton.

Campbell, A.V. (1984). *Moral dilemmas in medicine* (3rd ed.). London: Churchill Livingstone.

Christie, R.J. & Hoffmaster, C.B. (1986). *Ethical issues in family medicine.* New York: Oxford University Press.

Dagi, T.F. (1990). Letting and making death happen: Is there really no difference? The problem of moral linkage. *The Journal of Medical Humanities, 11,* 81–90.

Daniels, N. (1987). Justice and health care. In D. Van De Veer & T. Regan (Eds.), *Health care ethics: An introduction* (pp. 290–325). Philadelphia, PA: Temple University Press.

Dempsey, D. (1975). *The way we die.* New York: Macmillan.

Donovan, P. (1983). When does personhood begin? *Family Planning Perspectives, 15,* 40–44.

Dworkin, G. (1971). Paternalism. In R.A. Wasserstrom (Ed.), *Morality and the law* (pp. 107–126). Belmont, CA: Wadsworth.

Fletcher, J. (1954). *Morals and medicine.* Princeton, NJ: Princeton University Press.

Fletcher, J. (1966). *Situation ethics: The new morality.* Philadelphia, PA: Westminister Press.

Fox, R.C. & Willis, D.P. (1983). Personhood, medicine, and American society. *Milbank Memorial Fund Quarterly/Health and Society, 61,* 127–147.

Gratton, C. (1990). Letting and making death happen, withholding and withdrawing life-support: Morally irrelevant distinctions. *The Journal of Medical Humanities, 11,* 75–80.

Grobstein, C. (1983). A biological perspective on the origin of human life and personhood. In M.W. Shaw & A.E. Doudera (Eds.), *Defining human life: Medical, legal, and ethical implications* (pp. 3–11). Ann Arbor, MI: AUPHA Press.

Harron, F., Burnside, J. & Beauchamp, T. (1983). *Health and human values: A guide to making your own decisions.* New Haven, CT.: Yale University Press.

Hegland, K.F. (1979). Unauthorized rendition of life saving medical treatment. In T.L. Beauchamp & S. Perlin (Eds.), *Ethical issues in death and dying* (pp. 194–203). Englewood Cliffs, NJ: Prentice-Hall.

Higgs, R. (1985). On telling patients the truth. In M. Lockwood (Ed.), *Moral dilemmas in modern medicine* (pp. 187–202). Oxford, NY: Oxford University Press.

Hundert, E.M. (1987). A model for ethical problem solving in medicine with practical applications. *American Journal of Psychiatry, 144,* 839–846.

Kantor, N.L. (1979). A patient's decision to decline life-saving medical treatment: Bodily integrity versus the preservation of life. In T.L. Beauchamp & S. Perkin, (Eds.) *Ethical issues in death and dying* (pp. 203–231). Englewood Cliffs, NJ: Prentice-Hall.

Kass, L.R. (1989). Neither for love nor money: Why doctors must not kill. *Public Interest, 94,* 25–46.

Knowles, J.H. (1977). The responsibility of the individual. In J.H. Knowles, (Ed.), *Doing better and feeling worse: Health in the United States* (pp. 57–80). New York: W. W. Norton.

Loewy, E.H. (1989). *Textbook of medical ethics.* New York: Plenum.

Macklin, R. (1983). Personhood in the bioethics literature. *Milbank Memorial Fund Quarterly/Health and Society, 61,* 35–57.

Morison, R.S. (1977). Death: Process or event? In R.F. Weir (Ed.), *Ethical issues in death and dying* (pp. 57–69). New York: Columbia University Press.

Munson, R. (1988). *Intervention and reflection: Basic issues in medical ethics* (3rd ed.). Belmont, CA: Wadsworth.

Orentlicher, D. (1989). Physician participation in assisted suicide. *Journal of the American Medical Association, 262,* 1844–1845.

Pinkus, R.L. (1981). Medical foundations of various approaches to medical-ethical decision-making. *Journal of Medicine and Philosophy, 6,* 295–307.

Ramsey, P. (1978). *Ethics at the edges of life.* New Haven: Yale University Press.

Rosenblum, V.G. & Forsythe, C.D. (1990). The right to assisted suicide: Protection of autonomy or an open door to social killing? *Issues in Law and Medicine, 6,* 3–31.

Schaffner, K.F. (1988). Philosophical, ethical, and legal aspects of resuscitation medicine. II. Recognizing the tragic choice: Food, water, and the right to assisted suicide. *Critical Care Medicine, 16,* 1063–1068.

Self, D.J. (1979). Philosophical foundations of various approaches to medical-ethical decision-making. *Journal of Medicine and Philosophy, 4,* 20–31.

Slade, R.M. (1971). Medical care as a right: A refutation. *New England Journal of Medicine, 285,* 1288–1292.

Sontag, S. (1978). *Illness as metaphor.* New York: Farrar, Straus and Giroux.

Susser, M. (1974). Ethical components in the definition of health. *International Journal of Health Services, 4,* 539–548.

Thomasma, D.C. (1984). The context as a moral rule in medical ethics. *The Journal of Bioethics, 5*, 63–79.

Tormey, J. & Brody, E.B. (1978). Values and ethics in medicine. In G.U. Balis, L. Wurmser & E. McDaniel (Eds.), *The behavioral and social sciences and the practice of medicine* (pp. 655–671).

Unger, P. (1979). Why there are no people. *Midwest Studies in Philosophy, 4*, 177–222.

Veatch, R.M. (1981). *A theory of medical ethics.* New York: Basic Books.

Veatch, R.M. (1983). Definitions of life and death: Should there be consistency? In M.W. Shaw & A.E. Doudera (Eds.), *Defining human life* (pp. 99–113). Ann Arbor, MI: AUPHA Press.

Wanzer, S.H., Federman, D.D., Edelstein, J.J., et. al. (1989). The physician's responsibility toward helplessly ill patients: A second look. *The New England Journal of Medicine, 320*, 844–849.

Wasserstrom, R. A. (Ed.) (1971) *Morality and the law.* Belmont, CA: Wadsworth.

Wikler, D. (1983). Concepts of personhood: A philosophical perspective. In M.W. Shaw & A.E. Doudera (Eds.), *Defining human life: Medical, legal, and ethical implications* (pp. 12–23). Ann Arbor, MI: AUPHA Press.

Waitzkin, H. & Stoeckle, J.D. (1972). The communication of information about illness: clinical, sociological, and methodological considerations. *Advances in Psychosomatic Medicine, 8*, 180–215.

World Health Organization. (1976). *Health aspects of human rights with special reference to developments in biology and medicine.* Geneva, Switzerland.

SUGGESTED READINGS

Albernethy, V. (Ed.). (1980). *Frontiers in medical ethics: Applications in a medical setting.* Cambridge, MA: Ballinger.

Bandman, E.L. & Bandman B.H. (Eds.). (1978). *Bioethics and human rights.* Boston: Little, Brown.

Beauchamp, T.L. & Childress, J.F. (1983). *Principles of biomedical ethics* (2nd ed). New York: Oxford University Press.

Beauchamp, T.L. & Perlin, S. (Eds.). (1978). *Ethical issues in death and dying.* Englewood Cliffs, NJ: Prentice-Hall.

Clark, E.J., Fritz, J.M. & Rieker, P.P. (Eds.) (1990). *Clinical sociological perspectives on illness & loss: The linkage of theory and practice.* Philadelphia, PA: Charles Press.

Eys, J.V. & McGovern, J.P. (Eds.). (1988). *The doctor as a person.* Springfield, IL: Charles C Thomas.

Gillon R. (1986). *Philosophical medical ethics.* New York: John Wiley & Sons.

Ginzberg, E. (1990). *The medical triangle: Physicians, politicians, and the public.* Cambridge, MA: Harvard University Press.

Graber, G.C., Beasley, A.D., & Eaddy, J.A. (1985). *Ethical analysis of clinical medicine: A guide to self-evaluation.* Baltimore-Munich: Urban and Schwarzenberg.

Haddon, P.A. (1985). Baby Doe cases: Compromise and moral dilemma. *Emory Law Journal, 34*, 545–615.

Humphry, D. (1984). *Let me die before I wake.* Los Angeles: The Hemlock Society. (Distributed by Grove Press, New York.)

Kenyon, E. (1986). *The dilemma of abortion.* London: Faber & Faber.

Kluge, E.W. (1975). *The practice of death.* New Haven: Yale University Press.

Lammers, S.E. & Verhey, A. (Eds.). (1987). *On moral medicine: Theological perspective in medical ethics.* Grand Rapids, MI: William B. Eerdmans.

Mori, M. (1987). The philosophical basis of medical ethics. *Social Science and Medicine, 25,* 631–636.

National Academy of Sciences. (1975). *Experiments and research with humans: Values in conflict.* Washington, DC.

Rawls, J. (1971). *A theory of justice.* Cambridge, MA: Harvard University Press.

Regan, T. (Ed.). (1986). *Matters of life and death: New introductory essays in moral philosophy* (2nd ed.). New York: Random House.

Rodman, H., Sarvis, B. & Bonar, J.W. (1987). *The abortion question.* New York: Columbia University Press.

Shelf, E.E. (Ed.). (1981). *Justice and health care.* Holland/Boston: Dorddrecht.

Stein, J.J. (1978). *Making medical choices: Who is responsible?* Boston: Houghton Mifflin.

Sumner, L.W. (1987). Abortion. In D. Van De Veer & T. Regan (Eds.), *Health care ethics: An introduction* (pp. 162–183). Philadelphia, PA: Temple University Press.

Walton, D.N. (1979). *On defining death.* Montreal, Canada: McGill-Queen's University Press.

Warren, M.A. (1987). The abortion issue. In D. Van De Veer & T. Regan (Eds.), *Health care ethics: An introduction* (pp. 184–214). Philadelphia, PA: Temple University Press.

Waymack, M.H. & Taler, G.A. (1988). *Medical ethics and the elderly: A case book.* Chicago, IL: Pluribus Press.

Wikler, D. (1987). Personal responsibility for illness. In D. Van De Veer & T. Regan (Eds.), *Health care ethics: An introduction* (pp. 326–358). Philadelphia, PA: Temple University Press.

Winslade, W.J. & Ross, J.W. (1986). *Choosing life or death: A guide for patients, families, and professionals.* New York: Free Press.

Younger, S.J. (1986). *Human values in critical care medicine.* New York: Praeger.

Chapter 12

PROFESSIONALISM: WHAT IS IT?

Professionalism is a state of mind, not a reality. Neither statute nor regulation, neither code or shibboleth will make a . . . professional.

F.J.C. Seymour

What sort of doctor is he? Oh, well, I don't know much about his ability; but he's got a very good bedside manner.

Punch Magazine, 1884

What makes a professional and what constitutes professional behavior are too often left to chance learning by the student in the health professions. Faculty expectations are that the receipt of a degree will transform the student into a professional. While health professions graduates can recite their professional oaths at graduation, there is little previous formal effort to educate the graduates about expectations and responsibilities that their peers and the public will use in judging their competence, performance, and professionalism. As is the case with many of the behaviors in our society that call for an examination of our values and their priorities, educators feel more comfortable in letting students discover the meaning of professionalism on their own. Since behavior modeled by professionals is the major way in which professionalism is learned by neophytes, it is left up to the recent graduates to sort and select the models they wish to emulate. Every profession entertains a stereotype of the ideal colleague. Every profession sets out the conditions and the stringency for professional status. Ideas about what is good/bad, right/wrong, and appropriate/inappropriate are established within one's profession. Ethical codes are important for what they say, but the character of the person which the codes accredit and the nature of the world the codes portray are the essence of what constitutes professionalism.

The Professional Model

"Profession" was historically a vow made upon entrance to a religious order. It is still customary to speak of the time when novitiates will make their profession and, thereby, become fully initiated into an order. The word formally identified three classic professions (divinity, law, and medicine), but was broadened to include any vocation or occupation in which some branch of learning is used in application to a clientele, performs a service on a client, is self-regulating and is cloaked in the mystique of language and apparel (Smith & Churchill, 1986). Cogan (1953) has traced the definition of the word "profession" historically and examined its various meanings in detail.

A profession's mandate lies in a service perceived as needed by society, but the profession's license to act lies in a knowledge and skill base which it alone controls. Society looks to a profession for specialized knowledge, special resources, and special responsibilities. In return, the profession is granted special authorities and powers. The prestige of the professions, their economic and political independence, derive not only from the special expertise of their members, and from their control over acquisition and application of this knowledge, but also from the group solidarity that is reinforced and expressed in special ethics and codes of behavior, set apart from the morality of the common person (Goldman, 1980).

Because self-organization and self-regulation are essential aspects of a profession, it follows that accountability to professional peers is a critical element. This self-imposed accountability to peers constitutes the basis for collegiality within the profession as it functions to set standards for "good" professional practice and the development of career lines within the profession.

Francis Bacon once said that every man is held a debtor to his profession. The obligations of professionals to their professions approach an allegiance which is religious in its depth of commitment.

Profession Defined

Sieghart (1982) has provided a clear, concise definition of "profession." "A profession is composed of people who are experts in a discipline that confers power to do both good and harm, who practice that discipline for the benefit of others, who choose to give the interests of those others consistent precedence over their own, and who seek to limit the harm they might otherwise do by submitting themselves to a set of ethical rules designed to serve the paramount interest of some noble cause" (p.27).

Engelhardt and Callahan (1977) note three conditions for professional status in order of stringency: (1) professionals engage in their chosen activities "for a living" rather than "for fun"; (2) there is a recognized body of skills, constituting the "state of the art" and a network of guild-type institutions; and (3) there are statutory bodies which confer on professionals privileges attached to the exercise of the profession. All professions seem to possess: (1) systematic theory; (2) authority; 3) community sanction; (4) ethical codes, and (5) a culture (Greenwood, 1957).

Because understanding of theory is so important to professional skill, preparation for a profession must be an intellectual as well as a practical experience. On-the-job training becomes inadequate for a profession. There are a number of free-lance professional pursuits (acting, painting, writing, composing) wherein academic preparation is not mandatory. However, an occupation becomes a profession when apprenticeship and informal learning yield to formal education.

Extensive education in the theory of one's discipline imparts to the professional a type of knowledge that highlights the layman's comparative ignorance. This is the basis for the professional's authority. A non-professional occupation has customers; a profession has clients. Customers determine what services or commodities they want and shop around until they find them. In a professional relationship, professionals dictate what clients need. Clients cannot diagnose their own needs or discriminate among the range of possibilities for meeting them because they do not have the necessary background. Therefore, clients often have no choice and are often unable to evaluate the quality of the services received.

Every profession strives to persuade the community to sanction its authority by conferring a series of powers and privileges. Among its powers is the profession's control over its training. This is achieved through an accrediting process exercised by the profession. Through accreditation, the profession acquires control over admission into the profession. One of the most important of professional privileges is that of confidentiality. The community regards this as privileged communication, shared solely between client and professional, and protects the latter legally from encroachments upon such confidentiality.

A profession's ethical code is part formal and part informal. The formal part is the written code to which the professional usually swears upon being admitted to practice. The informal part is the unwritten code, whereby the profession makes it public knowledge that it commits itself to the welfare of society. While the specifics of ethical codes vary among the professions, the essentials are uniform. These may be described in terms of client-professional and colleague-colleague relations.

Finally, every profession has an informal and a formal culture. There are organizations through which the profession performs its services, e.g., hospitals, clinics, offices, social agencies. There are organizations whose functions are to replenish the supply of the profession's talent and expand its knowledge, e.g., educational and research centers. There are also organizations which emerge to promote professional interests, e.g., professional associations, lobby groups. In addition to these formal expressions of a profession's culture, there are numerous informal groups, e.g., professionals with interests in specific specialties within their profession. The social values of a professional group are its basic and fundamental beliefs. Foremost among these values are the essential worth of service and the commitment to objectivity in theory and technique. One of the central concepts of a profession is that of a career.

At the heart of the career concept is a certain attitude toward work that is uniquely professional. Menke (1969) notes that professional service is not and cannot be standardized; it is highly personal and unique. Professional persons give not only of their skills; they give of themselves. Their whole personalities enter into their work. Professional work is never viewed solely as a means to an end; it is the end. Treating the sick, educating the young, and advancing science are values in themselves. Professionals perform their services primarily for the psychological satisfactions and secondarily for the monetary rewards. Self-seeking motives are supposed to be only minimally evident among professionals (Greenwood, 1957).

The attributes of a profession and professional person just discussed are ideal. Ethical standards and codes of conduct, in reality, rest in the individual professional.[1] As Evans (1981) has stated, "ethical standards are the product of conscience, and if a man offends his own conscience, he is the first to know his own guilt."

Professionalism Defined[1]

A *profession* is an occupation that has gained its status by meeting certain criteria. *Professionalism,* however, is an attitude that motivates individuals to be attentive to the image and ideals of their particular professions. Professionalism was discussed first by Carr-Saunders in a lecture he delivered at Oxford University in 1928 (Carr-Saunders, 1933).

VanZandt (1990) noted that professionalism means different things to different people. To some, professionalism is merely a label used by occupations to win power and prestige (Ritzer, 1973). To some, it may mean altruism or dedication to service or a high level of competence in their work. To others, professions are conceptualized as occupations with core characteristics. The *-ism* suffix suggests that professionalism includes behaviors and attitudes that are characteristic of "true" professionals. Freidson 1970(a) points out that the professional's ideals and career are expressed in attitudes, ideals, and beliefs which, together, are called professionalism. Professionalism is composed of three major sets of attitudes, values, or orientations. One set is addressed to the professional ideals of knowledge and service; a second set to the professional occupation and the life-career it provides; and the third set to the character of professional work.

Professionalism is the intrinsic motivation that helps build on the foundation of a health professional's education. The concept of professionalism must be individualized or personalized; no one has control over that attribute but oneself. Whether or not an occupation has attained the status of a profession, an individual can attain the attribute of professionalism.

Professionalism is a complex attribute. Several factors, which consistently emerge in the literature on professionalism, are: (1) the way in which a person relies on a high personal standard of competence in providing professional services; (2) the means by which a person promotes or maintains the image of the profession; (3) a person's willingness to

---

[1]Though many people have attempted to distinguish between the terms *ethics* and *morals,* the distinction has never been entirely satisfactory. Both describe rules of conduct, and both are concerned with differentiating between right and wrong. We sometimes intend to convey another meaning if we say an action is immoral rather than unethical—the former description connotes some contravention of religious law, while the latter indicates a departure from traditional or customary behavior. But the difference can only be subjective since the two words, one Latin (*moralis*) and the other Greek (*ethikos*), are interdependent and historically synonymous (Evans, 1981).

pursue professional development opportunities that will continue to improve skills within the profession; and (4) a person's sense of pride about the profession (Van Zandt, 1990).

Learning Professionalism

One becomes labeled a professional person upon mastering the knowledge and skills required for entrance into a specific profession. During the formal process of learning a profession, a person also learns professionalism. What professionals in a given profession believe, what they value, how they behave toward each other and toward clients, and understanding their career goals and priorities, is learned by listening to what bonafide professionals say, by observing how they behave, and by feeling the impact of events and situations they must deal with, especially those which are unclear or challenge one's own values. Students learn professionalism by selecting what they consider "good" or "desirable" characteristics from the spectrum of behaviors exhibited by their teachers. Students choose one or more persons to emulate and these models become the informal basis for learning professionalism. The students, then, through experience, test the compatibility of the modeled behavior with their own values and beliefs, and eventually evolve as "professional persons." This evolution is not necessarily complete at the time of graduation. Indeed, professionalism is not a static, single, or uniform characteristic. Rather, professional persons are constantly changing, by choice or due to changes in their professions which are beyond their control, and, as such, what they think, how they behave, and what they value, also is subject to change. Professional persons may have core values and beliefs which they may not change, but changes in societal values, beliefs, and expectations will impact on the professional's practice and behavior in some way; e.g., the AIDS epidemic has created the need for explicit sex information from health practitioners; similarly, some clients/patients demand family planning and abortion information.

Professionalism in the health professions is often learned by chance. An exceptional teacher or practitioner may become a serious mentor for a student. A mentor can be important in modeling professional behavior as well as imparting knowledge. Professionalism is usually not formally taught, but students are drawn to teachers they like and would like to emulate. There is a need for teachers involved in direct patient care to help students see the connection between how patients are cared for and being a professional person. Jonas (1978) relates the following vignette:

> Several years ago I posed the question, "Why should we be concerned with the quality of medical care and why should we want to deliver good care?" to a class of third-year medical students. The first answer was "to protect our incomes," and the second was "to fend off malpractice suits." A bit later in the discussion, a student did say there was something to good care in and of itself. Another brought up the issue of "professionalism." (p.141).

Providing quality health care and treating the sick person as a "whole person" are interrelated. Health professions educators express such cliches, but the failure of students to link quality care and treating the patient as a person with professionalism is apparently not modeled and, therefore, not learned (or if learned, not highly valued). The approach to health care that is most commonly seen and modeled is treatment for a specified complaint. Preventive care is seldom modeled unless it is the specific interest of the physician and is usually considered to be common sense and a distraction from the major goal of the physician, namely, to cure illness. Freidson 1970(b) points out that a review of data on the values of physicians showed that while physicians do not lack a service orientation, it does not seem to be as prominent a value as others. Furthermore, the value is addressed to helping individuals rather than to serving society.

The transformation of a neophyte into a professional is essentially an acculturation process wherein a person internalizes the social values, the behavior norms, and the symbols of the occupational group. It is a process whereby the neophyte learns how to blend incompatible values into a consistent and stable pattern of professional behavior. These values include those which relate to the professional's self-image, the professional's relations with clients/patients, and their relations to colleagues and to the community. Too often, the learning of professionalism does not follow a plan; professionalism is learned as situations arise. Hence, there are usually large gaps of knowledge regarding professionalism that are unexperienced and unlearned by students.

Characteristics of a Professional Person

Seymour (1966) has outlined seven characteristics of a professional teacher that are appropriate to other professions (Vollmer & Mills, 1966). These include:

1. possesses a body of knowledge and skills related to and essential to teaching;
2. is prepared to make judgments in the capacity of a teacher and to take appropriate action if necessary;
3. is responsible for the consequences of one's judgments and actions;
4. places primary emphasis on one's function to serve society;
5. works with colleagues in developing and reinforcing standards that are basic requirements for continuous improvement of one's profession and observes such standards in personal practice;
6. engages in a continuing search for new knowledge and skills;
7. practices one's profession on a full-time basis.

Cullen (1978) specifies some additional characteristics of a professional person. He includes the fact that professional persons should be tested for competency and licensed, to define for themselves and others the nature and boundaries of their profession's activities. In addition, he notes that the professional person should be person oriented.

Toulmin (1977) pointed out the necessity for a recognized body of skills, constituting the "state of the art," and for statutory bodies, which confer professional privileges, to exist before one can be called a professional. Therefore, even though persons who engage in professional sports might do so "for a living," and not "for fun," they would not be considered professional because they lack the two essential conditions for professional status—a recognized body of skills constituting a state of the art, and statutory bodies that confer professional privileges to those practicing the profession.

In addition to identifying what kind of work a person does and one's status, the word "professional" can be used to describe a person's behavior ("she related to that patient in a highly professional manner") or to judge a person's behavior ("he should not have revealed information that was considered confidential"). When we use the word "professional" in these ways, we call upon our own moral code, i.e., our own personal definition of professionalism, in describing or evaluating other people's degree of professionalism. Thus, there are conceptual boundaries which outline the limits of professional behavior for professions; there are also personal boundaries which further define acceptable or unacceptable behavior. As Durkheim (1958) pointed out, there are two kinds of rules. The first apply to mankind in general, the second apply to the individual: how each of us relates to our own self, and how each of us relates to other people. Between these two broad rules, lies the moral code related to one's profession, which Durkheim called professional ethics. The melding of our own ideals and beliefs with the ideals and beliefs of our profession exhibit themselves in a set of attitudes and behaviors, which we show to others as "professionalism." As Friedson 1970(a) has put it, ideals plus a professional career plus professional pride equal professionalism.

The Professional as a Person

Sometimes, professionals mistakenly equate professionalism with the refinement of knowledge and skills. The consummate professional is thought of as the specialist who is known for a special clinical expertise. The board certified specialist or subspecialist is viewed and envied as the person who has achieved the ultimate heights of his/her profession. As one medical school dean observed, "everybody has become so specialized that the only generalist left is the patient" (Ashworth, 1989).

DiMatteo (1979) says that the ability to communicate caring and concern to patients is essential, as is technical expertise. He emphasizes that a professional person has good manners, that he/she is sensitive to other people's feelings and is able to detect changes in how other people feel by observing affect. Good manners means the professional should not be so concerned with communicating what he/she wants that a patient's feelings are ignored. Wilmer (1987) has separated the world of feelings into pity, sympathy, and empathy. Pity is a feeling of tenderness aroused by suffering or misfortune in others which prompts a desire for its relief. Usually, pity is associated with the perception that someone or something is weak and in a "one down" position. Sympathy is the image of how we would feel if we were in his/her place. Sympathy is a step toward empathy. If there is real understanding, there is empathy. Empathy we feel for and with the other person. In empathy, it is as if: I were he/she.

Reiser and Rosen (1984) offer five aspects necessary in an effective interaction in a physician-patient relationship. Acceptance and empathy are essential for a healing partnership. The physician's ability to conceptualize is necessary in providing comprehensive care. Competence is necessary not only to convey trust to the patient, but a sense of ease and comfort on the part of the physician. Finally, there is the element of human spirit, or, as Osler (1906) said, "mix the waters of science with the oil of faith." Rapport is when the mix of feelings between a health

professional and patient results in a harmonious mutual working relationship. Both professional and patient feel an affinity for each other,
which is exhibited in mutual understanding (see Fig. 12-1).

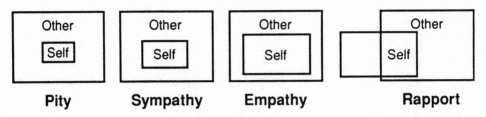

Pity   Sympathy   Empathy   Rapport

Figure 12-1. Four interrelated feeling states in a health professional-patient relationship.

Purtilo (1984) warns that we often draw a dichotomy between human
and professional qualities in considering professionalism. It is important
for professionals to see themselves as "whole professionals," not just
show emotion or express empathy only in crisis, such as caring for dying
patients. Sometimes health professionals feel that they have to control
their human side in order to maintain a practitioner-client distance.
Professionalism is not a matter of turning on or off certain behaviors;
rather, it is a matter of professionals being comfortable with whom they
are as persons. If their motivations are honorable, so will be their
behavior towards other people. Purtilo (1984) has pointed out that professionalism is often viewed as a dichotomy between the professional and
personal self. Calling patients by their first names might be viewed as
unprofessional, or patting a patient on the back might be too personal
and, hence, unprofessional. Certainly, the situation, the personalities of
the practitioner and the patient, and how well the practitioner and
patient know each other are variables which influence whether a pat on
the back, a hug, or holding a patient's hand are professional or unprofessional behaviors. For example, the phrase "you are in good health for a
person your age" could be considered offensive and unprofessional
depending upon the type of relationship the practitioner and patient
have. Since professional behaviors are learned through modeling and
not through textbooks, professionals have to evolve unique professional
selves according to their degree of personal comfort in revealing themselves as persons.

As Sarason (1985) notes in his examination of caring and compassion
in clinical relationships, most people consider themselves to be caring

and compassionate persons. It is socially desirable to admit to having these qualities. Yet, caring and compassion refer to relationships between people in certain situations. When we say a person is caring and compassionate, we do not mean that those qualities are evident in all relationships or that a person is caring and compassionate every day from the time of rising to the time of going to sleep. The acid test for caring and compassion comes when clinicians must deal with individuals or situations foreign to their experiences and values, e.g., abortion, attempted suicide, or adoption of a child with a severe medical problem. Caring and compassion are not things that can be taught in a course for graduates to learn and, in turn, become more caring and compassionate practitioners. Caring and compassion extend beyond treating a single person in distress. They are qualities that everyone has and should show to others irrespective of their health status. But, we must be realistic and acknowledge that there are health practitioners who are not caring and compassionate, just as there are people in the general public who do not possess these qualities.

One of the reasons we do not do a good job of modeling professional ethics and behavior in health professions schools is that the two goals to cure and to care are taught separately and mainly as technical interventions. Medical practice is designed to cure disease. In this regard, the sick person is seen as having a deficiency that care will technically set right. Whether the health problem is primarily physical or psychological, the tendency will be to see it as presenting a technical challenge. Thus, the nonphysical aspects of the problem are often regarded as analogous to the physical aspects, and students are instructed in techniques to manage the problem (that is, in techniques of how to care). The nonphysical aspects of the patient's problem, the loss of freedom, independence, job, income, prestige, etc. are not dealt with. If practitioners provide technical care for patients, they are regarded as responsible, caring professionals. Yet, it is *how* practitioners provide *total* care for patients that concerns us here. Therapeutic relationships imply a process in which wholeness is restored to the sick person. The integrity of the person, which is lost through sickness, is restored. The moral sense of caring and compassion should not escape us as citizens and as health practitioners (Agich, 1980).

The Apostolic Function and Professionalism

Balint (1957) discussed doctors' individual ways of dealing with their patients, especially doctors' ideas of how patients ought to behave when ill. This he called the apostolic mission or function. An especially important aspect of the apostolic function is the doctor's urge to prove to patients, to others, and to oneself that one is good, kind, knowledgeable and helpful. The apostolic function or "healer" evolved from a conception in which religious and medical functions were united in the same person. Most laymen, today, attribute great power to physicians because of their special knowledge and skills and, sometimes, their expectations of physicians are more appropriately attributable to a divine rather than a human healer (Loewy, 1989).

Most people who seek health care are people in trouble. They turn to someone whom they hope can help solve their troubles. Forming a relationship with a helper is an emotional experience. The professional with a heart is simply one who, by responding to the feelings of a person, is affirming that person's personal worth and individuality. A supportive, affirmative working alliance between the helper and the help seeker is what any professional relationship is for. The attributes that experienced clinicians seem to agree upon as desirable or even necessary are: warmth, acceptance, empathy, caring-concern, and genuineness (Perlman, 1982; Egan, 1990).

Egan (1990) has outlined five sets of values that he regards as important personal values in a professional helping relationship. These are:

1. *Pragmatism*
   - keep the client's agenda in focus
   - maintain a real life focus
   - stay flexible
   - develop a bias toward action
   - do only what is necessary
   - avoid generating resistance
   - do not offer help as a panacea
2. *Competence*
   - become good at helping
   - continue to learn
   - use modeling
   - be assertive
   - find competence, not in behaviors, but in outcomes

3. *Respect*
- do no harm
- treat clients as individuals
- suspend critical judgment
- be "for" the client
- be available
- understand and communicate understanding to clients
- assure the client's good will
- be warm within reason
- help clients utilize their own resources
- help clients through the pain

4. *Genuineness*
- do not overemphasize the helping role
- be spontaneous
- avoid defensiveness
- be consistent
- be open
- work at becoming comfortable with behavior that helps clients

5. *Client's Self-responsibility*
- do not limit clients' ability to exercise self-responsibility
- let clients make choices
- empower clients to act
- use participative rather than directive modes of helping
- encourage client to use self-help groups

Professionalism is perfecting the art of helping. A professional respects clients' values, attitudes, and feelings. This does not mean that the professional who has values which differ from those of the client should not express them so that the client knows where the helper stands. If the values of professional and client clash to such a degree that it inhibits communication and trust, the professional should refer the client to another helper. Professionalism is knowing the limits of one's competence as well as recognizing the negative effect of one's values and beliefs on others.

Norman Cousins (1983) has summarized the apostolic function of the physician as follows:

> There are qualities beyond pure medical competence that patients need and look for in their doctors. They want reassurance. They want to be looked after and not just looked over. They want to be listened to. They want to feel that it

makes a difference, whether they live or die. They want to feel that they are in their doctor's thoughts. In short, patients are a vast collection of emotional needs. Psychological counselors, family, and clergy are helpful, but the patient turns most of all and first of all to the physician . . . It is the presence of the doctor just as much as what the doctor does that creates an environment for healing. The physician's words and not just his prescriptions are tied to restoration (p.136).

The physician is not the only healer and, in some cases, may not be the primary caregiver for a particular patient. A victim of a heart attack, stroke, head injury, or broken hip may find that physical and occupational therapists are his/her major caregivers. For many patients, the apostolic function is attributable to whomever the major caregiver happens to be. The discipline of the helper is not as important as the kind of person the helper is. Professionalism is not a function of one's discipline; it is a function of how one practices his/her discipline.

Professionalism and the Work Ethic

The number of hours spent working or the degree of dedication to one's job does not necessarily indicate professionalism. Professionals who work long hours are often thought of as being dedicated to their professions. But work can satisfy many personal and professional needs in addition to the altruistic needs of serving society (Ritchie, 1988). Aristotle said that any virtue applied in excess is no longer a virtue. Morrow (1988) has suggested that work commitment embraces five aspects: (1) value focus, e.g., where does work fit in an individual's value system; (2) career focus, e.g., how important is the present position in relationship to the individual's career goal; (3) job focus, e.g., degree to which work is a central focus in an individual's life (how ego involved is the person in his/her work); (4) organization focus, e.g., degree of commitment and loyalty to the organization; and, where applicable, (5) union focus, e.g., commitment or obligation to the union. These aspects of work may overlap and may constitute different ways of expressing an individual's involvement in his/her work.

Older employees and employees at higher levels of administration in an organization have been found to have a greater degree of commitment to the organization than other employees. Tenure and length of professional employment are also significantly related to commitment. As persons become more experienced in what they do, they become more able to cope with the negative and positive aspects of their jobs. However, educational level has not been found to be related to commitment. The tendency is for highly educated employees to be equal in commitment to less educated employees (Weisch & LaVan, 1981).

Weisch & LeVan (1981) found that only satisfaction with work and promotion were significantly related to commitment. Satisfaction with pay was not significant. This suggests that organizations cannot "buy" commitment from their employees. This also indicates that job satisfaction is transitory and that while day-to-day events may affect employees' feelings about their jobs, daily events do not cause employees to question their commitment to the organization.

Employees whose roles are not clear and whose jobs are not well integrated into the organization have a lower job commitment. Teamwork, on the other hand, is important in forming attachments to the organization. Power is also related to organizational commitment. People are more committed to an organization as their power increases. An organizational climate that is participative and in which lines of communication are open also is significantly related to organizational commitment. Of particular interest is the finding that professional behavior has no impact on organizational commitment. Professionalism is, indeed, a set of values unique to professionals, which they practice irrespective of their degree of commitment to the organization in which they work. Stated in another way, professionalism is related to personal security rather than to job security.

Professionalism and Change

Schon (1983) has written that professionals claim to contribute to social well-being, put their clients' needs ahead of their own, and hold themselves accountable to standards of competence and morality. But both popular and scholarly critics accuse the professions of serving themselves at the expense of their clients, ignoring their obligations to public service, and failing to police themselves effectively. Surveys of client populations reveal a widespread belief that professionals overcharge for their services, discriminate against the poor and powerless in favor of clients who can pay their bills, and refuse to make themselves accountable to the public. Many younger professionals find that the professions, in general, do not demonstrate a real interest in the values they are supposed to promote: there are lawyers who have no real interest in justice or compassion; physicians who have no interest in the equitable distribution of quality health care; scientists and engineers who have no interest in the beneficence and safety of their technologies (Schon, 1983).

Professionals have also been critical of their own failure to solve problems. Former Supreme Court Justice Warren Burger recently criticized the preparation and performance of trial lawyers, and David Rutstein reflected on the failure of the health care system to keep pace with the nation's research and technology. Some observers have also noted a trend toward deprofessionalization as evidenced in the decline of medical school applicants, shortage of nurses due to nurses leaving the field or applying to other professional schools, and a decline in the economic status of some professions. Some professions are unionizing in increasing numbers. Yet, professions do have an appeal because of their power, prestige, and autonomy, and predictions are that the number of professionals in the U.S. labor force could reach 25 percent by the year 2000.

The crisis in confidence in the professions seems to be rooted in a growing skepticism about professional effectiveness and the professions' actual contribution to society's well-being. Part of this skepticism is due to the rising costs of professional services, especially in the health sector, the growing influence of bureaucracy in the professions, and questions about self-interests. Part of this skepticism is due to societal change and the ability of the professions to direct change and keep abreast of its effects. A third aspect of this skepticism is due to changes within the professions themselves, the growth of knowledge and skills, the effects of societal change on the standards, codes, and procedures of practice, and the situations of practice that are changing in complexity. As Schon (1983) notes, "the situations of practice are inherently unstable." The professions are now confronted with the unprecedented need for adaptability. Professionals, today, must bridge the gap between the body of knowledge they must use and the expectations of society. Some health professional groups are reacting to change by expanding their boundaries of expertise, while others are retrenching to become more specialized and professional (Bruhn, 1987). To clients and consumers, turf battles and professionalization activities have little to do with the welfare of the public. Efforts by some professional groups to expand practices and become participants in the latest cost reimbursement mechanisms have placed more emphasis on earning than on serving (Hendrick, 1985). Shortages of health manpower in some professional groups have escalated starting salaries and made recruitment by hospitals analogous to recruiting in sports by offering large sign-on bonuses and other fringe benefits to young graduates, for example, those in the allied health professions. The young graduates are faced with reconciling the high salaries being paid for their services and the large choice of jobs available with a concept of professionalism that is supposed to put patient interests before self-interests.

Too much social change, too fast, can force people to retrench, to confine their concerns to their own interests, and to forget those of their clients. Retrenchment also helps to protect one's power, professional boundaries, and to fend off unwanted pressures to change. On the other hand, taking a more offensive approach to change often means that professions need to become involved in politics, and this weakens their authority as dispensers of value-free knowledge (Osiel, 1984). Within this range of possible behaviors, many professions, today, are renegotiating their contracts with society (Inglehart, 1988). Many contracts with society in the past, especially in the health professions, were based on the *status quo.* Everyone knew most of the key players in health care and what their jobs were. Now there are a growing number of new types of health care professionals, each with special expertise, and the whole experience of hospitalization is fraught with emotional issues involving rights, power, authority, values, ethics, and the law.

The patient or client is a key player in professional codes of ethics. Codes of ethics usually represent the professional group's viewpoint and are rarely developed with help from the client who receives the professional's services. Professionals who work in a school system or mental health/mental retardation agency, for example, need a code of ethics which is practical, workable, and less vulnerable to litigation. Bersoff (1975) suggests that parents, agency representatives, and others who will be directly affected by the actions of certain professionals, be asked by these professionals to become mutual participants in evolving a code of ethics. When clients and professionals work together in search for solutions, it diminishes mistrust, conflict, and litigation.

An examination of the Hippocratic Oath (Appendix A) and the Principles of Medical Ethics (Appendix F), reveals their limitations in decision making in professional practice. Codes can be a helpful starting point in decisions, but they are not sufficient, by themselves, to guide decisions (The Code of Ethics for Nurses is shown in Appendix G and professional pledges for allied health professionals are shown in Appendix H). For example, in a case involving suspected child abuse, different codes may yield conflicting directives. The Hippocratic Oath regards confidentiality as important enough to forbid revealing this information. The Principles of Medical Ethics, on the other hand, place the obligation to obey the law above the principle of confidentiality. There are similar conflicts between provisions of the same code. For example, the AMA Principles contain injunctions to "deal honestly with patients" and to show "compassion." But what if a physician determines that telling a patient the truth about his/her diagnosis would be an act of cruelty? Sometimes, provisions in a code require interpretation before they can be applied. For example, the Hippocratic Oath prohibits "giving any deadly drug." Yet, what is a deadly drug? Sometimes the code provisions are clear, but some physicians may find them unacceptable on moral grounds. Especially controversial are the absolute prohibitions in the Hippocratic Oath against abortion and mercy killing by means of drugs. Finally, there are many ethical decisions on which the codes offer no advice at all. For example, the Hippocratic Oath speaks of three sorts of therapies, diet, drugs, and surgery; however, the ethical issues arising in connection with radiation therapy, genetic manipulation, or other new techniques are not addressed. Therefore, while professional codes are important tools in deciding what to do, they must be supplemented by more fundamental principles of ethics (Graber, et al., 1985).

Bolger (1987) notes that the Hippocratic Oath contains some statements that are not in agreement with most twentieth century physicians. The meaning of the Hippocratic Oath and its enduring value appear to be its highly personal quality, which reflects the basic concepts of devotion to people and a desire to serve them. Bolger suggests that if we select medical students more on the basis of their motivations, goals, and satisfactions, we will be able to produce more physicians who are truly concerned and vitally interested in their profession. This would be a big step toward resolving the problem of depersonalization.

Unprofessionalism

When health professionals perform in an outstanding manner, they are noticed and acknowledged. Similarly, when a health professional's behavior is unprofessional, it is noticed, and depending upon the extent of misconduct, patients may respond by not returning to that person for care and not recommending that professional to others, or they may go to the extreme of filing a lawsuit. Unprofessional behavior is not entirely in the "eye of the beholder." There are standards, codes, and pledges, as discussed earlier in this chapter, which serve as guides for professionals. Nonetheless, what constitutes unprofessional behavior can range widely, for example, from being treated impersonally to outright incompetence.

A. *Impairment*

There are many reasons why professionals act unprofessionally. Health professionals are human and experience the same problems of living as people who are not in professional occupations. But, professional work carries with it other risks that can result in the impairment of professionals. The American Medical Association (AMA) defines the impaired physician as "one who is unable to practice medicine with reasonable skill and safety to patients because of physical or mental illness, including deterioration through the aging process or loss of motor skill, or excessive use or abuse of drugs including alcohol" (Shortt, 1979).

Based on its definition, the AMA conservatively estimates that one of every ten physicians is at risk to impairing conditions. It is generally agreed that impaired physicians persist in their professional activities or do not perceive or deny their impairment, and if they do, they usually do not seek help (Scott & Hawk, 1986).

The work ethic in the health professions, especially in medicine, is one of overwork. Many health professionals have unrealistic expectations of their performance and endurance, which predispose them to burnout. Medical students commonly take drugs to keep them awake for long hours of studying, and the release of pent-up emotions following a block of tests often can be accomplished by the abuse of alcohol and other drugs. Baldwin and his colleagues (1988) surveyed a large, nationally representative sample of senior medical students (N = 2,047) in an attempt to establish reliable prevalence rates for substance abuse. They found that with the exception of alcohol and tranquilizers, medical students use fewer drugs than comparable groups of young people in the population. Furthermore, they established that the use of such substances began well before medical school. Physicians are highly susceptible to chemical and alcohol dependency. Talbott et al., (1980), found that 12 to 14 percent of physicians have had, currently have, or will have problems with alcohol or drugs. But Brewster (1986) stated that no one really knows how many practicing physicians are having problems with alcohol and other drugs. He notes that survey data suggest that the overall prevalence of problems with alcohol and other drugs among physicians may not be different from that found among the general population.

McAuliffe and his colleagues (1987) studied physicians, medical students, pharmacists, and pharmacy students to determine what factors were associated with the risk of drug impairment. They found that substantial proportions of drug abusers had suffered from family and marital problems, chronic fatigue, chronic pain, job stress, and emotional disorders. Medical students reported more life and job stress, sensation seeking, and emotional problems than did physicians; and both medical samples reported more job or school stress than did their pharmacy counterparts. The two professions did not differ with respect to other forms of stress. The question of why some health professionals who experience the same risk factors turn to drugs while others do not was not answered.

Physicians' attitudes toward drugs are closely tied to their prescribing practices and, therefore, to the addiction of their patients. Physician-induced addiction, or iatrogenic addiction, can be of three general types. Inadvertent addiction can occur with the prescription of drugs not yet suspected as addictive. Unintentional addiction can occur if the physician prescribes to meet the desires of a patient, prescribes to keep a patient, or gain a patient, or prescribes without thought of the consequences. The third type is intentional iatrogenic addiction in the case of a terminally ill patient or addiction to methadone in the attempt to cure another drug addiction. The addicted physician is more casual or enthusiastic about providing drugs without restraint to patients (Musto, 1985).

Physicians take their own lives with greater frequency and generally at an earlier age than do members of the general population. Suicides account for between 33 and 38 percent of all premature deaths among physicians. The suicide rate for female physicians is the highest reported for any occupational group of women and is four times greater than that for women in the general population who are 25 years of age and older. In reviewing the literature on the correlates of physician suicide, the most commonly described are: (1) a sense of hopelessness associated with their medical practice; (2) depression; (3) drug dependency; (4) chronic disease; (5) failure to cope with the loss of the physician role through retirement; and (6) being professionally successful but personally unsuccessful. These physicians often leave regular colleague contacts, retreating to a solo practice. Colleagues of physicians who have committed suicide often recall their indecisiveness, disorganization, and depression (Pfifferling, 1986).

As patients, physicians are poor role models. Many physicians are too harried and too busy to lead balanced and satisfying lives. The physicians' medical knowledge may also contribute to their anxiety and lack of cooperation. Physicians generally have strong feelings about knowledge and control and, as a group, are resistant to change (Robinowitz, 1983). According to Vaillant (1972), physicians are overburdened by perfectionistic, mythologized self-images and are slow to seek treatment for themselves.

B. *Malpractice*

Another end result of one form of impairment is malpractice. Very few malpractice cases arise from the sheer stupidity of the physician (Slavitt, 1987). Instead, there is the bright physician who doesn't care anymore, or who is too hurried and stressed to take the time that ought to have been taken. Or there is a kind of megalomania that drives a physician to practice beyond his competence. Drugs, alcohol, and depression are responsible for a fair number of malpractice suits.

The majority of malpractice claims are based on the tort of negligence. Tort law can best be understood as a creation of the common law meant to give rise to duties of conduct that are enforceable by law. Thus, a physician who deviates from a medically recognized standard of practice may be liable to an individual who is injured as a result of this deviation. Tort law protects the interests of society as a whole. To successfully prove a malpractice case, four things must be shown:

1. A physician-patient relationship was established and existed at the time the alleged malpractice occurred.
2. The physician breached one of the basic duties invoked upon him/her by the physician-patient relationship.
3. The breach of duty, hence the negligence of the physician, caused damages to the patient. This ties together two concepts, namely, that the negligent act was the cause of the damages and that damages did occur. If negligence occurs without damage, there is no malpractice. Also, if damage occurs but the negligent act did not cause the damage, there is no malpractice. This concept is referred to as "proximate cause," since it is necessary to prove that the physician's negligence is the proximate cause of the damages.
4. Freedom from contributory negligence. In certain jurisdictions,

the plaintiff must show that he/she in no way contributed to the causation of damage in order to make a claim for award based on malpractice.

All of the above must be shown to be true by a preponderance of the evidence in order for a court to decide against a physician (Harrison et al., 1985). Harrison and his colleagues state that from the physician-patient relationship evolves all the duties a physician has to a patient. These duties, as well as the relationship from which they arise, find their origins and history in key court cases.

Physician communication skills have been reported to be a major factor in malpractice claims. Adamson and her associates (1989) studied the relationship between patients' opinions about their physicians' communication skills and the physicians' history of medical malpractice claims. The sample consisted of 107 physicians and 2,030 of their patients who had had an operation or a delivery. Although patients tended to give their physicians favorable ratings, they were least satisfied with the amount of explanations they received. Patients gave higher ratings to general surgeons and obstetrician-gynecologists and poorer ratings to orthopedists and anesthesiologists. Women and better-educated patients gave higher ratings on explanations and communication to physicians with fewer malpractice claims. Men and patients with less education gave higher ratings on these dimensions to physicians with more claims. These findings suggest the need for physicians to tailor their communications to a patient's individual needs. McCaughrin (1979) also stresses that standard messages cannot be given to all patients.

The malpractice liability of allied health professionals is relatively new, but is of increasing importance as some professional groups engage in independent practice, e.g., physical and occupational therapists. Physical therapists and radiographers are the allied health professionals most frequently involved in published appelate court cases. Various types of technicians are sometimes mentioned, but their exact credentials and functions are not always clear (Peterson, 1985). Claims of negligent performance of specialized treatments arise in some cases. For example, this occurred in a suit brought for negligent performance of physical therapy in contradiction to the referring physician's orders and in a case where an x-ray technician's performance fell below the standard of care when failing to obtain a clear film of the cervical thoracic junction that would have revealed a fracture which, because undetected, later caused paralysis. Negligent use of equipment is another source of liability, e.g., a case involving burns from an electrical diathermy machine. In another case, a basket swing chain came apart as a physical therapy patient was lowered into a Hubbard bath, causing him to fall and suffer the reopening and contamination of his surgical wound.

More common are situations involving physical handling or support of patients receiving services. Injury from some kind of fall or jolt is relatively common. One case involved a physical therapy patient who, after having a total hip replacement, fainted while stepping back to the tilt table following parallel bars exercise. This was after the therapist inadequately heeded a complaint of weakness and dizziness. Slumps or slides during tilt-table use by physical therapists and radiographers have also presented problems. An example of this is the incident in which a sedated patient, inadequately supported by an x-ray technician during tilt-table raising for an upright position abdominal x-ray, slid down and broke an ankle (Peterson, 1985).

So far, nurses and physicians have been the focus of malpractice liability. Since the majority of allied health professionals are not independent practitioners and usually work in collaboration with physicians, nurses, and other practitioners, they will be increasingly involved in the issues of malpractice liability. Regardless of whether an allied health professional involved in a malpractice case was a defendant, the appropriateness of his/her professional conduct was usually adjudicated. Therefore, case law precedents involving allied health professionals' conduct have been established.

The "New" Professionalism

Professionals who follow their profession's code of ethics, "keep their noses clean," treat clients politely, "do the best they know how," and "mind their own business," are passé. This type of professionalism was based on the premise that professionals were responsible for their own behavior, were authorities and in charge in the professional-client relationship, and that the client acquiesced to their wishes and advice. Clients' expectations of professionals were relatively clear and straightforward, and there were few threats to a professional's autonomy, power, and prestige. This is what might be called "self-contained" professionalism.

Previously, professionals held their own values and paternally accepted the client's values in their decision-making. It is no longer accepted by clients that professionals know best (Spiegel, Rubin & Frost, 1981). Now professionals may find that their profession's code of ethics is too abstract to be helpful in cases of litigation; that they are legally responsible for students who work under their supervision; that they can be sued as a member of a team of professionals who provide services to a client; that "doing their best" is not sufficient in the face of clients' demands for second opinions and consultants; and that how they relate to clients on a personal level is scrutinized by the clients for evidence of discrimination, violation of one's rights, and offensiveness to one's values and beliefs. Expectations of what professionals are or do are not always clear to clients, and there are numerous threats and questions that challenge the professionals' competence.

Schon (1983) advocates a new type of professional accountability in which professionals can function as "reflective" practitioners. Practitioners' relationships with their clients take the form of reflective conversation. They attribute to their clients, as well as to themselves, the capacity to mean, know, and plan. They recognize an obligation to make their own understandings accessible to clients. For example, if they are physicians, they may urge their patients to stop smoking, but they may also be alert to discover *how* smoking plays a part in a patient's life and the other consequences in personal habits and life style that might occur when a patient stops smoking. If a practitioner has a patient with cancer who has been unable to accept the disease and its prognosis, and therefore is not cooperating in his/her treatment, the reflective practitioner discusses cancer, its forms, the meaning of disease in the patient's life, its impact on the family, and the fears and concerns the patient has about the future. These examples of reflective teaching and management are what could be called "shared" professionalism. While professionals are credentialed and competent, their claim to authority is based on their ability to manifest their special knowledge in interaction with their clients.

Reflective practitioners are more directly accountable to their clients than practitioners who remain detached and relegate accountability to the client. Schon notes that there are constraints in being "reflective." It is time consuming, difficult, and there may be types of clients who want nothing more than intervention with minimal conversation. There are also crisis situations when the practitioner can do little more than the task required and when a lot of conversation of any type may not be possible or appropriate. Indeed, for some practitioners who have a need "to be in control," it may be impossible to adapt to a reflective mode. However, Schon's approach is workable and worthwhile. It does take different kinds of skills than some practitioners have. And, it assures that clients can question and confront practitioners without defensiveness. Practitioners and clients shape their expectations of each other as they test the boundaries of expertise and knowledge.

Whether or not professionals try to adopt Schon's approach, someone else's, or modify their own, "professionalism," in the future, will take on new meaning. It will no longer mean only *how* professionals practice their profession, but *how* professionals practice *with* colleagues and clients. Professionalism will no longer be restricted to how effective one is in influencing the well-being of individual clients, but include, as well, the practitioner's willingness, as a citizen, to help effect a just health care system in our country.

In Retrospect

Professionalism is how you put yourself into the practice of your profession. It is more than being friendly and honest with your patients, and well-qualified to do what you do. Professionalism is a set of values and behaviors which emanate from our values. Professionalism involves a mandate to keep current and acquire new knowledge in one's profession, it implies a commitment to the community in which one lives and works to participate in projects, activities and decision-making; it requires advocacy for a safer and healthier environment and equity in the provision of health services, it presumes a "moral fiber" that will pervade one's personal attitudes and behaviors. Professionalism is not totally "in the eye of the beholder" as the ethical standards of each profession, as well as legal statutes, provide common boundaries for determining what is acceptable and what is unacceptable professional behavior.

There are many enticements for a professional to become unprofessional. Stresses associated with work and life itself, coupled with the availability of drugs, can ease a health professional into a life of substance abuse. Similarly, alcohol can be used as a stress reliever. Overwork can lead to burnout and depression, and one's profession can become merely a series of unsatisfying routine tasks. It is not easy to ask for help, especially for health professionals who are providers of help. Therefore, an important aspect of professionalism is an awareness of one's own strengths and weaknesses and the adoption of an agenda for living that enables a person to obtain satisfaction other than that provided by one's work. Professionalism is not a fixed trait or state. Rather, it is a quality that changes and can be gained or lost. Professionalism is a life-long task, which one has to work at to perfect and to teach by example.

REFERENCES

Adamson, T.E., Tschann, J.M., Gullion, D.S. & Oppenberg, A.A. (1989). Physician communication skills and malpractice claims: A complex relationship. *Western Journal of Medicine, 150,* 356–360.

Agich, G.J. (1980). Professionalism and ethics in health care. *The Journal of Medicine and Philosophy, 5,* 186–199.

Ashworth, K. (1989). Competency for service and for self. In *Proceedings and Conference on Physician Competence: Whose Responsibility?* (pp. 161–167). The Warwick, Houston, Texas, April 7–9, 1988, American Medical Association, 1989.

Baldwin, D.C., Conrad, S., Hughes, P., Achenbach, K.E. & Sheehan, D.V. (1988). Substance abuse among senior medical students in 23 medical schools. Proceedings of the Annual Conference on Medical Education, 1988.

Balint, M. (1957). *The doctor, his patient, and the illness.* New York: International Universities Press.

Bersoff, D.N. (1975). Professional ethics and legal responsibilities: On the horns of a dilemma. *Journal of School Psychology, 13,* 359–376.

Bolger, R.J. (Ed.) (1987). *In search of the modern Hippocrates.* Iowa City: University of Iowa Press.

Brewster, J.M. (1986). Prevalence of alcohol and other drug problems among physicians. *Journal of the American Medical Association, 255,* 1913–1920.

Bruhn, J.G. (1987). The changing limits of professionalism in allied health. *Journal of Allied Health, 16,* 111–118.

Carr-Saunders, A.M. (1933). *The professions.* Oxford: Clarendon Press.

Cogan, M.L. (1953). Toward a definition of profession. *Harvard Educational Review, 23,* 33–50.

Cousins, N. (1983). *The healing heart.* New York: W.W. Norton.

Cullen, J.B. (1978). The *structure of professionalism: A quantitative examination.* New York: Petrocelli Books.

DiMatteo, M.R. (1979). A socio-psychological analysis of physician-patient rapport: Toward a science of the art of medicine. *Journal of Social Issues, 35,* 12–33.

DeWitt, C.B., Jr., Conard, S., Hughes, P., Achenbach, K.E. & Sheehan, D.V. (1988). Substance use and abuse among senior medical students in 23 medical schools. *Proceedings of the Annual Conference on Research in Medical Education, 27,* 262–266.

Durkheim, E. (1958). *Professional ethics and civic morals.* Translated by Cornelia Brookfield. Glencoe, IL: Free Press.

Egan, G. (1990). *The skilled helper: A systematic approach to effective helping,* 4th edition. Pacific Grove, CA: Brooks/Cole.

Engelhardt, H.T., Jr. & Callahan, D. (Eds.). (1977). *Knowledge, value and belief,* Vol. II. The Foundation of Ethics and Its Relationship to Science. Hastings-on-Hudson, NY: Institute of Society, Ethics and the Life Sciences.

Evans, W.A. (1981). *Management ethics.* Boston: Kluwer-Nijhoff.

Freidson, E. (1970)(a). *Professional dominance: The social structure of medical care.* Chicago: Adline.

Freidson, E. (1970)(b). *Profession of medicine.* New York: Dodd, Mead.

Goldman, A.H. (1980). *The moral foundations of professional ethics.* Totowa, NJ: Rowman and Littlefield.

Graber, G.C., Beasley, A.D. & Eaddy, J.A. (1985). *Ethical analysis of clinical medicine: A guide to self-evaluation.* Baltimore-Munich: Urban & Schwarzenberg.

Greenwood, E. (1957). Attributes of a profession. *Social Work, 2,* 45–55.

Harrison, L.B., Worth, M.H. Jr. & Carlucci, M.A. (1985). The development of the principles of medical malpractice in the United States. *Perspectives in Biology and Medicine, 29,* 41–72.

Hendrick, H.L. (1985). Professionalism: The eye of the beholder. *Journal of Allied Health, 14,* 241–248.

Inglehart, J.K. (1988). Medicine and professionalism. In *Conference on the medical profession: Enduring values and new challenges* (pp. 149–154). The Baltimore Hotel, Los Angeles, CA., February 25–27, 1987, Medical Education Group, American Medical Association, 1988.

Jonas, S. (1978). *Medical mystery: The training of doctors in the United States.* New York: W.W. Norton.

Loewy, E.H. (1989). *Textbook of medical ethics.* New York: Plenum.

McAuliffe, W.E., Santangelo, S., Magnuson, E., Sobol, A., Rohman, M. & Weissman, J. (1987). Risk factors of drug impairment in random samples of physicians and medical students. *International Journal of the Addictions, 22,* 825–841.

McCaughrin, W.C. (1979). Legal precedents in American law for patient education. *Patient Counseling and Health Education, 1,* 135–141.

Menke, W.G. (1969). Professional values in medical practice. *New England Journal of Medicine, 280,* (April 24) 930–936.

Morrow, P.C. & Goetz, J.F., Jr. (1988). Professionalism as a form of work commitment. *Journal of Vocational Behavior, 32,* 92–111.

Musto, D.F. (1985). Iatrogenic addiction: The problem, its definition and history. *Bulletin of the New York Academy of Medicine, 61,* 694–705.

Osiel, M.J. (1984). The politics of professional ethics. *Social Policy, 15,* 43–48.

Osler, Sir W. (1906). *Aequanimitas.* London: Lewis.

Perlman, H.H. (1982). The helping relationship: Its purpose and nature, In H. Rubenstein & M.H. Bloch, (Eds.) *Things that matter: Influences on helping relationships* (pp. 7–27). New York: Macmillan.

Peterson, R.G. (1985). Malpractice liability of allied health professionals: Developments in an area of critical concern. *Journal of Allied Health, 14,* 363–372.

Pfifferling, J. (1986). Cultural antecedents promoting professional impairment. In

C.D. Scott & J. Hawk (Eds.) *Heal thyself: The health of health care professionals* (pp. 3–18). New York: Brunner/Mazel.

Preven, D.W. (1983). Physician's suicide: The psychiatrist's role. In S.C. Scheiber & B.B. Doyle (Eds.) *The impaired physician* (pp. 39–47). New York: Plenum.

Purtilo, R. (1984). *Health professional/patient interaction.* Philadelphia, PA: W.B. Saunders.

Reiser, D.E. & Rosen, D.H. (1984). *Medicine as a human experience.* Baltimore, MD: University Park Press.

Ritchie, K. (1988). Professionalism, altruism, and overwork. *The Journal of Medicine and Philosophy, 13,* 447–455.

Ritzer, G. (1973). Professionalism and the individual. In E. Freidson, (Ed.) *The professions and their prospects* (pp. 59–73). Beverly Hills: Sage.

Robinowitz, C.B. (1983). The physician as a patient. In S.C. Scheiber & B.B. Doyle (Eds.) *The impaired physician,* (pp. 137–144). New York: Plenum.

Sarason, S.B. (1985). *Caring and compassion in clinical practice.* San Francisco, CA: Jossey-Bass.

Scheiber, S.C. (1983). Emotional problems of physicians: Nature and extent of problems. In S.C. Scheiber & B.B. Doyle (Eds.) *The impaired physician* (pp. 3–10). New York: Plenum.

Schon, D.A. (1983). *The reflective practitioner: How professionals think in action.* New York: Basic Books.

Scott, C.D. & Hawk, J. (Eds.) (1986) *Heal thyself: The health of health care professionals.* New York: Brunner/Mazel.

Seymour, F.J.C. (1966). Occupational images and norms. In H.M. Vollmer & D.L. Mills, (Eds.) *Professionalization* (pp. 126–129). Englewood Cliffs, NJ: Prentice-Hall.

Shortt, S.E.D. (1979). Psychiatric illness in physicians. *Canadian Medical Association Journal, 121,* 283–288.

Sieghart, P. (1982). Professional ethics — for whose benefit? *Journal of Medical Ethics, 8,* 25–32.

Slavitt, D.R. (1987). *Physicians observed.* Garden City, NY: Doubleday & Co., Inc.

Smith, H.L. & Churchill, L.R. (1986). *Professional ethics and primary care medicine. Beyond dilemmas and decorum.* Durham: Duke University Press.

Spiegel, A.D., Rubin, D. & Frost, S. (Eds.) (1981). *Medical technology, health care and the consumer.* New York: Human Sciences Press.

Stoeckle, J.D. (Ed.) (1987). *Encounters between patients and doctors: An anthology.* Cambridge, MA: The MIT Press.

Talbott, G., Benson, D. & Benson, E. (1980). Impaired physicians — The dilemma of identification. *Postgraduate Medicine, 68,* 56–64.

Toulmin, S. (1977). The meaning of professionalism: Doctors' ethics and biomedical science. In H.T. Engelhardt, Jr., & D. Callahan, (Eds.) *Knowledge, value and belief,* Vol. II (pp. 254–278). The Foundation of Ethics and Its Relationship to Science. Hastings-on-Hudson, NY: Institute of Society, Ethics and the Life Sciences.

Vaillant, G.E., Sobowale, N.C. & McArthur, C. (1972). Psychological vulnerabilities of physicians. *New England Journal of Medicine, 287,* 370–375.

Van Zandt, C.E. (1990). Professionalism: A matter of personal initiative. *Journal of Counseling and Development, 68,* 243–245.

Vollmer, H.M. & Mills, D.L. (Eds.) (1966). *Professionalization*. Englewood Cliffs, NJ: Prentice-Hall.

Webster, T.G. (1983). Problems of drug addiction and alcoholism among physicians. In S.C. Scheiber & B.B. Doyle (Eds.) *The impaired physician* (pp. 27–38). New York: Plenum.

Weisch, H.P. & LaVan, H. (1981). Inter-relations between organizational commitment and job characteristics, job satisfaction, professional behavior, and organizational climate. *Human Relations, 34,* 1079–1089.

Wilmer, H.A. (1987). The doctor-patient relationship and the issues of pity, sympathy, and empathy. In J.D. Stoeckle (Ed.) *Encounters between patients and doctors: An anthology* (pp. 403–411). Cambridge, MA: The MIT Press.

SUGGESTED READINGS

Appelbaum, P.S., Lidz, C.W. & Meisel, A. (1987). *Informed consent: Legal theory and clinical practice.* New York: Oxford University Press.

Barber, B. (1980). *Informed consent in medical therapy and research.* New Brunswick, NJ: Rutgers University Press.

Beauchamp, T.L. & Childress, J.F. (1983). *Principles of biomedical ethics.* New York: Oxford University Press.

Bell, N.K. (Ed.) (1982). *Who decides? Conflicts of rights in health care.* Clifton, NJ: Humana Press.

Bok, S. (1978). *Lying: Moral choice in public and private life.* New York: Pantheon.

Brammer, L.M. (1979). *The helping relationship: Process and skills,* 2nd ed. Englewood Cliffs, NJ: Prentice-Hall.

Bruhn, J.G. (1978). The doctor's touch: Tactile communication in the doctor-patient relationship. *Southern Medical Journal, 71,* 1469–1473.

Bruhn, J.G. (1986). Time in therapeutic relationships: Myth and realities. *Southern Medical Journal, 79,* 344–350.

Callahan, J.C. (Ed.) (1988). *Ethical issues in professional life.* New York: Oxford University Press.

Dowie, J. & Elstein, A. (Eds.) (1988). *Professional judgment: A reader in clinical decision making.* New York: Cambridge University Press.

Fletcher, J. (1979). *Morals and medicine.* Princeton: Princeton University Press.

Gorovitz, S., Jameton. A.L. & Mocklin, R. *et al.* (Eds.) (1976). *Moral problems in medicine.* Englewood Cliffs, NJ: Prentice-Hall.

Gross, S.J. (1984). *Of foxes and hen houses: Licensing and the health professions.* Westport, CT: Quorum Books.

Hochschild, A.R. (1983). *The managed heart.* Berkeley: University of California Press.

Humber, J.M. & Almeder, R.F. (Eds.) (1979). *Biomedical ethics and the law.* 2nd. ed. New York: Plenum.

Kass, L.R. (1985). *Toward a more natural science: Biology and human affairs.* New York: Free Press.

Kimball, C.P. (1981). *The biopsychosocial approach to the patient.* Baltimore, MD: Williams & Wilkins.

Kultgen, J. (1988). *Ethics and professionalism.* Philadelphia, PA: University of Pennsylvania Press.

Maddison, D. (1980). Professionalism and community responsibility. *Social Science and Medicine, 14A,* 91–96.

Osterman, P. & Gross, R. (Eds.) (1972). *The new professionals.* New York: Simon & Schuster.

Pavalon, E.I. (1980). *Human rights and health care law.* New York: American Journal of Nursing Co.

Pelligrino, E.D. & Thomasma, D.C. (1988). *For the patient's good: The restoration of beneficence in health care.* New York: Oxford University Press.

Purtilo, R.B. & Cassel, C.K. (1981). *Ethical dimensions in the health professions.* Philadelphia, PA: W.B. Saunders.

Report of the Special Committee on Biomedical Ethics (1985). *Values in conflict: Resolving ethical issues in hospital care.* Chicago, IL: American Hospital Association.

Southby, R. McK. F. & Hirsh, H.L. (Eds.) (1989). *Health Care law and ethics.* Washington, DC: The George Washington University Press.

Veatch, R.M. (1977). *Case studies in medical ethics.* Cambridge, MA: Harvard University Press.

Weich, W.T. (Ed.) (1979). *Encyclopedia of bioethics.* New York: Free Press.

Wertz, R.W. (1973). *Readings in ethical and social issues in biomedicine.* Englewood Cliffs, NJ: Prentice-Hall.

APPENDIX A
OATH OF HIPPOCRATES

I swear by Apollo Physician and Asclepius and Hygeia and Panaceia and all the gods and goddesses, making them my witnesses, that I will fulfil according to my ability and judgment this oath and this covenant:

To hold him who has taught me this art as equal to my parents and to live my life in partnership with him, and if he is in need of money to give him a share of mine, and to regard his offspring as equal to my brothers in male lineage and to teach them this art—if they desire to learn it—without fee and covenant; to give a share of precepts and oral instruction and all the other learning to my sons and to the sons of him who has instructed me and to pupils who have signed the covenant and have taken an oath according to the medical law, but to no one else.

I will apply dietetic measures for the benefit of the sick according to my ability and judgment; I will keep them from harm and injustice.

I will neither give a deadly drug to anybody if asked for it, nor will I make a suggestion to this effect. Similarly I will not give to a woman an abortive remedy. In purity and holiness I will guard my life and my art.

I will not use the knife, not even on sufferers from stone, but will withdraw in favor of such men as are engaged in this work.

Whatever houses I may visit, I will come for the benefit of the sick, remaining free of all intentional injustice, of all mischief and in particular of sexual relations with both female and male persons, be they free or slaves.

What I may see or hear in the course of the treatment or even outside of the treatment in regard to the life of men, which on no account one must spread abroad, I will keep to myself holding such things shameful to be spoken about.

If I fulfil this oath and do not violate it, may it be granted to me to enjoy life and art, being honored with fame from among all men for all time to come; if I transgress it and swear falsely, may the opposite of all this be my lot.

Text taken from Edelstein, Ludwig. *The Hippocratic Oath: Text, Translation and Interpretation.* Baltimore: The Johns Hopkins Press, 1943.

APPENDIX B
VALUES CLARIFICATION AND VALUES SURVEY

Values clarification is an approach that attempts to help individuals select, analyze, and set the priorities of their own values. Values clarification is not concerned with the context of people's values but with the process of valuing. Raths, Simon, and Merrill (1966, p. 27) provide a useful description: "When we value something we chose freely from alternatives after consideration of the consequences of each alternative; are proud of and happy with the choice; are willing to affirm the choice publicly; and make the choice part of our behavior and repeat the choice."

In addition to using values clarification to consider personal values, health care professionals can use a similar strategy in helping patients deal with conflicts, evaluate and choose alternatives, set goals, and take action. Values clarification alone is not sufficient to help us determine what to value and how to behave. It does not provide a basis for value selection or moral choice. However, discovering what we in fact do value is as important as beginning to examine our values. The value survey which follows, which is an abbreviated and modified version of Rokeach's survey of values, is a simple exercise to sensitize the reader to his/her values and priorities as a first step in the process of clarifying one's values.

Raths, L., Simon, S. & Merrill, H. (1966). *Values and teaching.* Columbus, Ohio: Charles E. Merrill.

VALUE SURVEY
INSTRUCTIONS

Listed below, in alphabetical order, are 18 values. Please rank them in order of their importance to YOU, as guiding principles in YOUR life.

Study the list carefully and pick out the one value which is most important to you. Place a number 1 next to it.

Then pick out the value which is second most important for you. Place a number 2 next to it. Do the same for each of the remaining values. The value which is least important should have the number 18 next to it.

RANK   *VALUES*

_____ A COMFORTABLE LIFE (a prosperous life)

_____ AN EXCITING LIFE (a stimulating, active life)

_____ A SENSE OF ACCOMPLISHMENT (lasting contribution)

_____ A WORLD OF PEACE (free of war and conflict)

_____ A WORLD OF BEAUTY (beauty of nature and the arts)

_____ EQUALITY (brotherhood, equal opportunity for all)

_____ FAMILY SECURITY (taking care of loved ones)

_____ FREEDOM (independence, free choice)

_____ HAPPINESS (contentedness)

_____ HEALTH (physical and mental well being)

_____ INNER HARMONY (freedom from inner conflict)

_____ MATURE LOVE (sexual and spiritual intimacy)

_____ NATIONAL SECURITY (protection from attack)

_____ PLEASURE (an enjoyable, leisurely life)

_____ SALVATION (saved, eternal life)

_____ SOCIAL RECOGNITION (respect, admiration)

_____ TRUE FRIENDSHIP (close companionship)

_____ WISDOM (mature understanding of life)

Adapted from Ware, J.E., Jr., Young, J.A., Snyder, M.K. & Wright, W.R. (1974), *The measurement of health as a value: Preliminary findings regarding scale reliability, validity and administrative procedures.* (Tech. Rep. No. MHC 74-11). Washington, D.C.: National Technical Information Service, U.S. Department of Commerce, pp. 55–56. Reprinted with permission.

APPENDIX C
ROE V. WADE

Majority Opinion, Blackmun, Justice

It is . . . apparent that at common law, at the time of the adoption of our Constitution, and throughout the major portion of the nineteenth century, abortion was viewed with less disfavor than under most American statutes currently in effect. Phrasing it another way, a woman enjoyed a substantially broader right to terminate a pregnancy than she does in most States today. At least with respect to the early stage of pregnancy, and very possibly without such a limitation, the opportunity to make this choice was present in this country well into the nineteenth century. Even later, the law continued for some time to treat less punitively an abortion procured in early pregnancy. . . .

Three reasons have been advanced to explain historically the enactment of criminal abortion laws in the nineteenth century and to justify their continued existence.

It has been argued occasionally that these laws were the product of a Victorian social concern to discourage illicit sexual conduct. Texas, however, does not advance this justification in the present case, and it appears that no court or commentator has taken the argument seriously. . . .

A second reason is concerned with abortion as a medical procedure. When most criminal abortion laws were first enacted, the procedure was a hazardous one for the woman. This was particularly true prior to the development of antisepsis. Antiseptic techniques, of course, were based on discoveries by Lister, Pasteur, and others first announced in 1867, but were not generally accepted and employed until about the turn of the century. Abortion mortality was high. Even after 1900, and perhaps until as late as the development of antibiotics in the 1940s, standard modern techniques such as dilation and curettage were not nearly so safe as they are today. Thus it has been argued that a state's real concern in enacting a criminal abortion law was to protect the pregnant woman, that is, to restrain her from submitting to a procedure that placed her life in serious jeopardy.

Modern medical techniques have altered this situation. Appellants and various *amici* refer to medical data indicating that abortion in early pregnancy, that is, prior to the end of first trimester, although not without its risk, is now relatively safe. Mortality rates for women undergoing early abortions, where the procedure is legal, appear to be as low as or lower than the rates for normal childbirth. Consequently, any interest of the state in protecting the woman from an inherently hazardous procedure, except when it would be equally dangerous for her to forgo it, has largely disappeared.

The third reason is the state's interest—some phrase it in terms of duty—in protecting prenatal life. Some of the argument for this justification rests on the theory that a new human life is present from the moment of conception. The state's interest and general obligation to protect life then extends, it is argued, to prenatal life. Only when the life of the pregnant mother herself is at stake, balanced against the life she carries within her, should the interest of the embryo or fetus not prevail. Logically, of course, a legitimate state interest in this area need not stand or fall on acceptance of the belief that life begins at conception or at some other point prior to live birth. In assessing the state's interest, recognition may be given to the less rigid claim that as long as at least *potential* life is involved, the state may assert interests beyond the protection of the pregnant woman alone.

Parties challenging state abortion laws have sharply disputed in some courts the contention that a purpose of these laws, then enacted, was to protect prenatal life. Pointing to the absence of legislative history to support the contention, they claim that most state laws were designed solely to protect the woman. Because medical advances have lessened this concern at least with respect to abortion in early pregnancy, they argue that with respect to such abortions the laws can no longer be justified by any state interest. There is some scholarly support for this view of original purpose. The few states' courts called upon to interpret their laws in the late nineteenth and early twentieth centuries did focus on the state's interest in protecting the woman's health rather than in preserving the embryo and fetus. . . .

The Constitution does not explicitly mention any right to privacy. In a line of decisions, however, going back perhaps as far as *Union Pacific R. Co. v. Botsford* (1891), the Court has recognized that a right of personal privacy, or a guarantee of certain areas or zones of privacy, does exist under the Constitution. In varying contexts the Court or individual Justices have indeed found at least the roots of that right in the First Amendment, . . . in the Fourth and Fifth Amendments . . . in the penumbras of the Bill of Rights . . . in the Ninth Amendment . . . or in the concept of liberty guaranteed by the first section of the Fourteenth Amendment. . . . These decisions make it clear that only personal rights that can be deemed "fundamental" or "implicit in the concept of ordered liberty," . . . are included in this guarantee of personal privacy. They also make it clear that the right has some extension to activities relating to marriage, . . . procreation, . . . contraception, . . . family relationships, . . . and child rearing and education. . . .

This right of privacy, whether it be founded in the Fourteenth Amendment's . concept of personal liberty and restrictions upon state action, as we feel it is, or, as the District Court determined, in the Ninth Amendment's reservation of rights to the people, is broad enough to encompass a woman's decision whether or not to terminate her pregnancy. . . .

Appellants and some *amici* argue that the woman's right is absolute and that she is entitled to terminate her pregnancy at whatever time, in whatever way, and for whatever reason she alone chooses. With this we do not agree. Appellants' arguments that Texas either has no valid interest at all in regulating the abortion decision, or no interest strong enough to support any limitation upon the woman's sole determination, is unpersuasive. The Court's decisions recognizing a right of privacy also acknowledge that some state regulation in areas protected by that right is appropriate. As noted above, a state may properly assert important interests in safeguarding health, in maintaining medical standards, and in protecting potential life. At some point in pregnancy, these respective interests become sufficiently compelling to sustain regulation of the factors that govern the abortion decision. The privacy right involved, therefore, cannot be said to be absolute. . . .

We therefore conclude that the right of personal privacy includes the abortion decision, but that this right is not unqualified and must be considered against important state interests in regulation.

We note that those federal and state courts that have recently considered abortion law challenges have reached the same conclusion. . . .

Although the results are divided, most of these courts have agreed that the right of privacy, however based, is broad enough to cover the abortion decision; that the right, nonetheless, is not absolute and is subject to some limitations; and that at some point the state interests as to protection of health, medical standards, and prenatal life, become dominant. We agree with this approach. . . .

The appellee and certain *amici* argue that the fetus is a "person" within the language and meaning of the Fourteenth Amendment. In support of this they outline at length and in detail the well-known facts of fetal development. If this suggestion of personhood is established, the appellant's case, of course, collapses, for the fetus' right to life is then guaranteed specifically by the Amendment. The appellant conceded as much on reargument. On the other hand, the appellee conceded on reargument that no case could be cited that holds a fetus is a person within the meaning of the Fourteenth Amendment. . . .

All this, together with our observation, *supra,* that throughout the major portion of the nineteenth century prevailing legal abortion practices were far freer than they are today, persuades us that the word "person," as used in the Fourteenth Amendment, does not include the unborn. . . . Indeed, our decision in *United States v. Vuitch* (1971), inferentially is to the same effect, for we there would not have indulged in statutory interpretation favorable to abortion in specified circumstances if the necessary consequence was the termination of life entitled to Fourteenth Amendment protection. . . .

As we have intimated above, it is reasonable and appropriate for a state to decide that at some point in time another interest, that of health of the mother or that of potential human life, becomes significantly involved. The woman's privacy is no longer sole and any right of privacy she possesses must be measured accordingly.

Texas urges that, apart from the Fourteenth Amendment, life begins at conception and is present throughout pregnancy, and that, therefore, the state has a compelling interest in protecting that life from and after conception. We need not resolve the difficult question of when life begins. When those trained in the respective disciplines of medicine, philosophy, and theology are unable to arrive at any consensus, the judiciary, at this point in the development of man's knowledge, is not in a position to speculate as to the answer.

It should be sufficient to note briefly the wide divergence of thinking on this most sensitive and difficult question. There has always been strong support for the view that life does not begin until live birth. This was the belief of the Stoics. It appears to be the predominant, though not the unanimous, attitude of the Jewish faith. It may be taken to represent also the position of a large segment of the Protestant community, insofar as that can be ascertained; organized groups that have taken a formal position on the abortion issue have generally regarded abortion as a matter for the conscience of the individual and her family. As we have noted, the common law found greater significance in quickening. Physicians and their scientific colleagues have regarded that event with less interest and have tended to focus either upon conception or upon live birth or upon the interim point at which the fetus becomes "viable," that is, potentially able to live outside the mother's womb, albeit with artificial aid. Viability is usually placed at about seven months (28 weeks) but may occur earlier, even at 24 weeks. . . .

In areas other than criminal abortion the law has been reluctant to endorse any theory that life, as we recognize it, begins before live birth or to accord legal rights to the unborn except in narrowly defined situations and except when the rights are contingent upon live birth. . . . In short, the unborn have never been recognized in the law as persons in the whole sense.

In view of all this, we do not agree that, by adopting one theory of life, Texas may over-ride the rights of the pregnant woman that are at stake. We repeat, however, that the state does have an important and legitimate interest in preserving and protecting the health of the pregnant woman, whether she be a resident of the state or a nonresident who seeks medical consultation and treatment there, and that it has still *another* important and legitimate interest in protecting the potentiality of human life. These interests are separate and distinct. Each grows in substantiality as the woman approaches term and, at a point during pregnancy, each becomes "compelling."

With respect to the state's important and legitimate interest in the health of the mother, the "compelling" point, in the light of present medical knowledge, is at approximately the end of the first trimester. This is so because of the now established medical fact . . . that until the end of the first trimester mortality in abortion is less than mortality in normal childbirth. It follows that, from and after this point, a state may regulate the abortion procedure to the extent that the regulation reasonably relates to the preservation and protection of maternal health. Examples of permissible state regulation in this area are requirements as to the qualifications of the person who is to perform the abortion; as to the licensure of that person; as to the facility in which the procedure is to be performed, that is, whether it must be a hospital or may be a clinic or some other place of less-than-hospital status; as to the licensing of the facility; and the like.

This means, on the other hand, for the period of pregnancy prior to this "compelling" point, the attending physician, in consultation with his patient, is free to determine, without regulation by the state, that in his medical judgment the patient's pregnancy should be terminated. If that decision is reached, the judgment may be effectuated by an abortion free of interference by the state.

With respect to the state's important and legitimate interest in potential life, the "compelling" point is at viability. This is so because the fetus then presumably has the capability of meaningful life outside the mother's womb. State regulation protective of fetal life after viability thus has both logical and biological justifications. If the state is interested in protecting fetal life after viability, it may go so far as to proscribe abortion during that period except when it is necessary to preserve the life or health of the mother. . . .

To summarize and repeat:

1. A state criminal abortion statute of the current Texas type, that excepts from criminality only a *lifesaving* procedure on behalf of the mother, without regard to pregnancy stage and without recognition of the other interests involved, is violative of the Due Process Clause of the Fourteenth Amendment.

(a) For the stage prior to approximately the end of the first trimester, the abortion decision and its effectuation must be left to the medical judgment of the pregnant woman's attending physician.

(b) For the stage subsequent to approximately the end of the first trimester, the state, in promoting its interest in the health of the mother, may, if it chooses, regulate the abortion procedure in ways that are reasonably related to maternal health.

(c) For the stage subsequent to viability the state, in promoting its interest in the potentiality of human life, may, if it chooses, regulate, and even proscribe, abortion except where it is necessary, in appropriate medical judgment, for the preservation of the life or health of the mother.

2. The state may define the term "physician" . . . to mean only a physician currently licensed by the state, and may proscribe any abortion by a person who is not a physician as so defined. . . .

The decision leaves the state free to place increasing restrictions on abortion as the period of pregnancy lengthens, so long as those restrictions are tailored to the recognized state interests. The decision vindicates the right of the physician to administer medical treatment according to his professional judgment up to the points where important state interests provide compelling justifications for intervention. Up to those points the abortion decision in all its aspects is inherently, and primarily, a medical decision, and basic responsibility for it must rest with the physician. If an individual practitioner abuses the privilege of exercising proper medical judgment, the usual remedies, judicial and intraprofessional, are available.

Reprinted from 410 *United States Reports* 113, Decided January 22, 1973.

APPENDIX D
CHRONOLOGY OF THE ABORTION ISSUE, 1973-1990

1973

Jan. 22: In Roe v Wade, on a 7-to-2 vote, the court legalizes abortion nationwide for the first time. Basing its ruling on a woman's right to privacy, the Court says a decision to have an abortion during the first three months of pregnancy must be left to the woman and her doctor. States may interfere in that decision only to protect the woman's health during the pregnancy's second trimester and may take steps to protect fetal life only in the third trimester.

In Doe v. Bolton, on a 7-to-2 vote, the Court strikes down restrictions on facilities that can be used to perform abortions.

1976

July 1: In Planned Parenthood v. Danforth, the Court, 6 to 3, says states cannot give husbands of pregnant women veto power over the abortion decision. By a separate 5-to-4 vote, the Court says that neither can the parents of an unmarried young girl be given veto power.

Sept. 30: Congress imposes the Hyde Amendment, a spending restriction on Medicaid money made available for abortions. The appropriations measure is tacked onto the proposed budget for the Department of Labor and the then Department of Health, Education, and Welfare.

Oct. 1: Cora McRae, a 24-year-old Brooklyn woman who suffers from varicose veins and blood clots, files a lawsuit. In September, she had sought an abortion at a Planned Parenthood facility and was told no Medicaid money was available because of the impending Hyde Amendment.

Oct. 22: Federal Judge John F. Dooling, Jr. rules that the Hyde Amendment is unconstitutional and refuses to let the Federal Government enforce it. Mrs. McRae has her abortion, paid for by Medicaid, but meanwhile her lawsuit becomes a national "class action" with the rights of all women on welfare at stake.

1977

June 20: In Maher v. Roe, on a 6-to-3 vote, the Court says that states have no legal obligation to pay for "non-therapeutic" abortions, but a definition of that term is not fully provided. The Court also stops short of saying whether such a funding obligation exists for "therapeutic" or "medically necessary" abortions.

June 29: The Supreme Court sets aside Judge Dooling's injunction, telling him to restudy his ruling in light of the Justices' June 20 decision.

Aug. 4: The Congressionally mandated spending restriction resumes, and Mrs. McRae's case returns to Judge Dooling's courtroom in Brooklyn. The judge hears from dozens of witnesses, sifts through thousands of pages of testimony and submissions, then deliberates for 13 months.

1979

Jan. 9:   In Colautti v. Franklin, reached by a 6-to-3 vote, the Court reaffirms its intention to give physicians broad discretion in determining the timing of "fetal viability"—when a fetus can survive outside the mother. States may seek to protect a fetus that has reached viability, but that determination is up to physicians, not courts or legislatures.

July 2:   In Bellotti v. Baird, on an 8-1 vote, the Court elaborates on its parental consent decision of 1976, saying that states may be able to require a pregnant minor to obtain one or both parents' consent to an abortion if state law provides an alternative procedure, such as letting the minor seek consent of a judge instead.

1980

Jan. 7:   Federal Judge M. Joseph Blumenfield rules that Connecticut must pay for all abortions that a doctor declares "medically necessary," overturning a state regulation.

Jan. 15:   Judge Dooling issues a 622-page ruling once again striking down the Hyde Amendment.

Feb. 16:   Justice Thurgood Marshall issues a stay on Dooling's ruling.

Feb. 19:   The Court votes 6-to-3 to lift Marshall's stay on Harris v. McRae, saying it will review it during the current term along with three Illinois cases on the same issue.

June 30:   In Harris v. McRae, on a 5-to-4 vote, the Court rules that the Federal Government and individual states have no legal obligation to pay for even medically necessary abortions.

Sept. 17:   The Court denies petitions to rehear the cases of Medicaid funding limits decided June 30.

1981

Jan. 12:   The Court refuses Arizona's request to grant a stay of a lower court order that it continue to honor a contract with the state's Planned Parenthood organizations to provide family planning services.

Feb. 18:   The Massachusetts Supreme Court orders the state to pay for all "medically necessary" abortions for women on welfare, even if their lives are not in danger; it overturns a 1979 state law limiting public financing of abortions to life-threatening cases.

Mar. 15:   Georgia eliminates state payments for abortions except in cases in which the mother's life is endangered or for victims of rape or incest.

Mar. 23:   In H. L. v. Matheson, on a 6-to-3 vote, the Court rules that a state may require a doctor to notify the parents of a teenage girl before performing an abortion on her or face criminal penalties, at least when the girl is still living at home and is dependent on her parents.

Apr. 27:   In Gary-Northwest Indiana Women's Services v. Orr, the Court upholds without comment the constitutionality of an Indiana law that requires all abortions after the first three months of pregnancy be performed in a hospital.

May 21: The Senate, by a vote of 52-43, approves an amendment already approved by the House that places stringent restrictions on federal funding of abortions.

June 1: The House and Senate ratify the most stringent restrictions ever placed on Medicaid abortions after rejecting a House-passed measure that would have forbidden medical insurance payments for abortions for federal employees.

July 29: Massachusetts Appeals Court overrules a lower court's order that a 14-year-old must consult her parents before having an abortion.

1982

Aug. 25: Planned Parenthood files a federal court challenge to a new Indiana law that parents of underage girls requesting abortion be notified 24 hours in advance.

Dec. 22: California Superior Court Judge Eli Chernow rules that a state law banning abortions after the 20th week of pregnancy violates the Supreme Court's 1973 decision.

1983

June 15: In Akron v. Akron Center for Reproductive Health, on a 6-to-3 vote, the Court declares unconstitutional an Akron, Ohio ordinance that places obstacles in the path of access to abortion.

June 20: In Planned Parenthood Association of Kansas City, Missouri, Inc. v. Ashcroft, the Court refuses to hear an appeal from a ruling that it could not prohibit staff physicians from performing abortions at the city's public hospital.

Aug. 30: The U. S. Court of Appeals for the Seventh Circuit, Chicago, Illinois bars the enforcement of an Indiana rule requiring doctors to notify parents before performing abortions on minors.

1984

Oct. 12: Chief Justice Warren E. Burger lifts a stay on a ruling by a Maryland state court that the mother of a handicapped woman could obtain an abortion for her blind, deaf, and severely retarded daughter, the apparent victim of a rape.

1985

Apr. 15: The Court agrees to hear arguments on whether Pennsylvania's Abortion Control Act, which was substantially invalidated in 1984 by a United States Court of Appeals, is constitutional.

May 20: The Court agrees to hear a joint appeal by the State of Illinois and an antiabortion group, Americans United for Life, of a federal District Court ruling that elements of 1975 Illinois Abortion Law were unconstitutional.

July 11: A federal District Court in New Jersey voids a law requiring abortions after the 16th week to be performed in hospitals.

July 15: Acting Solicitor General Charles Fried files an amicus curiae brief asking the Court to overturn Roe v. Wade.

Aug. 31: The NARAL and other pro-Choice groups file an amicus curiae brief in the Supreme Court in new abortion cases. Eighty-one members of Congress file a brief opposing the government's position.

Sept. 18:   The Court denies the government's request to participate in oral arguments in the new abortion cases.

Nov. 6:   The Court hears oral arguments in two new abortion cases.

Dec. 18:   The New York Court of Appeals rejects Roman Catholic attempts to block abortion clinics in several New York localities.

1986

Apr. 30:   The Court dismisses Diamond v. Charles, the Illinois abortion case in which a physician challenged the lower federal court's declaration that those sections of The Illinois Abortion Act that require the physician to take action to preserve the life of a fetus if there is any possibility of survival and to advise patients that any prescribed post-conception birth control medications are abortifacients are unconstitutional. The Court holds the appellant lacking in standing to defend the law in court.

June 11:   In Thornburgh v. American College of Obstetricians and Gynecologists, by a 5-to-4 vote, the Court overturns six sections of Pennsylvania's Abortion Control Act, affirming its prior decisions that limit the power of the states to regulate abortion under the constitutional right of privacy.

1987

Dec. 14:   In Hartigan v. Zbaraz, by a 4-to-4 vote, the Court affirms and allows to stand the Illinois Circuit Court decision that invalidates the 24 hour waiting period after a minor notifies her parents of her intent to have an abortion.

1988

Feb. 22:   The Court denies a petition for a rehearing of Hartigan v. Zbaraz.

June 29:   In Bowen v. Kendrick, by a 5-to-4 vote, the Court upholds the Adolescent Family Life Act, stating that the act does not have the primary effect of advancing religion and would not lead to excessive entanglement of government in religion.

Dec. 7:   The Court grants a writ of certiorari in United States Catholic Conference v. Abortion Rights Mobilization, in which the tax-exempt status of the United States Catholic Conference of Bishops is challenged because of allegations that the Conference is engaged in impermissable political activities relating to support of anti-abortion candidates for office. The Court also allows the motion of the National Council of Churches of Christ in the U.S.A. to file a brief amici-curiae.

1989

July 3:   In Webster v. Reproductive Health Services, by a 5-to-4 vote, the Court upholds the constitutionality of the Missouri statutes which make it unlawful for public employees to perform or assist in the performance of an abortion (unless necessary to save the life of the mother) within the scope of the employees' employment and upholds the constitutionality of the statute prohibiting the use of public facilities to perform abortions, stating that the challenged provisions only restrict a woman's ability to obtain an abortion to the extent that she chooses to use a physician affiliated with a public hospital. The court declines to rule on the constitutionality of the statute prohibiting the expenditure of public funding for abortion counseling since the plaintiff in the case is a private clinic and is not affected by the statute, which is directed to state officials who control the use of public funds. The Court also declines to rule on the preamble to the Missouri statute, which contains a legislative finding that life begins at conception and that unborn children have protectable interests in life, health, and well-being, noting that the provision does not "by its own terms regulate abortion."

1990

April 30: The Court declines to review Abortion Rights Mobilization v. Baker (in Re United States Catholic Conference), holding that an abortion rights group and several individuals do not have standing to challenge the tax exempt status of the Roman Catholic Church.

June 25: In Hodgson v. Minnesota, by a 5-to-4 vote, the Court holds that states may by legislation require that both parents of a minor, under the age of 18, who seeks abortion be informed of that fact so long as the state provides a mechanism by which the minor can obtain state court approval for avoiding notification.

In Ohio v. Akron Center for Reproductive Health, the Court upholds an Ohio statute that requires the notification of one parent when a minor, under 18, seeks abortion, but has provision for the minor to avoid notification with permission of a state court judge. The Court holds that complete anonymity is not required as long as the general public is prevented from obtaining knowledge of the minor's identity.

References

1986–1990 Reporter on Human Reproduction and the Law. Boston, MA: Legal-Medical Studies, Inc.

Rubin, Eva R. Abortion, Politics, and the Courts: Roe v. Wade and Its Aftermath. Revised Edition (1987). New York: Greenwood Press.

APPENDIX E
A PATIENT'S BILL OF RIGHTS

American Hospital Association

The American Hospital Association presents a Patient's Bill of Rights with the expectation that the observance of these rights will contribute to more effective patient care and greater satisfaction for the patient, his physician, and the hospital organization. Further, the Association presents these rights in the expectation that they will be supported by the hospital on behalf of its patients, as an integral part of the healing process. It is recognized that a personal relationship between the physician and the patient is essential for the provision of proper medical care. The traditional physician-patient relationship takes on new dimensions when care is rendered within an organizational structure. Legal precedent has established that the institution itself has a responsibility to the patient. It is in recognition of these factors that these rights are affirmed.

1. The patient has the right to respectful and considerate care.
2. The patient has the right to obtain from his physician complete current information concerning his diagnosis, treatment, and prognosis in terms the patient can reasonably be expected to understand. When it is not medically advisable to give such information to the patient, the information should be made available to an appropriate person in his behalf. He has the right to know, by name, the physician responsible for coordinating his care.
3. The patient has the right to receive from his physician information necessary to give informed consent prior to the start of any procedure and/or treatment. Except in emergencies, such information for informed consent should include but not necessarily be limited to the specific procedure and/or treatment, the medically significant risks involved, and the probable duration of incapacitation. Where medically significant alternatives for care or treatment exist, or when the patient requests information concerning medical alternatives, the patient has the right to such information. The patient also has the right to know the name of the person responsible for the procedures and/or treatment.
4. The patient has the right to refuse treatment to the extent permitted by law and to be informed of the medical consequences of his action.
5. The patient has the right to every consideration of his privacy concerning his own medical care program. Case discussion, consultation, examination, and treatment are confidential and should be treated discreetly. Those not directly involved in his care must have the permission of the patient to be present.
6. The patient has the right to expect that all communications and records pertaining to his care should be treated as confidential.
7. The patient has the right to expect that within its capacity a hospital must make reasonable response to the request of a patient for services. The hospital must provide evaluation, service, and/or referral as indicated by the urgency of the case. When medically permissible, a patient may be transferred to

380

another facility only after he has received complete information and explanation concerning the needs for and alternatives to such a transfer. The institution to which the patient is to be transferred must first have accepted the patient for transfer.

8. The patient has the right to obtain information as to any relationship of his hospital to other health care and educational institutions insofar as his care is concerned. The patient has the right to obtain information as to the existence of any professional relationship among individuals, by name, who are treating him.

9. The patient has the right to be advised if the hospital proposes to engage in or perform human experimentation affecting his care or treatment. The patient has the right to refuse to participate in such research projects.

10. The patient has the right to expect reasonable continuity of care. He has the right to know in advance what appointment times and physicians are available and where. The patient has the right to expect that the hospital will provide a mechanism whereby he is informed by his physician or a delegate of the physician of the patient's continuing health care requirements following discharge.

11. The patient has the right to examine and receive an explanation of his bill regardless of source of payment.

12. The patient has the right to know what hospital rules and regulations apply to his conduct as a patient.

No catalogue of rights can guarantee for the patient the kind of treatment he has a right to expect. A hospital has many functions to perform, including the prevention and treatment of disease, the education of both health professionals and patients, and the conduct of clinical research. All these activities must be conducted with an overriding concern for the patient, and, above all, the recognition of his dignity as a human being. Success in achieving this recognition assures success in the defense of the rights of the patient.

APPENDIX F
PRINCIPLES OF MEDICAL ETHICS

American Medical Association

I. A physician shall be dedicated to providing competent medical service with compassion and respect for human dignity.

II. A physician shall deal honestly with patients and colleagues, and strive to expose those physicians deficient in character or competence, or who engage in fraud or deception.

III. A physician shall respect the law and also recognize a responsibility to seek changes in these requirements which are contrary to the best interests of the patient.

IV. A physician shall respect the rights of patients, of colleagues, and of other health professionals, and shall safeguard patient confidences within the constraints of the law.

V. A physician shall continue to study, apply and advance scientific knowledge, make relevant information available to patients, colleagues, and the public, obtain consultation, and use the talents of other health professionals when indicated.

VI. A physician shall, in the provision of appropriate patient care, except in emergencies, be free to choose whom to serve, with whom to associate, and the environment in which to participate in activities contributing to an improved community.

Adopted by AMA House of Delegates at annual meeting, July 22, 1980. Reprinted with permission.

APPENDIX G
CODE FOR NURSES

American Nurses Association

1. The nurse provides services with respect for human dignity and the uniqueness of the client unrestricted by considerations of social or economic status, personal attributes, or the nature of health problems.
2. The nurse safeguards the client's right to privacy by judiciously protecting information of a confidential nature.
3. The nurse acts to safeguard the client and the public when health care and safety are affected by the incompetent, unethical, or illegal practice of any person.
4. The nurse assumes responsibility and accountability for individual nursing judgments and actions.
5. The nurse maintains competence in nursing.
6. The nurse exercises informed judgment and uses individual competence and qualifications as criteria in seeking consultation, accepting responsibilities, and delegating nursing activities to others.
7. The nurse participates in activities that contribute to the ongoing development of the profession's body of knowledge.
8. The nurse participates in the profession's efforts to implement and improve standards of nursing.
9. The nurse participates in the profession's efforts to establish and maintain conditions of employment conducive to high-quality nursing care.
10. The nurse participates in the profession's efforts to protect the public from misinformation and misrepresentation and to maintain the integrity of nursing.
11. The nurse collaborates with members of the health professions and other citizens in promoting community and national efforts to meet the health needs of the public.

American Nurses Association, 1976. Reprinted with permission.

APPENDIX H
PROFESSIONAL PLEDGES*
FOR ALLIED HEALTH PROFESSIONALS

Pledge. . . . Physician's Assistant

As a physician assistant, I pledge my honor and conscience to the art of medicine, striving to promote the concept of comprehensive medical care which I uphold.

I pledge to act under the guidance, supervision and responsibility of a physician and will seek always to understand fully my own personal capabilities and limitations.

Pledge. . . . Occupational Therapy

In the belief that all humans can regain, retain, or attain function through means of occupation or purposeful activity, I pledge myself to the ethical and responsible practice of my profession.

Believing that all human beings are unique and have potential worthy of realization, I am committed to the value of human dignity.

While respecting the confidence of others, I vow to exchange pertinent knowledge with my colleagues and to use this knowledge for the advancement of the client in his environment.

For the betterment of the health and well-being of those receiving my services, I will ever strive to further my professional competence.

It is with honor and pride that I join my colleagues in Occupational Therapy in pledging to uphold the integrity of our profession.

Pledge. . . . Physical Therapy

Being cognizant of and ever committed to the premise that human dignity is each individual's undeniable right,

I will discharge the art and science of my profession with diligence and integrity, always striving to hold in highest esteem those individuals placed in my care.

I will practice physical therapy for the care of the sick using my abilities and judgement in the highest degree of which I am capable.

I will hold all confidence sacred, only using whatever is seen and heard for the betterment of the individual concerned.

I now join my colleagues to uphold and further the physical therapy profession, ever aware of my responsibilities, committing myself to continue learning and to share my knowledge with others who seek to practice the art and science of my profession.

---

*These professional pledges are administered at graduation by the Chairpersons of the respective disciplines at The University of Texas School of Allied Health Sciences at Galveston. They were written by faculty in the school in the early 1970s.

Pledge. . . . Medical Record Administration

I pledge myself to pursue the practice of my profession in a spirit of unselfishness, and of loyalty to the Association and to the institution which I am called to serve; to bear always in mind a keen realization of my responsibility; to seek constantly a wider knowledge of my profession through serious study and through interchange of opinion among associates; to consider carefully the interest and rights of my fellow professionals; and to seek counsel among them when in doubt of my own judgment.

Finally, I pledge myself to cooperate in advancing and extending the art and science of medical record administration.

Pledge. . . . Medical Technology

Being fully cognizant of my responsibilities in the practice of Medical Technology, I affirm my willingness to discharge my duties with accuracy, thoughtfulness and care.

Realizing that the knowledge obtained concerning patients in the course of my work must be treated as confidential, I hold inviolate the confidence placed in me by patient and physician.

Recognizing that my integrity and that of my profession must be pledged to the absolute reliability of my work, I will conduct myself at all times in a manner appropriate to the dignity of my profession.

APPENDIX I
MEDICAL ETHICS VIDEOCASSETTES

Please see the last page of this appendix for the addresses of companies listed with each videocassette.

1989

"Better Off Dead"—60 minutes, color. Fanlight Productions. (Saving Severely-Damaged Newborns)

"Crisis at General Hospital"—60 minutes, color. Fanlight Productions.

"Deception: A Program About Ethical Decision Making by Care Givers"—34 minutes, color. Fanlight Productions.

"Does Doctor Know Best?"—Columbia University Seminars: Ethics in America Video Series: Volume 4—60 minutes, color. Columbia University. (Intellimation, Inc.)

"Human Experiment"—Columbia University Seminars: Ethics in America Video Series: Volume 9—60 minutes, color. Columbia University. (Intellimation, Inc.)

"Nurses are the Difference: Caring, Healing Actions and Attitudes"—37 minutes, color. Wade Maurice & Associates.

"What About Mom and Dad"—60 minutes, color. Fanlight Productions.

1988

"The DNR Dilemma: Do Not Resuscitate with the Terminally Ill"—21 minutes, color. Carle Medical Communications.

"Is This Life Worth Living?"—30 minutes, color. Filmmakers Library.

"Let My Daughter Die"—60 minutes, color. PBS.

"A Matter of Life or Death"—20 minutes, color. Filmmakers Library.

"Quality of Mercy"—30 minutes, color. Filmakers Library. (Treatment of Pain and Fear of the Health Provider Concerning Patient Addicts)

"A Time to Die: Who Decides?"—33 minutes, color. Churchill Films.

"Who Lives, Who Dies?"—55 minutes, color. Filmmakers Library.

1987

"Doctors are People, Too"—30 minutes, color. Coronet/MTI Films.

"Last Right"—60 minutes, color. PBS Video. (The Ethics of Mercy Killing)

1986

"Cancer Disclosure: Communicating the Diagnosis to Patients"—40 minutes, color. Medcom, Inc.

"Code 10: Patients are Customers, Too"—20 minutes, color. Perennial Education.

"Death or Dying: The Physician's Perspective"—29 minutes, color. Fanlight.

"Final Choices"—60 minutes, color. Columbia University. (Managing Our Miracles: Health Care in America Series)

"For All the Good Intentions: Handicapped Newborns"—60 minutes, color. CBC Enterprises.

"No Heroic Measures"—23 minutes, color. Carle Medical Communications.

"Second Chance at Life"—60 minutes, color. Columbia University.

"Technology Rocks the Cradle"—60 minutes, color. Columbia University.

"To Hurt and to Heal: Parts I & II"—approximately 90 minutes for both parts, color. UCEMC.

"Truth and Confidences"—60 minutes, color. Columbia University.

1985

"Dax's Case"—60 minutes, color. Filmmakers Library.

"Right to Die"—19 minutes, color. Carle Medical Communications.

1984

"Professional Ethics in Nursing"—19 minutes, color. Medcom.

1983

"Code Gray"—This video examines the moral and ethical aspects of health delivery. Nurses confront dilemmas in four actual work situations. The video raises issues for discussion—30 minutes, color. Fanlight Productions.

1981

"The Theological Framework: Decisions About the Critically Ill"—61 minutes, color. Marshfield Regional Video Network.

1980

"Coping with Serious Illness"—6 parts (30 minutes each), color, Time-Life Video.

1978

"The Philosophical Basis of Biomedical Ethics"—60 minutes, color. University of Texas at Dallas.

Audio-Visual Company Addresses

Carle Medical Communications
510 West Main Street
Urbana, Illinois 61801

CBC Enterprises
Canadian Broadcasting Corporation
245 Park Avenue
New York City, New York 10167

Churchill Films
12210 Nebraska Avenue
Los Angeles, California 90025

Columbia University Seminars on Medicine and Science
Columbia University
Room 204—Journalism
New York, New York 10027

Concept Media Inc.
P. O. Box 19542
2495 DuBridge Avenue
Irvine, California 92741

Coronet/MTI Films
108 Wilmot Road
Deerfield, Illinois 60015

Fanlight Productions
47 Halifax Street
Boston, Massachusetts 02130

Filmakers Library, Inc.
133 East 58th Street
New York, New York 10022

Intellimation Inc.
2040 Alameda Padre Serra
P. O. Box 4069
Santa Barbara, California 93140

Marshfield Regional Video Network
1000 North Oak Avenue
Marshfield, Wisconsin 54449

Medcom Inc.
P. O. Box 3225
Garden Grove, California 92642

PBS Video
1320 Braddock Place
Alexandria, Virginia 22314

Perennial Education Inc.
930 Pitner Avenue
Evanston, Illinois 60202

Time-Life Video
777 Duke Street
Alexandria, Virginia 22314

UCEMC—University of California
Extension Media Center
2176 Shattuck Avenue
Berkeley, California 94704

University of Texas at Dallas
Health Science Center
5323 Harry Hines Boulevard
Dallas, Texas 75235

Wade Maurice & Associates
1919 American Court
Neenah, Washington 54956

INDEX